BRIGHTON'S COUNTY HOSPITAL, 1828 – 2007

By the same author:

A Guide to Hospital Careers
(Museum Press)

The Strongest Enemy
(A Novel: Alvin Redman)

Out of the Shadows: A History of Newhaven Downs, 1836 – 1996
(South Downs Health NHS Trust)

A Lingering Fear: The Workhouse Legacy and East Sussex Hospitals, 1930 – 1974
(In preparation)

Brighton's County Hospital
1828 – 2007

HARRY GASTON
BA (Hons), MHSM, DipHSM, D.Phil

Southern Editorial Services
2008

2008
Published by
SOUTHERN EDITORIAL SERVICES
34 Hillcrest Road,
Newhaven, East Sussex BN9 9EG

ISBN 978-0-9558467-0-0

Typeset in Garamond 12/14 pt by Southern Editorial Services, Australia,
28 Herbert Street, Albert Park, Melbourne, VIC, 3206
Printed by RPM Print and Design,
2-3 Spur Road, Quarry Lane Industrial Estate,
Chichester, West Sussex PO19 8PR

CONTENTS

ILLUSTRATIONS

Photos 1-82 from the hospital archives; Photos 83-117, Bulletin archives 118, the Friends of Brighton and Hove Hospitals; Photos 119-165, Bulletin archives.

Bulletin photos include 93, 99 originally published courtesy of the Editor of the *Evening Argus*; 97 orinally published in the *Nursing Mirror* courtesy of the *Nursing Times;* 92, 100, 102-3, 117, 156 (Department of Medical Photography); 94-96, 172, 175, 178-187 (Sybil Gaston); 113-116, 126, 137, 146-155, 157-165 (the author); 119, 122-126, 128-136, 138-145 (Sarah-Anne Morley).

ACKNOWLEDGMENTS

First and foremost, I must acknowledge the unstinting help given to me by my colleague Sarah-Anne Morley throughout the entire course of what we called the RSCH History Project. We worked together on much of the initial research at East Sussex County Records Office, she scanned and catalogued all the hospital archive photographs and she was responsible for many of the photographs originally taken for the hospitals' *Bulletin.*

Once he became aware of the project, Lee Soden, one of the Brighton and Sussex University Hospitals NHS Trust executive directors, was a constant source of support and encouragement. Lee also arranged for funding to support the project and to provide copies of the book to be sold in aid of their funds by the Friends of Brighton and Hove Hospitals.

I am grateful too to former trust chief executive Stuart Welling, who gave me permission to access the hospital's records and photographs (although he accompanied this by the thought that I might undertake similar work for the other trust hospitals, an enormous task that I doubt could ever be accomplished!).

As with previous hospital research projects, I received great help from the staff of East Sussex County Record Office and I must thank them and also the staff of Brighton History Centre for their help in the later stages of the research into 20th century local newspapers and also to Judy Lehmann and her staff in the library at the Audrey Emerton Centre.

I am also grateful to Baroness Cumberlege for the kind words in her foreword and for their help in various ways to Janet Cheesman, Kerry Dearson, Dr John Duncan, Dr Martin Fisher, Maud Gill, Suzy Horne, Kate Goddard, Rae Lee, James Lewis, Scott Marlow, Kevin Mayers, Kenneth Ross and especially Irene Sankey MBE.

Inevitably I will inadvertently omit some of those who gave various kinds of assistance since we set out on this project in the spring of 2003. It's been a long, hard haul. Please accept my apologies and thanks.

FOREWORD

The history of a hospital could be a dull read. Not this one.

This is the fascinating story of a great enterprise, conceived two hundred years ago and still thriving today. Thanks to Dr Russell who 'invented' the sea and Dr Relham who invented the Brighton 'air, it was considered essential to have a dispensary in the town, and the Sussex County Hospital and Sea Bathing Infirmary was established. It was a charitable concern for poor people living in the town who possessed as letter of recommendation from a subscriber to the charity.

Today, the Royal Sussex County Hospital serves rich and poor alike. It is remarkable that its early charitable tradition lives on through committed volunteers, fund raising, and the Friends of Brighton and Hove Hospitals.

Harry Gaston's historical account is full of marvellous vignettes – glimpses of a different social order, behaviours and tensions between professional groups. Some themes are constant, others thank goodness, have totally changed, not least through the introduction of the National Health Service.

For those of us who have worked in or for the hospital, it will bring back a host of memories. It will be a journey full of delights, with photographs and illustrations to remind us of forgotten events and people with whom we have enjoyed working.

For others it will be a rare insight into the vision and determination of generations of dedicated men and women who cared for the health and wellbeing of their local community. These staff also found the time, energy and inspiration to constantly develop the hospital site and introduce cures and treatments that were new and to the forefront of scientific discovery.

Hospitals, although brimming with information, are not always the most diligent in keeping full and accurate records, However, with huge determination and great skill, Harry Gaston and his associate Sarah-Anne Morley have raided every possible source and the result of their researches makes this history an enchanting read. Without Harry and his lovely wife Sybil, editor and photographer of the monthly hospital *Bulletin*, we would not have had such a richly researched volume.

For 40 years any noteworthy event was covered by Harry and published in the *Bulletin*. His editorials were often controversial, and for those of us in management, frequently challenging – but always worth a read. We respected and tolerated his editorial freedom recognising the importance of a high quality publication to inform and strengthen the collegiate effect on the organisation.

This history is equal to the *Bulletin* in its ability to captivate and charm the reader. It is not only a record of interest for those whose working life was spent at the Royal Sussex County Hospital but is also a story for the casual reader who will enjoy many hours of fascinating health and social history.

Baroness Julia Cumberlege, CBE, DL, Hon. FRSP, Hon FRSGPs.

Chairman 1981-1988

PREFACE

Looking back, I realise that the publication of this history is the result of two events in 1999. The first of these was the annual scientific meeting of the Surgeons of Great Britain and Ireland, held that year in Brighton's Hotel Metropole.

Retired consultant surgeon Philip Somerville had been asked to mount an exhibition depicting the history of medicine in Brighton and to achieve this he sought the help of the team responsible for producing the monthly house journal of Brighton Health Care, Sarah-Anne Morley and myself. The six large A1 posters we produced attracted considerable interest and were subsequently displayed at the Royal Sussex County Hospital.

At about the same time, I was asked to by Lee Soden, then the trust's director of facilities, to undertake the archive research for a major permanent display, the Millennium Walk Exhibition, *Images*, which was opened by the chairman during the evening of 31st December 1999. The historical section on the development of Brighton hospitals was set up along both walls of the corridor leading up past the Sussex Throat and Ear Department. This too attracted a great deal of interest, so much so that enquiries regarding the history of the hospital tended to be referred to me.

However, mindful of the fact that there were considerable gaps in my knowledge, I eventually set out, again with the help of Sarah-Anne, to undertake detailed research of its history. Hospital archives showed evidence of at least two attempts to write a history, neither of which had produced any tangible results. It was then that I decided to embark on what we called the RSCH History Project, aiming to produce an addition to the academic literature on the development of the voluntary hospital system in Great Britain. As the news of the project spread, however, it became clear that there was a demand for a history from present and former members of staff and from people interested in local history. Hopefully, this volume will be of interest to all three audiences.

My collection of hospital histories reveals no common denominator. Some are written by academics for the benefit of the institution, some by retired clinicians or others who have worked at the hospital, others by people researching local history. Some have a medical bias, most endeavour to present a balanced account. My background is more than 30 years in hospital administration and forty years in hospital house journalism. Nevertheless, non-nurse readers might argue that nursing occupies a disproportionate amount of space. If this is a valid criticism, there are good reasons why it should be so: nurses constitute the largest proportion of staff in a hospital and nurse recruitment ranks second only to finance as one of the principal factors affecting the smooth running of the institution; secondly, in the case of the County, its role as a leading nurse training school established during the late nineteenth century merits special attention.

Any hospital history depends very much on the availability and accessibility of its records. In the case of the Royal Sussex County, the records for the period when it was a voluntary hospital – minutes and annual reports especially, and photographs – have been well preserved. Backed by additional research into other sources – especially newspapers – it becomes possible to produce a fully rounded history. The problems begin from 1948 with the start of the National Health Service. The records of the Brighton and Lewes Hospital Management Committee in the period to 1974 are far from complete. The management committee's minutes, although available, are usually no more than confirmation of the acceptance of recommendations from its sub-committees. Unfortunately, many of their minutes, which would have contained more detail, do not appear to have been preserved.

The existence of press reports would have been helpful here but press reporting had undergone a significant change. During the nineteenth century and the early part of the twentieth, reports of meetings tended to be detailed, often verbatim, and peppered with *'hear, hears'*. Paper rationing during and immediately after the Second World War meant detailed reports were no longer possible. Later, the move from broadsheet to tabloid newspapers meant that reports became briefer and more selective. Just as nationally, parliamentary reporting was in decline, locally, court reporting for example (except in a number of the remaining regional broadsheets) was confined to the more sensational or newsworthy cases and the same applied to reports of hospital management meetings.

Post 1948 there was another problem. Individual hospitals had now become merged into groups. In Brighton, for example, those records that exist relate to the group of some 13 hospitals administered by the committee and it is not always easy to extract material pertaining solely to the County Hospital. Fortunately, in 1967, I was asked to introduce and edit what became a national award winning group house journal, *Brighton Hospitals Bulletin*, and for the next forty years, until its demise early in 2007, we recorded the development of the local hospitals and the work of their staffs. Throughout, the *Bulletin* had access to committee papers and from 1982 attended all board meetings at which local newspaper reporters were not always present. Not surprisingly, perhaps, the East Sussex County Record Office values its collection of copies of the *Bulletin* as one of the best sources of local hospital history.

For the historian of the future, it is to be hoped that board papers, at least, will be preserved but it is not easy to see what other sources will be available to produce a fully rounded record of the development of our local hospitals.

1. Introduction

For most people living in Sussex some two hundred or so years ago, becoming ill posed a major problem: medical care was something they simply could not afford.

Admittedly medical knowledge in the early nineteenth century was not very advanced, although the suggestion that it consisted of 'nurses gossip' and 'sick men's fancies' was perhaps a little extreme. Surgery was largely limited to fractures and amputations, usually the result of accidents or tubercular infections. It involved excruciating pain, any relief depending on the surgeon's skill and speed with his knife-and-saw work. Because of the risk of infection in hospitals, it was believed to be safer carried out at home, which was certainly the preferred option for the well-to-do. For the very poor, the paupers, there was an alternative in the form of the workhouse. But for the vast majority, there was no real provision.

A change had begun to take place in the middle of the eighteenth century with the establishment of voluntary hospitals, firstly in London, then in the provinces, especially in the county towns like Winchester and Bath.

Lewes at this time was a market town, one of the largest in the county. It was the social centre for the gentry, wealthy farmers and professionals. Until the coming of the railways, it was the main artery through which nearly all the traffic between the east and west of the county flowed. But it was not really large enough to support a hospital.

However, this was also the time when Brighton, or Brighthelmstone as it was then called (the spelling varies), was developing from a poor fishing village into a seaside resort, thanks in no small part to a doctor from Lewes, Richard Russell, and also to two other doctors, Anthony Relhan and John Awsiter.

Although sea bathing had become popular earlier in the century, it was Russell's advocacy of the curative powers of sea water that was the spur for Brighton's new prosperity. Russell sent his patients there and in 1750 built himself a house in the Steine on the site of the present Royal Albion Hotel. The publication of his dissertation on the use of sea water in diseases of the glands two years later enhanced his reputation although, interestingly, he had to encourage businessmen from Lewes to invest in impoverished Brighton because capital was unavailable locally.

Prosperous Lewes inhabitants, including Samuel Shergold, who developed the Castle Inn, and two doctors Poole and Relhan[1], who wrote the first history of Brighton, provided the resources the village of Brighthelmstone did not possess. They lent money on mortgage to householders there and thus helped play an important part in Brighton's development as a resort during the 1750s and 1760s.

Almost immediately patients eager for the new cure came thronging from London by post chaise and family coach.

According to an account written in 1766:

> Brighthelmstone in the County of Sussex is distant from London by 57 miles, is a small ill-built town, situated on the sea coast at present greatly resorted to in the summertime by persons labouring under various disorders for the benefit of bathing and drinking sea water, and by the gay and polite on account of the company which frequent it at that season. Until a few years ago it was no better than a mere fishing town, inhabited by fishermen and sailors, but through the recommendation of Dr Russel [sic], and by the means of his writing in favour of sea water, it is become one of the principal places in the kingdom for the resort of the idle and dissipated, as well as the diseased and infirm.[2]

Dr Relhan's role in this respect also deserves acknowledgement. Clifford Musgrave has described Relhan's history as 'the first guide to Brighton [that] attracted many and fashionable visitors ... with his enthusiastic descriptions of the place, which he compared more than favourably with the ancient resort of Baiae in Campania, where wealthy Romans retired for bathing and pleasure.' According to Musgrave, if Dr Russell 'invented' the sea, then it was Dr Relhan who invented the Brighton air[3]

Dr Awsiter's role was no less important.[4] He had the idea of mixing seawater with milk to make it more palatable for drinking and cited its value in cases of barrenness. Because of the unwillingness of private speculators, to overcome the problem of Brighton's pebbly beach for invalids and to enable the cure to be made available all the year round, he personally undertook the erection of a small single storey building near Pool Valley. This offered hot and cold baths in water pumped up through pipes from the sea.

Roads in Sussex were notoriously bad but by 1780 coaches could travel from London in five hours bringing with them people of distinction and fashion. In the mid-1860s poets and writers were attracted to the town and later Fanny Burney, 'the mother of English fiction', and Hester Thrale were among the visiting literary and intellectual set during the bathing seasons.

In September 1783, invited by his uncle the Duke of Cumberland, the Prince of Wales (later Prince Regent and subsequently George IV) paid a visit to try a sea water cure for swollen glands. It was to be the first of many visits, and not only for his health: during his second visit he attended Brighton Races which had been established the year before by a group of leading inhabitants including the Earl of Egremont. By now the Steine was a popular promenade and the centre of Brighton had grown complete with theatres, coffee houses, baths and libraries. The number of houses more than doubled in the latter part of the century and almost trebled itself again by 1820. Accompanying this growth, however, behind the façade of opulence, there were many people living in dire poverty.

It was against this background that the first purpose built hospital in Sussex was conceived, not just to cater for the medical needs of the local poor, but also to provide the benefits of seawater treatment for people from any part of the country.

It was to be called the Sussex County Hospital and Sea Bathing Infirmary.

2. *From Dispensary to Hospital*

According to a report in the *Sussex Daily News*, Brighton in 1809 with a population of 9,000 was 'in the glow of its first success, and ambitious to become a town by itself and not a mere adjunct to Lewes.' It continued: 'The sudden access of prosperity which had caused the "little fishing village" to begin to assume the position of "a fashionable watering place" seems to have beneficially affected but a small proportion of the inhabitants.'

The report appeared in the paper on the 26th November 1909 and marked the centenary of the founding of Brighton's first medical charity, the Brighthelmstone Dispensary under the patronage of the Prince of Wales.

Dispensaries provided the services of doctors and surgeons to the poor, either free or in return for a modest fee. A few had been established in the eighteenth century, but it was not until after 1800 that they were set up in considerable numbers in large towns across the country. The Brighthelmstone Dispensary was one of the first of these.

The reasons for setting up the charity were spelled out in the first annual report by the president, the Earl of Chichester. As the town had grown, he said, the number of poor had increased 'in more than equal ratio' with the result that 'opulence had drawn round it a circle of poverty'. Where there were many poor, diseases of various kinds, and especially epidemics, would be a very frequent occurrence. The increasing extent of misery of the lower orders produced by sickness and the consequent inability to procure the necessaries of life, he explained, convinced the medical gentlemen 'that nothing short of a dispensary could meet the exigencies of the case.'

The dispensary opened in January 1810 in three rooms over a warehouse near the market in Nile Street where it provided medical care for poor people living in the town who possessed a letter of recommendation from a subscriber to the charity. Anyone unable to attend in person could be visited at home.

In 1811 the dispensary moved to larger premises at 112 North Street. The following year, the Earl of Chichester evolved a scheme for adding an infirmary and accident ward and in November the Sussex General with ten beds was added. However, this was only a stepping stone to what the earl thought was really needed: a sea bathing and county hospital.

On 1st November 1813 an advertisement appeared in the *Brighton Herald* and *The Courier* giving details of a public meeting in the Castle Tavern with the Earl of Chichester in the chair 'to promote the Sussex General Hospital for Sea bathing and general purposes'.

> The benefits to be derived from a General Hospital are so obvious, that it may be sufficient to say, that there is no Hospital in the county of Sussex, and that Brighthelmstone has the peculiar advantages for the situation of such an establishment. Medical aid can be procured there with less inconvenience to the Faculty, and more benefit to the patients; and sea-bathing for the poor, a remedy long sought after by the Hospitals in London can be obtained more easily than in any other place.

The meeting approved a plan for the new hospital at a cost not exceeding £12,000. It was also estimated that the cost of maintaining sixty patients and a proportionate number of outpatients would not exceed £1,800 per annum. Although the hospital was intended for the treatment of the poor, it was agreed that those a little better off could be admitted on payment of a moderate sum for their maintenance to enable them to receive the benefits of sea bathing.

The list of subscribers to the proposed hospital was headed by the Earl of Egremont who offered £1,000 and included the Earl of Chichester and Lord Gage and a £500 legacy from E. Goff Esq.

However, in spite of generous offers of support from many Sussex residents, because the country was still at war with France which was immediately followed by a period of economic depression and popular unrest, no further progress was made with the proposal until 1824.

Then, at a meeting at the Old Ship Tavern on December 11 1824, with the Earl of Egremont in the chair, it was agreed:

> That the present area of profound peace and general prosperity is a proper season for renewing the efforts of the affluent and benevolent Inhabitants of the County of Sussex and town of Brighthelmstone[1] for the establishment of a County Hospital and General Sea Bathing Infirmary.

The meeting also agreed unanimously:

> That the town of Brighthelmston is admirably adapted by its central position and by the facility of access to it from all parts of the County, by its contiguity to the sea; by its means of obtaining pecuniary resources and the number as well as talent of Medical Practitioners resident in it for the establishment and support of such an Institution; while its vast and increasing population affords a wide field for diffusing the benefits of so benevolent a design among the labouring poor.

A county hospital with 72 beds for the reception of 'the sick and lame and poor of every county and nation' was proposed and a fund was established with gifts from the Earl of Egremont and Thomas Read Kemp and supported by other residents in Brighton and Sussex.

Next, a committee was appointed consisting of the committee of the dispensary and infirmary and some subscribers to the proposed new hospital. Those named were the Earl of Egremont and the Earl of Chichester together with Sir M.J. Tierney M.P., Thomas Read Kemp M.P., Thomas Attree, S.F. Milford, Rev. Dr Hooker, Rev. Dr Holland, Rev. T. Scutt, John Hall, Dr Blair, Nath. Kemp, Charles Elliott, J. Mills, R. Tamplin, G. Chapman, Isaac Bass, Major Allen and J. Mortlock. Attree and the Rev. Edward Everard, one of the curates of the parish church, were requested to undertake the office of honorary secretaries to the hospital.

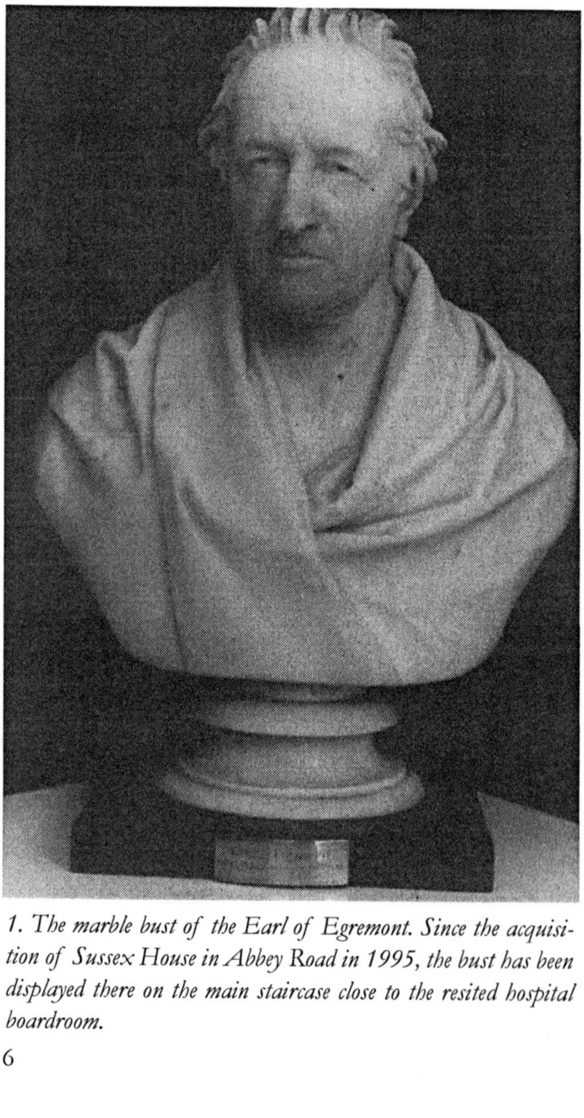

1. The marble bust of the Earl of Egremont. Since the acquisition of Sussex House in Abbey Road in 1995, the bust has been displayed there on the main staircase close to the resited hospital boardroom.

Finally, the meeting expressed 'the warmest gratitude of the friends of humanity' to the Earl of Egremont for his donation of £2,000 and for 'his actively benevolent exertions on this and all occasions to alleviate distress and to promote general welfare.'

The list of committee members illustrates the fact that the development of voluntary hospitals owed much to the nobility, the well-to-do and the church. The influence of the medical profession was to develop later as the scientific awakening of the eighteenth century made its impact upon the teaching and practice of medicine. Thomas Attree was an influential figure locally, a solicitor in a practice set up by his father, which at the time enjoyed a virtual monopoly of the most important legal business and had carried out negotiations on the purchase of land for the Prince of Wales. As Clerk to the Town Commissioners and Vestry Clerk he became known as 'the King of Brighton'[2]. Thomas Read Kemp was the son of a wealthy Lewes family who added to his fortune and property when he married a daughter of the banker Sir Francis Baring. He owned most of the land now known as Kemp Town. Under the influence of his wife's sister, an ardent evangelical, he became the minister of a dissenting religious sect and preached in his chapel in Ship Street for six years until 1823 but later returned to the established church.

A week later, on 18th December, the committee met at the Old Ship to draw up a list of possible sites for the new hospital. Initially, five were suggested. The committee stressed that four important objects should be kept in view. These were: two to four acres of ground in a healthy situation with easy approach from good roads; to be as near the centre of population making it convenient for outpatients and the attendance of physicians and surgeons; to be near the sea for the convenience of sea bathing; and, all things being equal, the comparative expense of the ground.

Four sites were then selected, preference being given to three, which were close to the Pavilion and the sea, and in two cases, within easy reach of the majority of the 'labouring population'. However, in a letter to the committee, Kemp offered a piece of land at the bottom of Whitehawk Hill, adding 'then you will have a broad road to a view of the sea, plenty of space, a southern aspect, and will not likely to be surrounded with trumpery buildings.'

Following a visit to the site by several members, the committee unanimously agreed that it was the best available. Kemp then arranged for the land to be conveyed to the trustees stipulating that no part of it should ever be let or sold and that no buildings should be erected near the boundary walls that would be a nuisance or affect the future sale of the surrounding land. He also offered £1,000 to the charity.

Finally, at a public meeting held in the County Hall at Lewes, it was agreed that 'a general hospital for the service of the county be created in Brighton.' It was also decided to reappoint the committee with additional members 'with full powers to adopt all such measures as they may think needful to facilitate the completion of the work.'

The new members included Viscount Gage, Sir G. Schiffner, M.P., the Rev. J.P. Crofts and Dr William King, who had studied medicine at St. Bartholomews and moved to Brighton after his marriage to the daughter of the vicar of Rottingdean.

Later in the month the committee submitted plans for the new building by Charles Barry ranging in price from just over £8,000 to £12,000. The prices varied according the number of beds – 70 or 80 were suggested – or the building materials used, either stone or less expensive bricks.

Charles Barry, later to become Sir Charles Barry who subsequently built the Houses of Parliament, was then at the beginning of his career and had won a competition to design St. Peter's Church, Brighton. Apparently the Earl of Egremont had him in mind as the prospective architect (but did not name him) at the first public meeting held to consider the erection of the hospital.

However, in a letter to the *Brighton Herald* Charles Busby claimed that the idea of constructing the hospital had been formed a year earlier between him and Everard and that later, jointly with Attree, that it should be entrusted to him and his partner Amon Wilds. (If this was so, Everard, a friend of Barry's, made no mention of it at the public meeting). Wilds and Busby, the principal architectural and building firm in Brighton, had earlier lost the commission to build St. Peter's Church to Barry, their design being voted second best of the eighty plans received in a public competition.

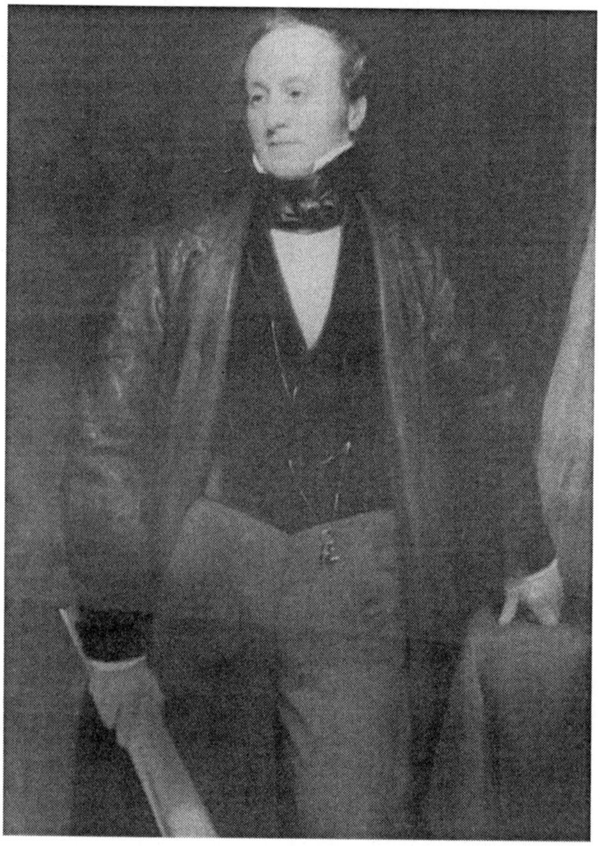

2. A photographic portrait of architect Sir Charles Barry displayed in the main entrance to the Barry Building. Taken from an oil painting reposing in the Houses of Parliament, Barry's most famous work, this portrait and another of his statue also on display, were acquired through the good offices of retired consultant anaesthetist Dr Rex Binning and presented to the hospital in 1982.

As a result of Busby's letter, it was decided to advertise a competition for plans and estimates for building the hospital. However, at a meeting held on 9th April, the committee preferred Barry's plan and he was written to and appointed architect.

Possibly there were people in Brighton who disliked the 'bold, robust style' of Wilds and Busby's buildings and wished to favour a promising young architect of about only thirty years of age[3]. However, the amount raised by public subscription did not allow for more than the bare minimum and, despite Barry's later reputation, the rather stolid building is not regarded as a work of architectural distinction.

At meetings held on the 25th and 26th April, the committee approved Barry's sketch plan for the interior of the building but removed the plan for a fever ward on the grounds of cost.

Tenders for the erection of walls and excavations for the building and drains were considered at a meeting on the 28th June when the tender for £8,121 from William Ranger, one of Brighton's most important builders, was accepted.

In September, following advertisements in Brighton and Lewes newspapers, the tender for erecting the 'intended Sussex County Hospital and General Sea Bathing Infirmary', also submitted by Ranger, was accepted.

Following a service in nearby St. George's Church (built for Kemp after he obtained a special Act of Parliament in 1824), the Earl of Egremont laid the foundation stone on 16 March 1826. A year later a sub-committee was appointed to fit up and furnish the building at an estimated cost of £1,370. The governors of the Sussex General Infirmary by then established at 25 Middle Street, which was to close, agreed to transfer '12 iron bedsteads together with several blankets, utensils, etc.' The total cost of the building, including boundary walls, a new road to the sea and digging a well came to £14,000.

In April 1828, a special Court of Governors elected 18 subscribers to serve on a committee to manage the affairs of the hospital. At the same meeting a subscription list was set up to defray the cost of a marble bust of the Earl of Egremont 'to be placed in the boardroom or some other conspicuous part of the hospital'. Individual subscriptions were limited to 10 guineas but the fund was immediately over-subscribed by more than £150.

The Statutes, Rules and Orders of the hospital were adopted at a meeting of subscribers in January 1828. At this meeting Viscount Gage was requested 'to respectfully solicit' His Majesty King George IV to transfer his patronage of the Sussex General Infirmary to the new hospital while the Earl of Egremont was elected President for Life 'as a small token of profound gratitude.' The medical officers of the Infirmary – physicians Drs Gibney, Blair and Yates, and surgeons, Mr Harry Blaker, Mr Robert Taylor and Mr William Attree – were requested to accept the same offices in the new hospital.

At the following meeting in March, Mr Benjamin Vallance was elected as resident house surgeon and Mrs Mary Comport as matron. Later the Rev. J.S.M. Anderson was appointed chaplain and W.H. Reed as secretary to the hospital.

All was now ready for the hospital to receive its first patients.

3. The Early Years

The first six patients were admitted on 11th June 1828. Three were aged 21 or under, one aged 27 and two in their sixties. Two were later recorded as 'relieved', three were 'cured' and one died. Their length of stay in the hospital ranged from nine to 180 days, and averaged almost exactly two months.

There were two main requirements to secure admission to the new hospital. Patients had to be too poor to pay for their treatment and they needed a letter of recommendation from a benefactor or subscriber to hospital funds.

Subscribers of one guinea a year or a single donation of ten guineas could recommend two outpatients for a treatment each year. For a two guinea subscription, and for a benefactor of 25 guineas, one person could be recommended for inpatient treatment. Thereafter the number of letters available to subscribers and benefactors rose in accordance with the sum involved: for example, in the case of a three guinea subscription or a thirty guinea donation one inpatient and two outpatient letters were allowed. The numbers were doubled for a four guinea subscription or a forty guinea donation, although only one inpatient and two outpatients could be recommended at the same time. Subscribers of twenty guineas and benefactors donating 200 guineas had no limit on the number of letters available to them, although they were restricted to two inpatient and ten outpatient letters at any one time.

In common with other voluntary hospitals, however, there were restrictions on the prospective patients for whom letters of admission could be given.

Wives, children and apprentices of people able to afford treatment were excluded. So too were children under the age of seven except for surgery, consumptives, 'women big with child', persons 'disordered in their senses, or suspected to have the small pox, itch, or any other infectious diseases'.

Patients who remained in hospital after eight weeks had to go before the weekly board meeting to determine whether treatment should be allowed to continue for up to a further eight weeks when the process would be repeated if necessary.

The rules of the hospital also made it clear 'that when Patients are cured, they be enjoined by the Chairman to return thanks to Almighty God in their respective places of public worship'.

Admissions normally took place on a Wednesday. Priority was given to urgent cases, secondly to those living furthest from the hospital, then to those recommended by a subscriber who had not made a recommendation for admission during the previous year and finally to patients recommended by 'the greatest Subscribers or Benefactors to the Charity'. Every week, two beds were reserved for accidents occurring during the following week.

In the first three months, a total of 84 patients were admitted, the admissions and discharges register recording, in addition to the usual details, the names of those who had recommended the patients for admission and the 'securities for burial or removal' which was another essential requirement for eligibility for admission. The majority of patients lived locally; others were admitted from various parts of Sussex including Shoreham, Lancing, Cuckfield and Fletching. Some patients were admitted from further afield, including Deal and Tonbridge in Kent, Bath, and Chelsea and Soho in London.

A total of 240 in-patients were treated during 1828. The number rose steadily during the following three years: to 350 in 1829, 417 in 1830 and 540 in 1831.

By 1831 the number of beds in the hospital had increased from the original 72 to 113, the figure including the detached fever wards, which opened in August 1829. Although it had originally been intended to build a detached block for fever cases, this was not included in the plans because of expense. However, thanks largely to a donation of £1,000 from the Earl of Egremont, work eventually went ahead and the wards containing ten beds were built at a cost of £1,610.

According the Rules and Regulations of the hospital, the wards provided for cases that included typhus fever, scarlet fever and measles. Each patient was required to bring two changes of linen and pay 5s. per week and £1 on admission, 'the whole to be guaranteed by a responsible person.' For patients living within the parish, a small carriage or chair 'fitted with moveable linen furniture' was made available for conveying them to the hospital, with the stipulation that the patient's friends or recommender were responsible for the cost of horse hire.

A 13 bed 'spacious female ward' had also been erected at a cost of £500 and additional beds were purchased and placed in various parts of the hospital. Nevertheless, it was reported that the new ward was constantly occupied and in spite of these additional beds patients were being rejected 'for want of room.'

The situation was apparently no better in 1834 when the annual report noted: 'several poor and wretched objects have most reluctantly and painfully been refused admission, till vacancies should arise and the funds be increased.'

By 1834 the number of patients treated during the year had risen to 604. Of these, 94 remained in hospital at the end of the year, 245 were discharged cured, 166 relieved, 49 were referred to the outpatient department, 35 died and 15 were discharged 'for irregularity.'

Rules and Regulations

There were strict rules for patients' behaviour. Those set out in 1828 were read over every Friday morning in every ward: patients had to constantly attend prayers, were not allowed to swear or curse, use abusive language, or behave indecently 'or in any other way'. Rule 232 also forbade patients 'to play cards, dice or any other game' as well as the use of tobacco within the House. Patients were not allowed to go in any other ward except their own. If they were able to work, they had to assist with the nursing of other patients or undertake tasks, which included washing and ironing and cleaning the wards.

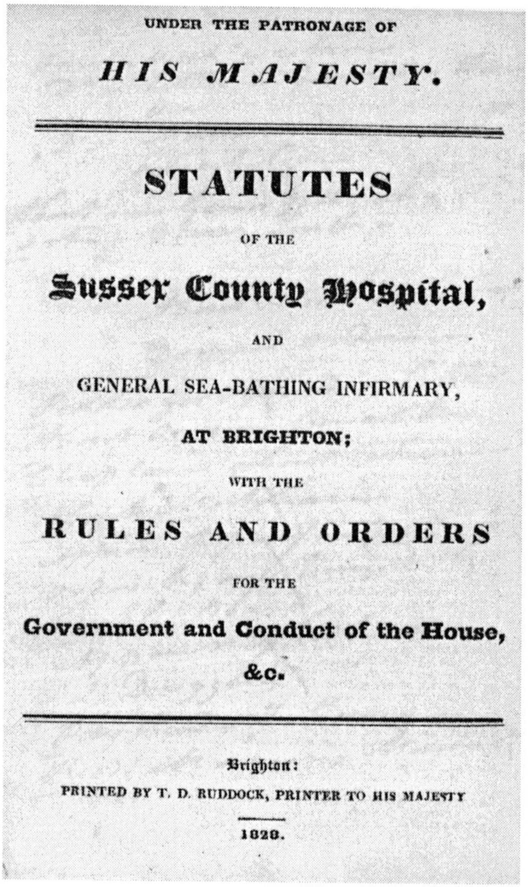

UNDER THE PATRONAGE OF

HIS MAJESTY.

STATUTES

OF THE

Sussex County Hospital,

AND

GENERAL SEA-BATHING INFIRMARY,

AT BRIGHTON;

WITH THE

RULES AND ORDERS

FOR THE

Government and Conduct of the House,

&c.

Brighton:

PRINTED BY T. D. RUDDOCK, PRINTER TO HIS MAJESTY

1828.

3. The Statutes, originally published in 1828. They contained detailed rules and orders concerning almost every aspect of life in the hospitals affecting patients and staff and were regularly updated.

Misbehaviour not only led to immediate discharge from the institution but also to entry in the Black Book, which meant permanent exclusion in the future.

Hospital records list the names of offenders as well as details of their offences. Alfred Chadwick was 'unruly, absented himself from chapel, got up a fight in the grounds on Sunday afternoon'. Ephraim Harmer was discharged for kissing a scrubber, a ward cleaner, and John Smith dressed in the scrubber's crinoline and made a disturbance in the ward.

Altogether, the Black Book contained 176 entries in its sixty-year existence. In the early years absconding was the principal reason for entry. After 1860 the most frequent reasons were insubordination, intoxication and, to a lesser extent, smoking.

It was not only the patients who were governed by the rules and orders contained in the hospital statutes. The house surgeon, for example, could not entertain anyone in the house 'either for pleasure or any other purpose'. If he was absent for more than two hours he had to arrange for a proper person to take care of the patients. He could not be away at night without the express permission of the committee and whenever he was absent he had to let the matron know where he could be found.

The matron herself had always to sleep in the hospital and was never allowed to be away at the same time as the house surgeon. Every evening she was responsible for locking the doors dividing the men's from the women's wards.

The house surgeon, matron, nurses and servants all had to be unmarried and 'not burdened with children or the care of a family'.

Two of the house surgeon's duties were the supervision of the brewery including the purchase of best pale malt and Kent or Sussex hops and the control of machinery to the water well. The matron was directed to see that 'the following limit in respect of beer' was enforced: 'nurses 2 pints, porters and washerwomen 2 pints each; the cook, housemaid and scullery maid 1½ pints each per day'. Beer was administered to patients only under strict instructions from the doctors.

In 1840, the hospital brewed 7,000 gallons of beer at a cost of a little over 9d per gallon compared with a purchase price of 10d. The following year the retail price of beer fell and the brewery was used for other purposes, consequently relieving the house surgeon of this particular responsibility. Another of the house surgeon's duties was engaging the porters and domestic servants. The porters received £16 per annum with a suit of clothes and two guineas per annum in lieu of tea and sugar. Domestic servants received only £8 per annum and also a tea and sugar allowance.

The House Visitors

The committee appointed two house visitors every month and it was their responsibility to visit the hospital together or by turns once a week. One of their tasks was to examine the bread and beer. Another was to ensure that none of the many rules and regulations had been breached, not only those already referred to, but others such as whether the porter had let any of the patients, nurses or servants leave without permission, or whether any liquor or provisions had been brought in to the patients.

In May 1829, one of the visitors reprimanded the under porter for allowing the secretary's horse to be kept in the hospital stable. But this was part of a much more serious issue. The month before the secretary had been reprimanded for employing the under porter as his groom for four or five weeks without permission and feeding his horse with provender provided by the charity for their own engine horse. Despite being ordered to remove the horse, the secretary had obviously failed to do so and in consequence was severely reprimanded.

The earliest surviving records of the house visitors provide a detailed description of their work and some of the best examples of what went on within the hospital walls in its earliest years.

The first entries record that the wards visited were clean and comfortable, gave details of any complaints by patients or nurses, and also the internal and external temperatures at the time of the visits.

In 1845, there is a record of dissatisfaction in No. 2 Ward where a nurse had given one patient 'a larger slice of bread than he deserved'. This same ward was the subject of a report two years later when the board requested the visitors to look into the circumstances surrounding the discharge of the upper nurse. This recorded:

> Being by her own admission pregnant, Matron dismissed her without ascertaining from her to whom her condition was to be ascribed. We have questioned the Under Nurse and the Scrubber on the same ward – and also the Porters – but without eliciting any information which would inculpate any person in the House though suspicion attaches to the Gate Porter arising from an intimacy, which for some time past has existed between him and the said nurse, which he utterly disclaims ever having been carried to an improper extent.

There are other examples of alleged sexual misdemeanours and of theft by an under nurse of several articles of a patient's clothes. However there were more frequent references to leaking taps, lack of hot water, smoking chimneys, leaks in the roof, poor food, smells (from patients, drains and water closets) and water closet blockages, 'some wilful'. The action of a patient who put his crutch through a water closet in Ward 10 appeared to the visitors to be connected to two nurses 'guilty of culpable negligence' for ignoring the fact that the WC had been blocked for the previous two days.

Ward 10 was the subject of another report in 1850 when a young man was seen rushing out of the nurses' room and back to the ward. He had been alone in the room with the nurse but claimed he had gone to purchase bullseyes, a practice that the visitors discovered had been going on for many years.

Some of the matters dealt with by the visitors have a not unfamiliar ring: smoking in bed, for example, (although perhaps not in more recent times, having lighted candles in bed), the discharge of a patient in Ward 10 for threatening another patient with a knife and lengthy waiting by outpatients. The latter was brought to the visitors' attention because male patients waiting for their medicines were said to be defacing the walls with 'indecent writing and caricatures'.

The longest entry in the earliest volume of house visitors' reports still in existence contained nine recommendations. Made in 1850, the report noted the need for a study room for the pupils; there was a long, detailed report on fire precautions and also a report of water seeping through the basement floor. There was also a reference to patients in Ward 10 who were in the habit of closing the windows as soon as the nurses' backs were turned. 'The charge I gave the patients upon the subject, will I hope remedy the evil', the visitor added.

The nurses

1500 to 1850 has been described as the Dark Age of hospital history and nursing. Following the dissolution of the monasteries, the thousands of nursing nuns who worked sixteen hours a day without pay were replaced by nurses who had to be hired and paid weekly.

According to one writer, 'Because the work was hard, the hours long, and the wages a pittance, the only available workers were women from the refuse heap of society, dirty, drunk and contemptuous of their charges.'[1] Possibly a rather harsh generalisation, but there is evidence to underpin this assessment: Dickens' Sarah Gamps certainly existed in hospitals in the nineteenth century, and the Sussex County was no exception.

In an interview in 1934, the hospital's matron, Miss Young, looking back a hundred years, believed 'nurses' to be 'women of the Gamp type, ignorant, untaught, often dirty, ill-fed, overworked and underpaid. They were frequently on duty 12 to 24 hours at a stretch, and went to sleep at night leaving the patients to look after themselves.'

Florence Nightingale has recounted how in the mid-eighteenth century a very large number of patients were under the care of one nurse – in one case a single night nurse had charge of four wards. From a Visitor's Report in 1862, this was certainly known to occur at the Sussex County Hospital.

Wishing to draw attention to the 'great amount of night work' the report stated that for Ward 2 (accident) 30 beds, wards 4 and 10, each 24 beds and Ward 6, 20 beds, there was only one established nurse for all the wards. Under committee minute 5295 a scrubber (mostly young inexperienced persons, the visitor noted) could be called upon to assist in periods of great pressure and although the house surgeon was authorised to call on additional night nurses, these could rarely be obtained when they were needed.

The Rev. R.B. Matson, writing in 1923, looked back 60 years to the time when he was a 12-year-old patient in the men's ward.

> There were only two nurses for the whole ward – the matron a stout sort of Mrs Gamp woman who had a room at the end of the ward and who went about with a bunch of keys and a pair of scissors – and to get on the right side of her the friends of patients gave her something. The other nurse was Sally – a good-hearted girl who got up very early, cleaned the grates, lit the fires, then helped dress the wounds.

However, although good-hearted, Sally was rough dressing wounds and the young Matson begged the doctors to be allowed to wash and dress his own wound.

A list of hospital servants compiled in 1871 shows that most wards were staffed by a nurse, an under nurse and a scrubber. The longest serving nurses received £25 a year. Nurse Huggett in the 21-bedded Ward 1 had 35 years service and nurse Mary Hilton in Ward 4 (26 beds) 25 years. The other nurses were paid from £22 to £24. Under nurses received £15 and scrubbers £12. Interestingly the cook received £30 a year and the head laundry woman £27. Even the second laundry woman, who was paid £16 a year, received more than the under nurses.

In this respect, the Sussex County was no different from any other voluntary hospital at the time. The matron and nurses were employed as servants, not medical attendants. The main requirements for a matron, who was really the housekeeper, were usually respectability, middle age and, of prime importance, no family ties.[2] Even Florence Nightingale subscribed to the view that nurses were the worst sort of women who were 'too old, too weak, too drunken, too dirty, too stolid, or too bad to do anything else'.[3]

However, it is probably fair to say that only the bad cases were referred to in committee minute books and reports and that diligent, hard-working nurses were rarely mentioned, but there are, in fact, examples of both in the Sussex County Hospital records. These records also give examples that show that the work undertaken by the nurses could be both onerous and unpleasant. A Visitor's report in 1862 drew attention to the great amount of work undertaken by a night nurse, the only person on duty to cover three wards with a total of 74 beds. Five years earlier, another house visitor reported on a visit to the fever ward. The condition of a venereal patient on the ward, it was reported, had been steadily getting worse. He was restless at night causing a great deal of extra work. The smell or stench of the sores covering his body, not only in the bath but also in the ward, was very offensive to the other patients – besides which he consumed eight ounces of port wine daily and was very fastidious about his diet. 'Although the poor nurse has an allowance of gin to sustain her in her disagreeable duties, she would rather attend twelve ordinary patients than this one,' the report continued, adding 'I feel it is my duty to report her case to the Board.'

The medical staff

One of the most important features of the voluntary hospital movement was that the medical staff made no charge for their services. Every hospital had one or more honorary appointments for physicians and surgeons. They gave their services free (or for a nominal honorarium) as an act of public generosity. In this way, too, they gained prestige and the opportunity, in the words of one eminent medical historian, 'to hobnob with the governors and gentry, and therefore gain powerful patrons and wealthy private patients.'[4]

At this time, of course, society was in the firm grip of the class system and medicine was no exception. The relative positions of medical men in Britain were firmly established: physicians were at the top of the order followed by the surgeons (a rivalry which can be seen to persist even today), then the apothecaries, later to become the general practitioners.[5]

According to Cameron in his history of Guy's Hospital:

> The physicians moved discreetly and quietly about the wards and always took their hats off; the surgeons stamped noisily to the bedside, hat on head, accompanied by crowds of chattering, jostling pupils. It was then the mode for a surgeon to be a rough, foulmouthed fellow ... without polish.[6]

It seems possible that the early medical men described by Cameron were by no means confined to Guy's. What is certain is that the physicians ruled and that a deep-rooted antagonism existed between them and the surgeons. The rift between the two has existed throughout history: the legislation of Henry VIII, for example, which was intended to bring some sort of order to the chaos then existing in the practice of medicine, actually widened the rift between physician and surgeon. Surgeons developed from barber surgeons and the Barber Surgeons' Company was formed in 1540. However the surgeons were refused a doctorate by the Royal College of Physicians, who considered their training and education had not reached a satisfactory standard. When eventually the physicians offered them a doctorate, the surgeons responded by retaining the title Mister as, in their eyes, almost a superior degree, much to the confusion until the present day of the general public.

It seems certain, that in the early days of the Sussex County, the physicians were the undisputed leaders medically. In early nineteenth century Hastings, for example:

> Physicians were the most respected and brought learning rather than technology to bear on their patients' problems. Surgeons worked with their hands and had only just received the respectability of a profession. The apothecaries were really druggists who were later allowed to order the remedies they dispensed.[7]

At the newly opened Sussex County Hospital the medical staff, physicians and surgeons, all held honorary appointments except the house surgeon, Benjamin Vallance, who received a salary. His professional work was frequently praised in the minutes of the board of management and Vallance Ward was later named after him.

He was succeeded in 1831 by Mr E. J. Furner. It was largely through Furner's efforts that the library and museum were founded in 1833 and the hospital was recognised as a School of Practical Medicine and Surgery in 1834 by the Court of Examiners of the Royal College of Surgeons in London and by the Examiners of Apothecary Hall in London.

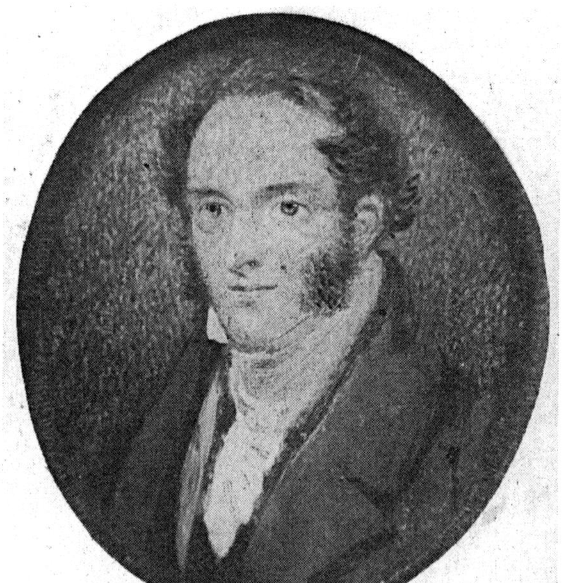

4. The first house surgeon: Benjamin Vallance. Vallance Ward was named after him.

The procedure for electing a house surgeon was set out in an advertisement in the *Brighton Gazette* in October 1842.

> Candidates must be unmarried, or in such circumstances as not to be burdened with children, or the care of a family; above 23 years of age, members of the College of Surgeons of London, or of the Colleges of Dublin, Edinburgh or Glasgow, and likewise Licentiates of the Apothecaries Company.
>
> Testimonials of good character, and of being such members of College and Licentiates as above mentioned, must be sent (post-paid) to the Secretary of the Sussex County Hospital, Brighton, on or before Monday the 21st November next.
>
> The emoluments of the office are as follows, viz:
>
> The House Surgeon shall have his board and lodging in the house, with a yearly salary of

> £80, exclusive of £10 per annum of each of his apprentices.
>
> The Election to be by ballot, commencing at Half-past Two precisely, and closing at four by St George's Chapel Clock and the succeeding Ballot to commence on the conclusion of the preceding one. Every Ballot after the first is to close as soon as the Chairman shall declare that all the Governors present have voted.

The procedure for electing a house surgeon was simplified three years later when it was decided that no second ballot should be held, the candidate having the highest number of votes being declared elected.

A similar procedure was followed for electing consultants to a vacant office and produced an interesting result in 1842 when Dr William King and Dr Jenks were admitted as candidates for the vacant office of physician.

Dr King is perhaps best known as a leading figure in the establishment of the Cooperative Movement. His interest in relieving poverty and improvement through education led him to establish an infants' school in 1823 and in 1825 he became vice president of the Mechanics Institute. Possibly because of his concern for the poor and destitute, he did not at first have an extensive medical practice among the rich. However, he was to admit later, in a letter, that his interest in co-operation 'severely injured me professionally'[8] although by 1842 he appears to have put this behind him and no less than the Earl of Chichester himself proposed him for the office of Physician.

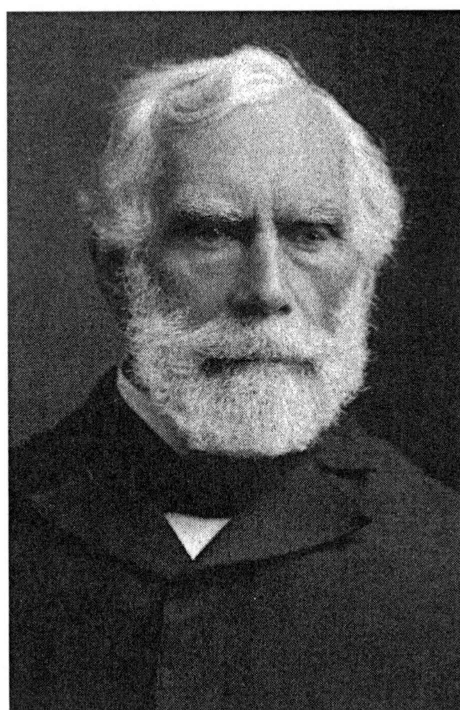

5. E.J. Furner succeeded Vallance as house surgeon in 1831. Like his predecessor, his responsibilities included the supervision of the hospital brewery.

The ballot proceeded in the usual way and at three o'clock by St George's Chapel clock the chairman, scrutineers and governors present 'proceeded to examine and cast up the number of votes'. The result: For Dr King 180; for Dr Jenks 179. A majority of just one vote would normally have been sufficient to secure Dr King's election but Mr Attree, one of the scrutineers, suggested that one of his votes was from Mrs Walker of Herne Hill who had died recently. If this was so, the chairman said, the votes would be equal and as he declined to give a casting vote the election would be null and void. Fortunately for Dr King, however, a letter later placed before the Board from Mary Farncombe of East Street confirmed that Mrs Walker was alive: 'I am happy to inform that I left Mrs Walker at Denmark Hill, Camberwell at 9 o'clock this morning as well and as comfortable as she has been for some time past' and Dr King was therefore confirmed as Physician to the hospital, a post he held until his retirement in 1861.

In the meantime, in 1847, the medical officers of the Dispensary resolved to form a medical society. Following a meeting held in Brighton Town Hall, the Brighton and Sussex Medico-Chirurgical Society was formed and Dr King became its first president. During the early years of its existence, clinical evenings were frequently held, and a discussion of cases treated at the Sussex County Hospital during the past year, and a description of specimens added to the hospital museum, featured in the annual programme.

Possibly the reason for the closeness of the vote for the office of Physician can be found in the writing of consultant surgeon Nathaniel Paine Blaker.[9] Dr King had the advantage of the support of the Earl of Chichester although, according to Blaker, '[he] was a man of gentlemanly manners, and very well informed, but his professional knowledge was rather antique'. On the other hand, 'Dr Jenks had been an army surgeon, and was in the Peninsular War, and had amputated at the shoulder joint at the Battle of Toulouse. He was a man of considerable ability.'

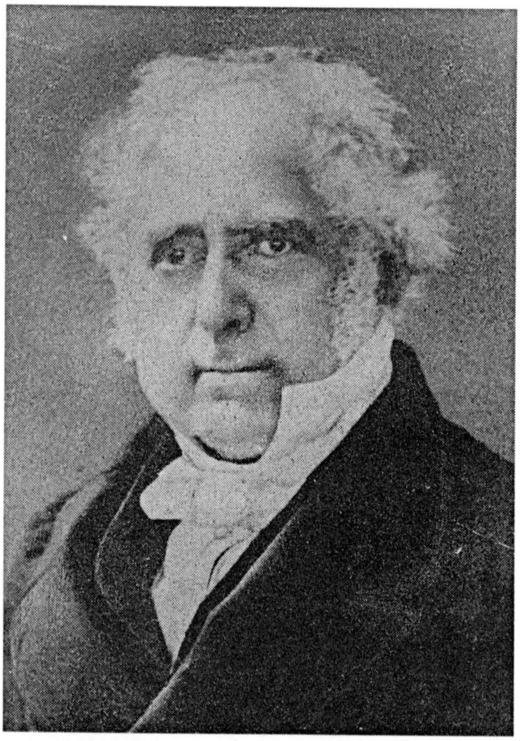

6. Dr William King, best known perhaps as a leading figure in the Co-operative movement, was elected as Physician by a majority of one vote in 1842. In 1847 he became the first president of the newly formed Sussex Medico-Chirurgical Society.

Nathaniel Blaker had a distinguished surgical pedigree; his great-uncle Harry Blaker was one of the 300 original surgeons of the Royal College of Surgeons. His first cousin, Harry Mills Blaker, was also a surgeon at the hospital. His second cousin Edgar Shaw Blaker later became a surgeon at Knapp Hill.

Nathaniel commenced his professional education as a resident pupil on one month's probation in 1852. An advertisement for a medical pupil two years later, for a fee of 100 guineas per annum, stated that the pupil would 'live in the House and board at the Matron's Table.' Interestingly, Nathaniel Blaker's book provides a pen portrait of the matron, Mrs Comport who had been in post since the hospital opened in 1828.

> She was a charming old lady, and was looked on as part of the Institution, in which she still took the greatest interest. She always spoke of the pupils as 'her boys,' and though we used to tease her, and play small practical jokes on her, we did not much fear her anger, which usually ended in an oyster supper.

The resident staff at the time of his first appointment consisted of the house surgeon, matron, three or four pupils and the dispenser

> The House Surgeon, besides having care of the patients and the supervision of the wards, was answerable for a good deal of the executive work, and being, by statute, resident master of the establishment, all cases of difficulty were referred to him. The Dispenser was responsible for the dispensing, which however was done chiefly by the resident pupils. Besides these resident pupils there were a number of non-resident pupils, who in those days were apprenticed to various medical men in the town, and were allowed to see the practice at the hospital on payment of £10 per annum.

Nathaniel Blaker's *Reminiscences* also give more information about some of the other surgeons and physicians at the Sussex County Hospital during its early years. Referring to the first three surgeons appointed, he said Harry Blaker was surgeon to the royal family and received £300 a year for attending the household at the Royal Pavilion; Robert Taylor 'was always looked on as an excellent surgeon' and so, he believed, was Mr Lawrence. The three all resigned on the same day and Benjamin Vallance, E.J. Furner and John Lawrence junior were appointed to succeed them.

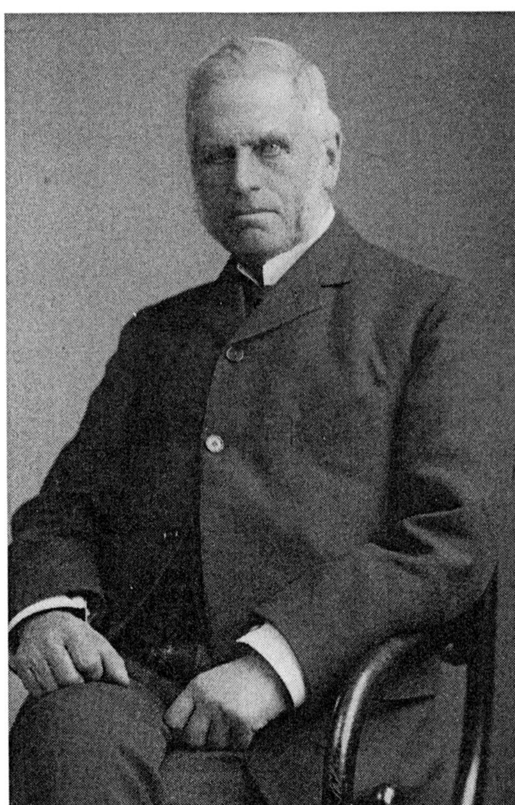

7. Consultant surgeon Nathaniel Paine Blaker (1869-1899) was originally a resident pupil at the hospital in 1852. His published Reminiscences *provide a picture of conditions there in his early days.*

Dr Edward Ormerod was one of the most celebrated of the hospital's physicians and published papers on medicine and natural history. He was appointed a few months after Nathaniel Blaker commenced his pupilage. Nathaniel described him as a man of great intellect, highly cultured, of great industry and up-to-date.

Dr Ormerod had left Barts Hospital a few years earlier when his health broke down and told Nathaniel he had come down to Brighton to die. If this was so, it did not prevent him from making his mark in Sussex and, in fact, he lived to serve the hospital for twenty years. During his admission week he came in to the hospital punctually at 9 a.m. and took histories of his cases, which he dictated to his clinical clerk, one of the apprentices who received medical education at the hospital before moving on to one of the London medical schools.

These case histories provide a roll call of many of the hospital's surgeons and physicians in its early years. In addition to those already mentioned were house surgeon G. Lowdell who was appointed surgeon in 1854 and died in office in 1871; the physicians included Drs. Thomas Blair, George Hall, Henry Moon, W. Withers Moore, Joseph Rutter, W.A. Hollis and William Kebbell.

Dr Kebbell, as chairman of a charitable trust, was responsible for building the Model Dwellings at the corner of Jew Street and Church Street in about 1852 as housing for the poor of the town. In 1848 he had issued a report containing damning comments on the town's poorer districts. These were characterised by open cesspits near drinking wells, sewers which ran above basement level and crowded tenements lining the tiny streets and courtyards, all of which contributed to the poor health of their inhabitants. In fact, the slums in this area were reputed to be as bad as any in London or the industrial north.

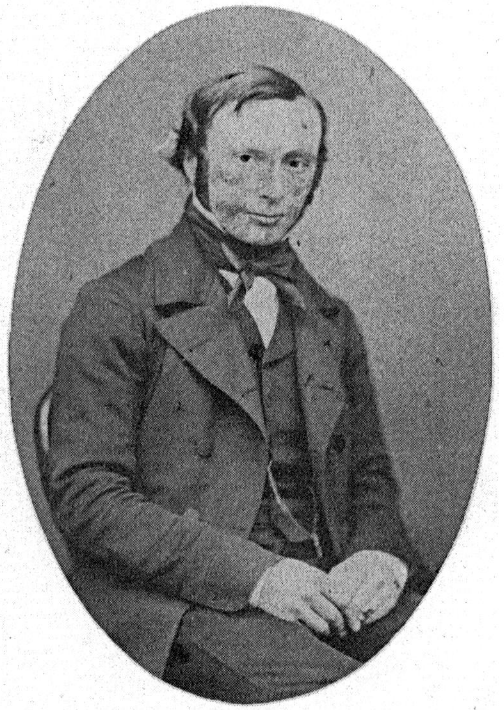

8. Dr Edward Ormerod, one of the most celebrated nineteenth century hospital physicians. His case histories can be seen at the East Sussex County Record Office.

In 1873, following the death of Dr Ormerod, the medical staff formed a committee to administer a memorial, the Ormerod Exhibition Fund, so that 'his name and good works should be kept alive'. The interest on this fund was then used to enable the most deserving student about to leave the hospital to complete his professional studies in London.

Sea Bathing

Although Dr Russell's work was largely responsible for Brighton's reputation as the place to visit for sea water cures, the distinction of establishing the first sea bathing infirmary actually fell to Brighton's seaside rival, Margate. Founded in 1791, the Royal Sea Bathing Infirmary opened five years later to treat the diseased poor from London with sea

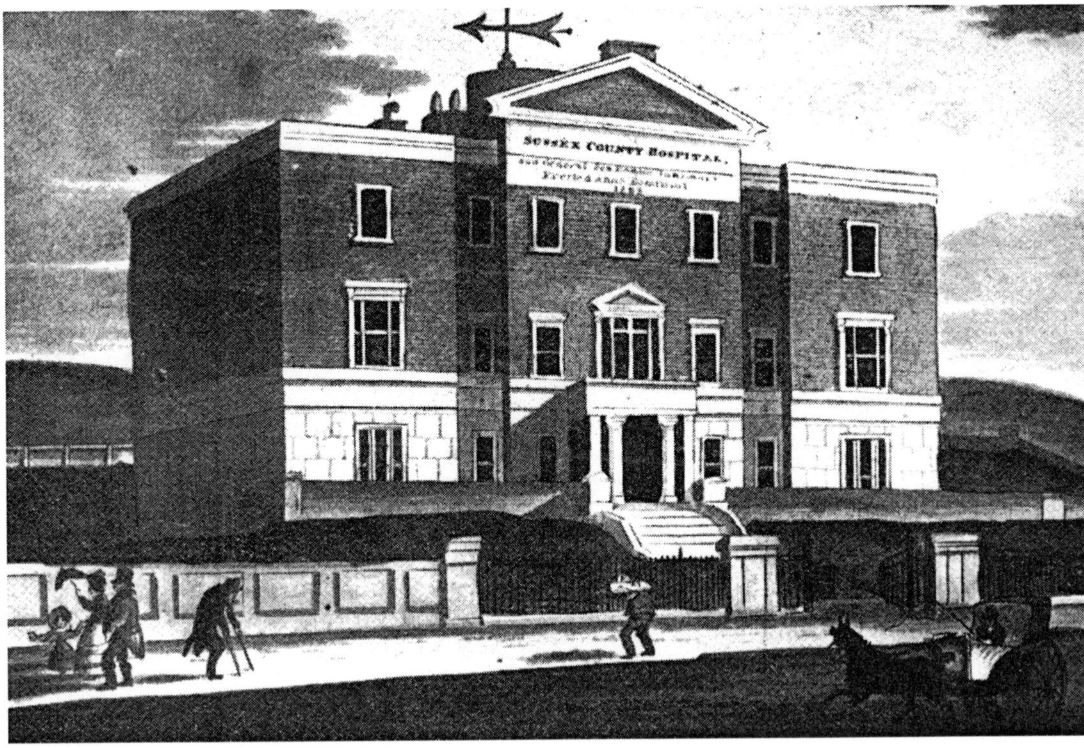

9. The Sussex County Hospital and Sea Bathing Infirmary, Brighton 1828.

air and sea bathing in the summer months. Internal baths were also built so that treatment might continue through the winter. In addition patients' treatment included drinking two pints of salt water in milk every day.

Although there is no record of drinking salt water as a treatment in the Sussex County, in the early years great importance was attached to sea bathing. Thousands of bathing tickets were issued and probably about half the patients were taken down to the sea each day while others were able to use a sea bathing pool in the basement.

One of the first acts of the board of management was to investigate the best way of bringing a supply of salt water to the hospital. A dray and butt were obtained and water was brought from the Old Steine Hotel to the hospital. However, the cost of supplying this obviously caused financial problems. In June 1836 a sub-committee appointed to consider the matter reported that salt water bathing had been 'left to cases of extreme urgency'. A special General Court was called for the 29th June to consider a report on the matter and accepted a recommendation to obtain water directly from the sea. Accordingly an application was made to the town commissioners for an arch to be constructed in the sea wall at the bottom of what is now

Paston Place. This was to house machinery for pumping 250 gallons of water daily directly to the hospital through pipes laid under the road.

The importance that many subscribers attached to sea bathing was illustrated in July 1838 when a subscriber declined to renew his subscription in the belief 'that it does not answer my expectation as a *Sea-bathing* Infirmary for which purpose I became a Subscriber.' Nevertheless this did not dissuade the board from changing the name of the hospital: they dropped the words 'General Sea Bathing Infirmary' and placed the emphasis on 'County Hospital'. A decision to place these words on the stone facing in front of the hospital 'in as large letters as the upper space will admit' was taken but almost immediately altered, the wording then read 'Sussex County Hospital. Established 1828'.

It is unclear whether the installation of the pump and the laying of pipes to the hospital ever went ahead. What is certain is that the practice of sea bathing gradually diminished.

4. Growth and Development, 1830 – 1856

The sixty years from 1839 to the end of the nineteenth century witnessed the growth of the major part of the hospital developed from the original Barry Building.

The Victoria Wing to the west of the Barry Building was built to celebrate the coming of age of Princess Victoria and subsequently to commemorate her first visit to Brighton. The wing opened on 19th June 1839. The eastern wing was named the Adelaide Wing by permission of Her Majesty Adelaide the Queen Dowager. Because of the pressure of urgent cases, the opening of the upper floor was brought forward and made available on the 15th September 1841. Extensions to the east and west wings were completed in 1853 and, after some delay, the hospital chapel was built in 1856.

The other major developments, the Jubilee Building, the outpatient department and the nurses home were completed during the latter part of the century.

Patronage by the reigning monarch and continued support to the present day by other members of the royal family is acknowledged in plaques on the walls of the Barry Building . King William IV donated £800 and subscribed £100 annually. Her Majesty Queen Adelaide subscribed £20 annually, Queen Victoria made a donation of £1,000 – sums which, of course, would be worth considerably more in present day prices.

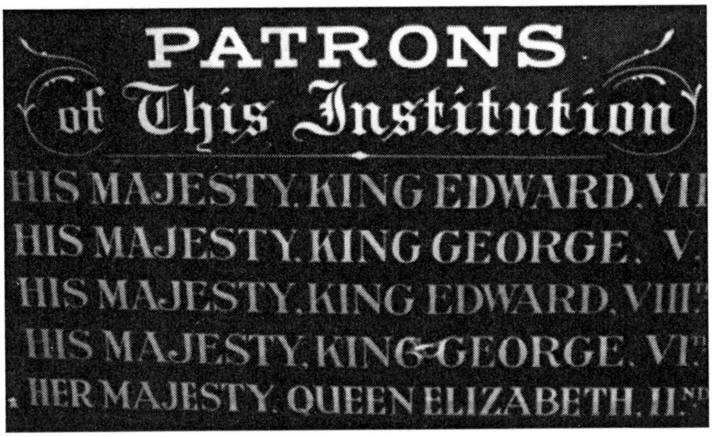
PATRONS
of This Institution
HIS MAJESTY KING EDWARD VII
HIS MAJESTY KING GEORGE. V.
HIS MAJESTY KING EDWARD VIII
HIS MAJESTY KING GEORGE. VI
HER MAJESTY QUEEN ELIZABETH. II

10. Three plaques on the staircase in ther Barry Building illustrate the envolving royal patronage of the hospital. An earlier plaque named King William and Queen Victoria

Hospital finance

By the end of 1830, two years after it opened, the Sussex County Hospital was £330 in debt, something which was to become a recurring feature over the following years. However, it was not alone in experiencing financial difficulties. The problem of securing sufficient funds to support their activities afflicted the entire voluntary hospital system. It was one of the major factors that led to its eventual demise in Britain in 1948 with the introduction of the National Health Service.

Once the initial impetus had been given to a hospital, it had to achieve financial stability. A major source of income came from subscriptions from interested members of the community. In return they were able, depending on the size of their subscription, to nominate patients for admission, to exercise a vote at general meetings and were eligible to serve as a house visitor and be involved in the day to day running of the institution. Donations, benefactions and bequests were also important sources of income, often saving the hospitals from closure.[1]

The church was also involved in helping to raise money to help the hospitals, no doubt reinforcing the view that the subscriber would be helping his cause on the Day of Judgement. Although in the early nineteenth century there is evidence that the church sermon in aid of hospital giving was in decline,[2] fortunately this was not the case in Sussex. In 1826, the Bishop of Chichester had issued a pastoral letter soliciting the clergy to preach sermons in parishes to promote the success of the institution.

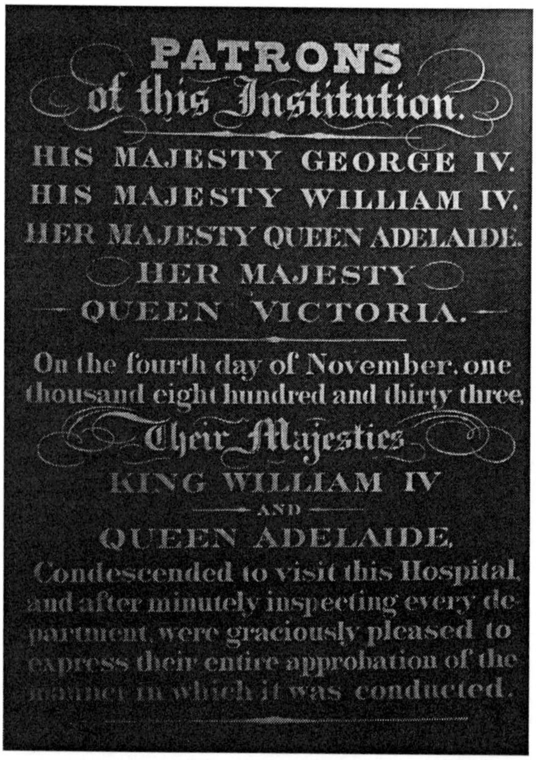

11. The plaque that commemorates the day King William and Queen Adelaide 'condescended' to visit the hospital.

In September 1828, local newspapers carried announcements that annual sermons were to be preached in aid of funds for the hospital. St Peter's Church, the Chapel Royal, St James' Chapel, St Margaret's and Trinity chapels were among those in Brighton 'where no money was to be paid for seats, or given to pew openers': clearly there was every incentive to the public to attend on these occasions. Copies of a sermon by the Rev. J.S.M. Anderson, the hospital chaplain, given in St George's Chapel in 1829, were even printed and made available for sale, the profits being donated to the hospital.

In 1832, the governors resolved that where the collections from their places of worship amounted to £10 or more, all clergymen and ministers should be entitled to the privileges of annual subscribers of five guineas.

In 1836, because of the increasing number of patients being received from Lewes and the eastern part of the county, the public appeal for congregational collections and subscribers was extended to the clergy and people of Lewes. At the same time, another source of income was developed. Workmen in the cabinet factory of Patching and Wood in Ship Street, Brighton, decided that from the 1st January 1837 they would put a penny a week in a box placed in the workshop towards funds for the hospital. Two of their employers, Mr Hunt and Mr Marchant, added 6d per week hoping that the scheme would be copied by workmen in the town and in the county. Other cabinet makers followed: Cheesman and Son of Kensington Street and Beves of West Street, Mr Beves himself contributing 3d a week.

The Court of Governors responded by agreeing to publish a list of subscribers in a range of newspapers at the end of the year. Moreover, they decided that where the sum collected in a workman's box equalled the amount qualifying a subscriber to recommend patients for treatment, the workshop concerned would enjoy corresponding privileges of recommendation.

By the end of the year, fifteen places of employment had collected sufficient amounts giving them the right to make recommendations. Five of these, including ironmongers. Attwood and Wimble were based in Lewes, the remainder in Brighton. They included the *Brighton Gazette*, Beves & Co. and the builders Cheesman & Son.

The continuing success of the scheme is illustrated by the list published in the *Guardian* in 1841. Collections in Brighton during 1840 totalled over £76. The list was headed by the workmen of Cheesman & Son – £10 4s 7d from the brickmakers' and £9 6s 10d from the carpenters' boxes. Other prominent contributors included Capt. Marsh's coastguardsmen (£9), the compositors and apprentices of the *Brighton Gazette*, the gas company at Black Rock, and the brewers Tamplin & Son.

Eight boxes in Lewes raised just over £23 while the £27 4s 0d from 'other places' included £13 10s 0d from the labourers on the railway at Preston and Patcham. Although significant, these were by no means the only way in which funds were raised to support the charity. Gideon Mantell gave a lecture in aid of the hospital at the Old Ship in February 1834. Tickets were priced at 2s 6d for the lecture on 'geology and the remains of a former world discovered in Sussex'.

The governors, meanwhile, had instituted an annual fundraising event, also at the Old Ship. They decided that the 8th October 1828 was to 'be kept according to the rules as the anniversary of the foundation of the Institution'. Subscribers and friends were invited to dine together, tickets one guinea including wine, 'dinner on the table at precisely five o'clock.' Later innovations included the Hospital Saturday Fund. Its principal aim was to collect small weekly collections from people who could not afford to give considerable sums at one time. The Hospital Sunday Fund was a centrally organised body that aimed to stimulate church collections and distribute the funds received to hospitals.

Music festivals and evening entertainments were a popular form of fund-raising for many voluntary hospitals. For the Sussex County, balls were popular. A concert and ball in Lewes in 1830 raised £46 10s for the charity. A ball organised by the High Constable of Brighton in 1832 realised £32 4s 8d. But the major fundraiser at this time was the sale of fancy work held over three days in the town hall in November 1833. Held under the patronage of their majesties King William IV, Queen Adelaide and Princess Augusta the sale raised over £1,380. The King and Queen had earlier paid a private visit and 'very minutely inspected the Hospital, expressing their high and decided appreciation at the manner in which it was conducted.'

The number of patients treated at the hospital continued to rise. By 1834, 604 inpatients, the highest number since the hospital opened, and 250 outpatients were treated when, according to the annual report, 245 inpatients were cured, 166 relieved and 35 died. 15 patients were discharged 'for irregularity'.

The following year, with the debt still in the region of £300, a resident surgeon was engaged to 'ensure utmost economy and constant superintendence of the Institution.'

The need for an additional wing

Meanwhile, in spite of its financial problems, the hospital contunued to develop. In 1834 gas lighting had been installed and a museum and other buildings had been erected for the surgical department intended to facilitate the studies of the medical students.

In 1837, the hospital embarked on the next major stage of its development. That year, the president, the Earl of Egremont, had died. Shortly before he had donated a further sum of £1,000 to the institution, emphasising that it was his wish that the wards should be extended. This would provide adequate accommodation for convalescent patients because, he believed, separating them from serious cases would accelerate the recovery of both.

Within a short time of his death, sufficient support was received from the public for progress to be made with a scheme to build a wing, to be known as the Victoria Wing. The fund was founded with a £500 donation from Mr Lawrence Peel and £401 4s 7d from a committee appointed by Brighton townsfolk for celebrating the coming of age of Princess Victoria and subsequently for commemorating her first visit to Brighton.

Support was also received from the Directors and Guardians of the Brighton Poor. They appointed a committee to superintend the employment of workmen receiving poor relief who were put to work excavating and removing earth from the site and shooting it over the cliff at Marine Parade. According to the annual report for 1838, this apparently included sloping away the hill surrounding the hospital to 'afford additional light and ventilation to the whole hospital, especially the Fever Ward.'

The architect responsible for the new wing was Mr William Hallett of the Bristol Hotel and Mr Penton contracted to undertake the building for £2,615 19s 3d. With the hospital's books balanced and sufficient donations received, work commenced earlier than anticipated and Mr Lawrence Peel laid the corner stone at noon on 17th August 1838, the birthday of the Duchess of Kent.

However, a report by the Victoria Wing Sub-Committee the following April revealed that there were financial problems. The wards on the three floors were nearly three times as large as the existing ones containing ten patients,

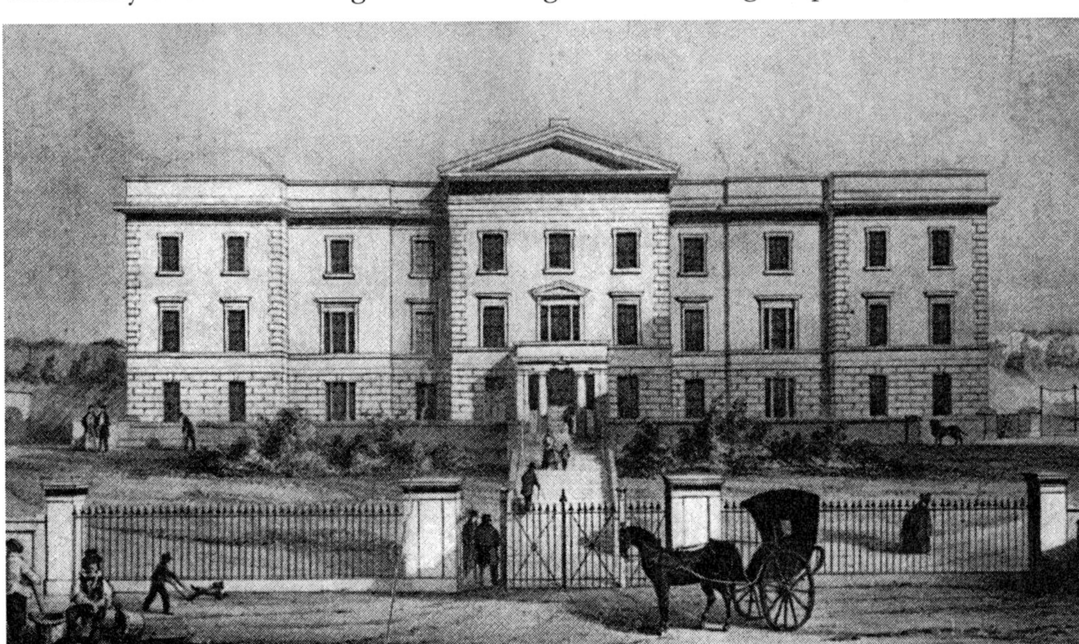

12. The Barry Building pictured after the addition of the Victoria and Adelaide wings.

the report explained, but there were insufficient funds and the committee appealed to the public for more donations in order to complete the work.

The appeal was obviously successful. In September, the *Sussex Express* reported that there was a balance that would be used towards the foundation of a fund to build a second wing. The final report of the committee in October recorded that contributions had amounted to £2,970 17s 9d leaving a balance of £354 18s 6d which included a reserve of small sums for painting and other work. In addition to extra beds, the report continued, a spacious dormitory had been provided in the basement for eight female servants. A room in Ward 4 had been converted to a library and museum for the use of the medical officers and students, 'an advantageous place for the preservation of specimens,' and which included facilities 'for medical pupils and others in the prosecution of their studies.'

Although many additional beds became available when the Victoria Wing opened on 19th June 1839, it was evident that even more were required to cope with increasing demand. 728 patients were admitted during the year, 56 more than in 1838. 195 accident cases were admitted, more than 70 coming from work on the railway under construction in the vicinity of Brighton. Outpatient numbers, too, were on the increase, the total of 865 being 175 greater than the previous year.

The surplus in the fund subscribed to build the Victoria Wing having been set aside to form the nucleus of a fund to build another wing to the east of the Barry Building, permission was given by the Queen Dowager for it to be known as the Adelaide Wing. Work on the extension commenced in May 1840 under the supervision of the architect, Mr Herbert Williams of Bloomsbury.

The corner stone of the building was laid on the 13th August, the anniversary of the Queen Dowager's birthday. Contemporary reports of the occasion noted that for two hours before the ceremony was due to take place, the town was alive 'with bustle and excitement'. The military band of the 11th Hussars led a procession to the hospital. They were followed by 'the Brethren of the Mystic Sign, the Freemasons of the York and Clarence Lodges who, being decorated with all the signs and trappings of their Order, gave additional éclat to the grand and imposing appearance of the ceremony.'

Addressing the 300 people attending the ceremony, the chaplain, Mr Anderson, explained that the applications for admission were greater than they could accommodate. The reason for this, he suggested was 'the salubrity of the air of Brighton and the high reputation which its physicians and surgeons have obtained, have been a great inducement to have the sick and infirm from other parts of the country brought to this place'. He continued:

> The many casualties to which human nature was subject, should lead them to feel some commiseration for this class of person, so that when they came here for relief, they should not refuse to receive them; neither should they rest satisfied in bestowing a transient glance upon their wretchedness and then, without further notice, pass them by; No, they should exert themselves to furnish fresh means of accommodation.

Lord Chichester, who presided at the ceremony, then presented an inscribed silver trowel with an ivory handle (made by Lewis & Son of Ship Street) to Mr Cordy, Grand Master of the Clarence Lodge, deputising for the Earl of Munster, who was 'severely indisposed.'

The cost of the Adelaide Wing, which included expenditure on equipment, was estimated to be in the region of £4,000. The list of subscribers included Lawrence Peel (£105) and Lady Jane Peel (£52 10s 0d). Another Fancy Fair held in the Town Hall during November 1839 under the patronage of the Queen Dowager provided major support for the project. Half the proceeds of the fair, nearly £930, were donated to the building fund.

The proprietors of the Shoreham Branch of the London and Brighton Railway announced that they, too, were to support the fund. They proposed to give the gross receipts of passenger traffic on the 28th September 1840 (or the following day if the weather was unfavourable) to the Sussex County Hospital. The proprietor of the Swiss Gardens at Shoreham also announced that he would devote the net receipts of admission on the day, which would also include 'sundry amusements ... for the gratification of the visitors'.

A few weeks earlier, details of the plans for the new wing had been announced in local newspapers stating that the upper ward had been completed and giving details of the two remaining wards.

> Upon the basement floor ... additional rooms for servants have been constructed, and also a new laundry and wash-house with rooms adjoining, all of which are large and more conveniently arranged than could be effected within the dimensions of the buildings formerly appropriated with these offices. The first, second and third storeys of the Wing consist of three separate Wards for patients presenting each of them an uninterrupted area of 1520 square feet.

It had been thought the two new wings would be ample to meet demands on the hospital for many years to come but within six years the Board of Governors was once again drawing up plans for further extensions.

The Arrival of the Railway

There were a number of factors accounting for the growth of the Sussex County Hospital, not the least of these was the ever-increasing number of people living both locally and in other parts of the county.

The need for a medical charity in Brighton in 1809 was ascribed to the town's rapid growth, which was accompanied by a disproportionate rise in the numbers living in poverty whose wretched living conditions made them subject to illness, disease and epidemics. During the intervening years before the establishment of the County Hospital, and immediately after, the problem had continued to grow. During the Napoleonic Wars, for example, the soldiers based in the town acted as 'a magnet for their families and young ladies seeking marriage',[3] which was seen as one of the factors which swelled the increasing numbers in the population. Whatever the reasons, by 1831 Brighton ranked fourth in the South East behind only Southwark, Dover and Woolwich for the density of its population.[4] Despite this, there were signs that this growth would be arrested, which it was believed might affect the development of the hospital and its sustainability.

During the 1820s, royalty began to desert the town, threatening the loss of royal patronage. George IV, fed up with gawping commoners, stopped visiting in 1827, and the fashionable set transferred their allegiance to Margate and Ramsgate. It became harder to let houses in Kemp Town and the development of Adelaide Crescent in 1830 was halted four years later with only ten houses built.

Brighton was saved, and the future development of its County Hospital assured, by the coming of the railway. Although a town meeting had been held at the Old Ship three years before the hospital opened to support the building of a railway line between Brighton and Shoreham, it was not until 1840 that the line actually opened. The link with London was completed the following year and this, according to Musgrave, 'marked the beginning of the modern age for Brighton.'[5]

Between 1851 and 1911, the population doubled, rising from 336,844 to 633,378. Commercial activity had already been growing in the county's ports and harbours bringing further increases in population in Shoreham, Southwick and Newhaven. Still more rapid growth took place after 1851 in both Shoreham and Newhaven.

The railway led to increasing demands on the hospital from the very beginning. The Bill giving Royal Assent to the building of the London to Brighton line by the most direct route was passed in 1837. This, and the associated branch lines from Brighton to Shoreham and Lewes, meant its construction would involve building viaducts, driving cuttings through hillsides and tunnelling underground. Clayton Tunnel provided the greatest challenge, over 2,200 yards long and 270 feet deep, with the 1841 census recording a large encampment of men at Pyecombe who were working on the project. Cutting into the chalk at Dyke Road Ridge to build Brighton Station required an army of 3,500 men. The effort to complete the Shoreham branch, which also involved driving a tunnel under Dyke Road, was reportedly pursued with feverish activity, day and night, by large teams of Irish navigators who were said to be addicted to drinking and fighting at the weekends.[6]

All this activity inevitably put pressure on the County Hospital. In 1839, 728 patients were admitted, 56 more than the year before. Of these, 195 were accident cases, more than 70 of whom were working on the construction of the railway in the neighbourhood. In 1840, the number of patients treated rose again, by 146 to 874. According to the annual report, the increase was partly due to the 'extraordinary amount of casualties, 116 from the railroad alone.'

Whilst these numbers were never as great again, the completion of the railway meant accidents to employees continued and were at a higher level than the national average. The main causes were engines running off the lines and boiler explosions, possibly the result of men working overlong hours or in fear of the notorious locomotive superintendent, John Craven.

Accidents to passengers and others provided another new demand on the hospital. Nathaniel Blaker, in his *Reminiscences,* describes two such cases while he was a pupil. The first was on the evening in 1852 after Lady Jane Peel had laid the foundation stone for the east and west wings, when he witnessed the amputation of both legs of a woman from Pyecombe who had been brought in after a railway engine had passed over them. The second case in 1855, the last he saw as a pupil before going to Guy's Hospital, involved a man who had been knocked down by an engine at the station, which ran over him as he lay between the rails, compressing his pelvis.

Fortunately the hospital had to deal with only one major disaster on the railway. This was on a Sunday morning in August 1861 in what has been described as 'the most gory and horrific accident in LBSC [London and Brighton South Coast railway] history'[7] when 23 people were killed, 22 of them and three children instantly, and 176 injured when two trains collided in Clayton Tunnel. According to the annual report nine cases were admitted 'without inconvenient pressure on the resources of the Institution or any interruption of its ordinary work.' Despite many serious injuries, only one case terminated fatally due to the advanced age of the patient and a great loss of blood, which 'rendered recovery all but hopeless from the beginning'.

The need for further extensions

At first four main requirements were considered to be essential, but these did not include extending the provision for in-patients. A chapel was needed for inpatients and staff who, since 1828, had used the boardroom for church services. The need for a hospital chapel had been raised in a letter to the board of management in 1847 by the vicar of Brighton, the Rev. H.M. Wagner, who was also a hospital governor. He was later to play an influential role when, as a measure of economy, it was suggested that the fever ward could be converted for the purpose.

Secondly, there were no waiting rooms for patients, which led to problems on receiving day. Enlarged facilities were also needed so that the physicians and surgeons could receive and examine their patients. Finally, by enlarging the inadequate dispensary it was believed it would be possible to reduce the cost of the department.

Although Mr Thomas Atkinson, an original contributor to the hospital, bequeathed £100 for these developments in his will, the committee of management concluded that 'many reasons existed which rendered it un-advisable to take immediate steps upon this matter.'

However, in June 1851, the committee were 'fully persuaded that the evils to which they have adverted are too great to allow of their being any longer permitted to exist.' In a public appeal issued in November, the chairman, the Earl of Chichester, drew attention to the fact that since 1841 the number of inpatients had risen from 861 to 1,065 and the number of outpatients had more than doubled from 1,274 to 2,734. £4,000 was required, therefore, to provide a waiting room, a chapel, a larger dispensary, larger and better ventilated fever wards and, significantly, increased accommodation for general patients.

The appeal was successful and raised more than £4,300, possibly helped by a decision to extend to all contributors of twenty-five guineas or more the privileges of Life Governors. Among the principal donors were the Marquis of Bristol and Mr William Catt, who donated 100 and 200 guineas respectively. Herbert Williams was again appointed as architect. He drew up plans for extensions to the east and west wings and the first stone was laid on the 21st September 1852 by Lady Jane Peel following divine service in nearby St George's Chapel.

However, even at this stage it was clear that the sum contributed was not sufficient to meet the cost of building a chapel, the total costs of the developments having escalated to about £7000. Priority was given to improving the facilities for the reception of patients who were 'compelled, most inconveniently, to throng all the passages of the hospital'. But the idea of providing a chapel was not lost sight of. Guests at the stone-laying ceremony were assured: 'it was scarcely postponed for a short time.'

In its report of the occasion, the *Brighton Gazette*, referred to an address by Dr William King, whose association with the hospital began with the first meeting of the committee called to consider its foundation. Dr King, after paying tribute to its founder, the Earl of Egremont, said one great object the establishment of the hospital had always been, in addition to taking care of the poor for the time being, to form a school of medicine, which it had gradually become. The new buildings, he said, were partly to provide for the increasing number of students. The *Gazette's* report of Dr King's address continued:

> At present there were 40 inmates, besides the patients. Of these 24 were nurses; and to show how well the Hospital had been conducted and superintended, he mentioned that the Hospital, having been in existence for 24 years, one of the nurses there had been employed there 22 years, another 18, another 14, another 12, another 10 and so on. In fact, the conduct of the nurses had been such as everybody could approve of. The matron had a great deal of business to do. Her books were complicated and laborious; and she had to perform this arithmetical part of housekeeping, as well as superintend the *morale* of the institution.
>
> At present the Board Room was used as a chapel; it was not large enough, and it was therefore desirable that it should be increased. But he looked forward to the day, when so large a hospital as this, and with so many patients in it, as well as servants and pupils, would be able to afford a resident chaplain, to conduct a daily religious service, and be, in some sense, the instructor of pupils. The study of medicine involved, not merely a high scientific education, but the cultivation of the finer feelings of human nature. When science and skill had done their all, there often remained nothing for the physician, but to sympathise with sufferings which he was unable to relieve. The cultivation of the heart and the affections must, therefore, be at basis of medical education. And in this view, a resident chaplain would be most desirable.

Despite the views expressed by Dr King, there was no immediate progress in building the chapel. The delay was debated during the following year, when it was suggested the money involved (nearly £2,000) would be better spent on 'more pressing things.'

Although the debt incurred in building the new extensions completed in 1853 was liquidated within a year, for the first time the governors experienced great difficulty in meeting current expenses on maintenance. In 1854

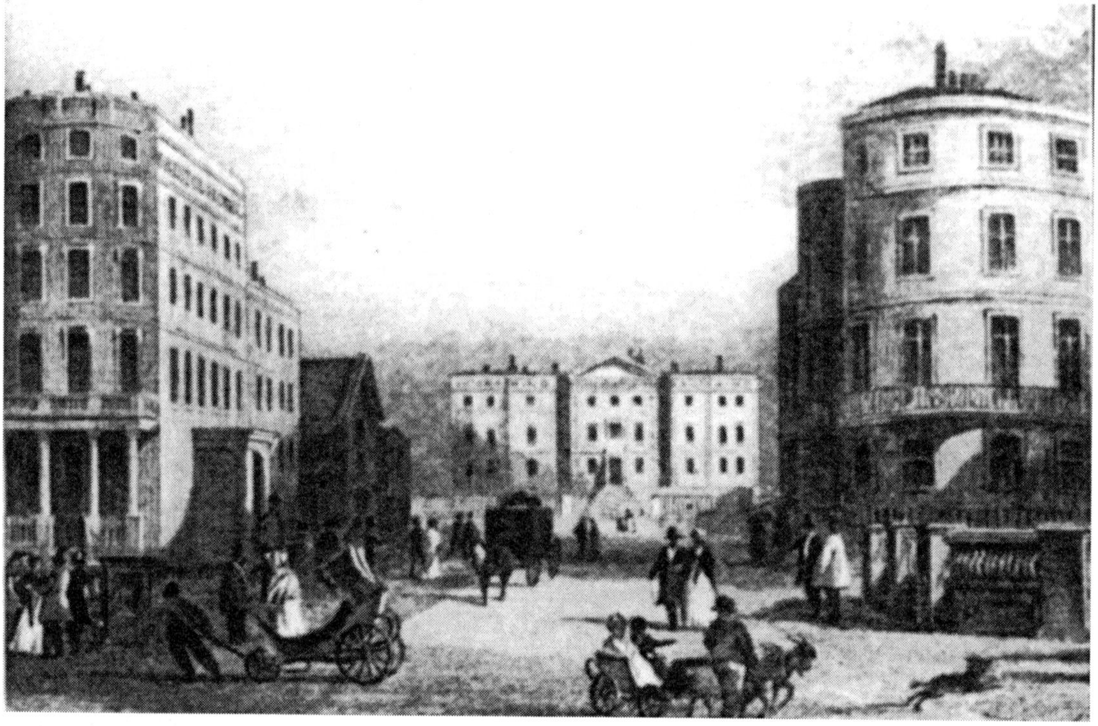

13. The hospital seen from the bottom of Paston Place in 1860. The extensions to the east and west wings had been completed in 1853.

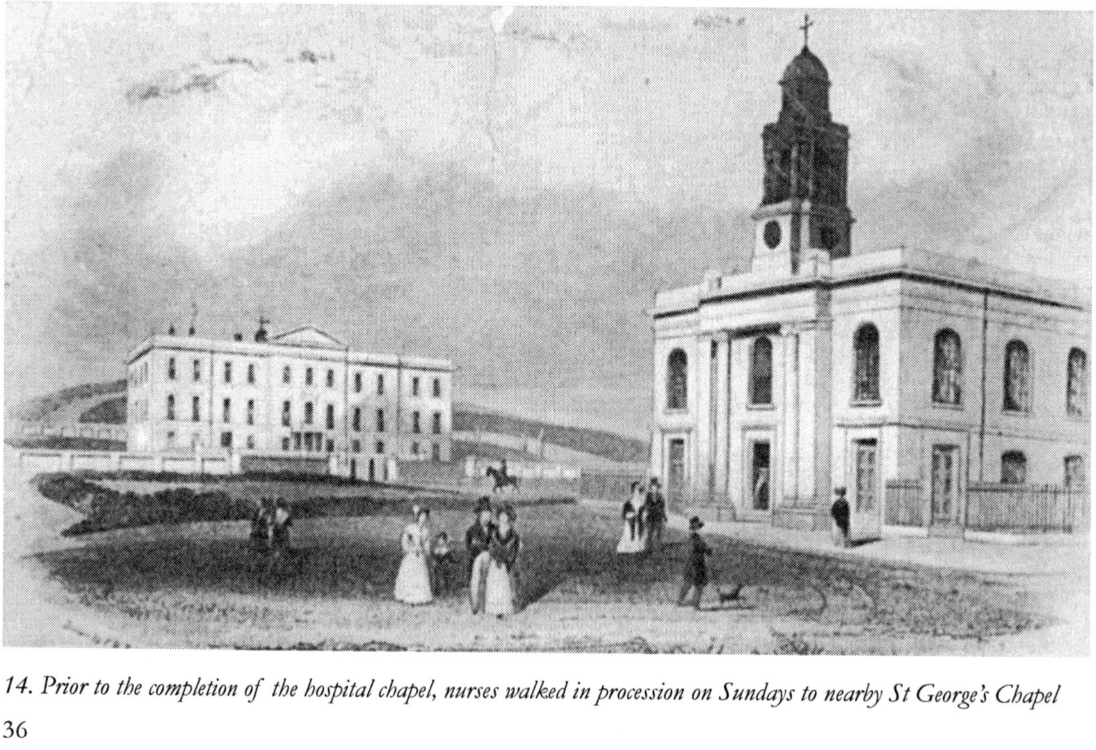

14. Prior to the completion of the hospital chapel, nurses walked in procession on Sundays to nearby St George's Chapel

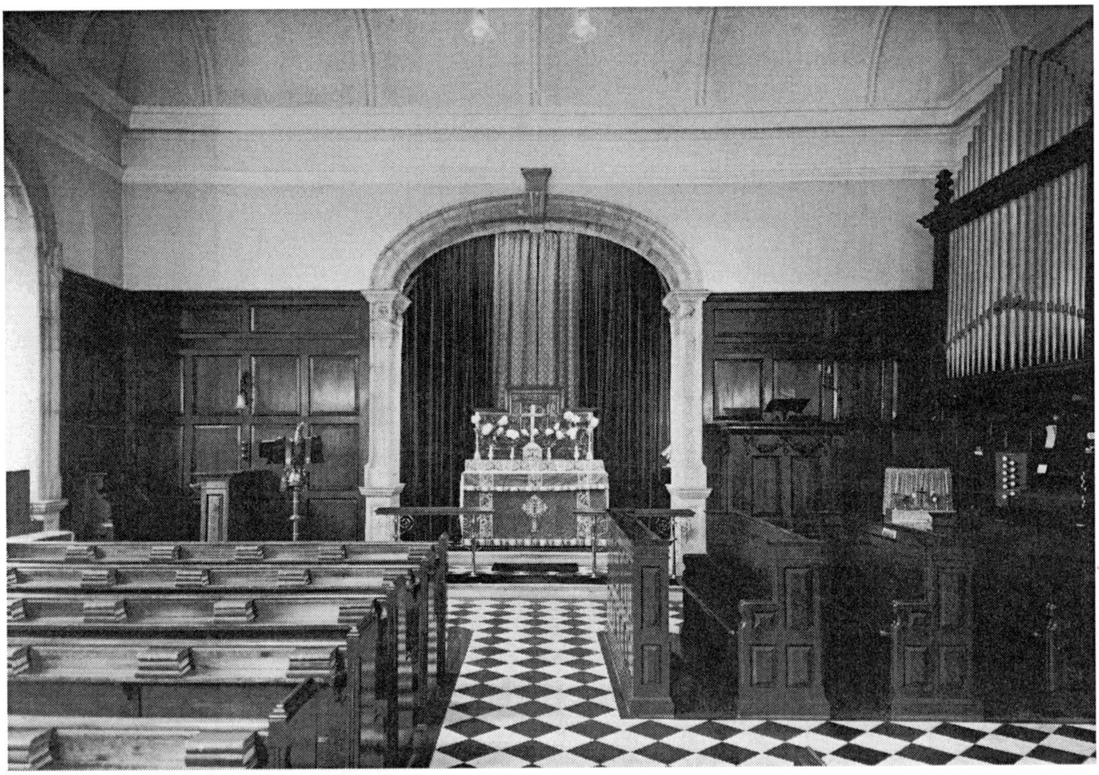

15. An early picture of the hospital chapel.

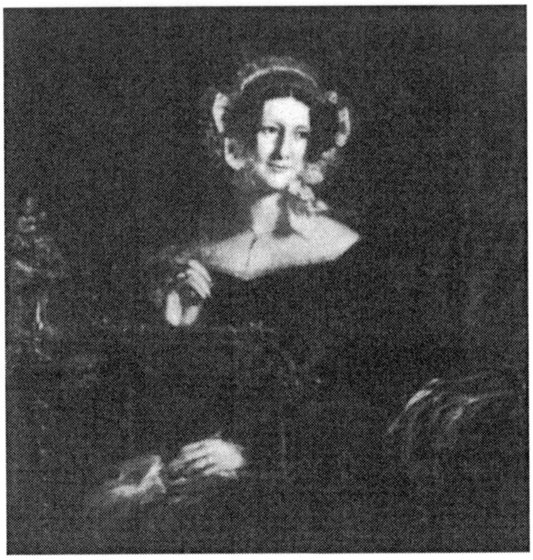

16. A portrait of Lady Jane Peel that was presented to the hospital by her son, Colonel Cecil Lennox Peel in 1899. The painting was restored in 1973 and hung in he boardroom together with a portrait of he husband, Mr Lawrence Peel.

the deficiency had arisen to nearly £1,300 leading to the sale of stock valued at £2,000. Despite these difficulties, the board acted generously towards the matron, Mrs Comport, who had been forced into retirement by advanced age and failing health. She was awarded a pension equal to the full amount of her salary 'in testimony of the zeal and vigilance with which she had discharged her duties from [the hospital's foundation.'

In the following year the deficit was reduced to £346 12s 8d, in part due to reducing the number of patients 'not without regret and only in a sense of urgent necessity.' Three new wards, which the committee was anxious to open, remained closed. According to the annual report, total liabilities at the end of the year amounted to more than £1,200 and an appeal was made for financial support so that the 'large space within its walls, now unoccupied, shall be filled with those who need … its benefits.'

The report also recorded that thanks to the Marquis of Bristol the long-running saga of the hospital chapel was almost at an end. The Rev. H. M. Wagner had successfully argued against a proposal to convert the fever ward to a chapel. He spoke of four incongruities: the metamorphosis of the fever ward, the fact that the chapel would be placed over that 'which it is unseemly in me even to name' (it is not clear what exactly this was) and the unseemliness flanked by a death house and post mortem examination room.

The vicar won the day and work on the chapel was completed in 1856, the cost being defrayed by the Marquis. Lady Jane Peel paid for the original furniture and Mr P.C. Cazalet presented the stained glass window at the eastern end of the building. Although the original idea had been to provide the chapel for the patients, it now became available for the nurses who since the foundation of the hospital had walked in procession every Sunday to nearby St. George's Chapel to attend morning service.

5. *The Jubilee Years*

In November 1856 a Fancy Fair was held over three days, which raised almost £2,500. Because much of this was used to cancel the hospital's liabilities, there was no significant change in the financial position in 1857. The number of patients continued to be restricted and three wards remained closed.

In a public statement, the committee pointed out that:

> the number of Sick Poor seeking admission to the hospital has much increased: a certain class of Patients have often waited for months before they can obtain relief, whilst others, who have been admitted, are most unwillingly to be discharged by the Medical Officers, to make room for urgent cases which will not admit of delay.

To admit from forty to fifty additional in-patients into the closed wards would cost about £1,000 per annum, including £250 for nurses. However, this could not be done without an increase in annual subscriptions, the committee warned.

> The population of Brighton now numbers about 280,000, whilst that of the County of Sussex, Brighton included, is computed at about 365,000. It will scarcely be credited, that of these thousands, exclusive of 350 Life Governors, only about 700 persons subscribe annually to the Sussex County Hospital.

In the hope of increasing the charity's income, a collector was appointed and a lower minimum subscription of half a guinea was introduced as an inducement to the recruitment of a larger number of subscribers. At the same time, a stringent investigation was ordered into the large increased consumption of 'meat, wine and other stimulants (erysipelas and phlebitis then prevailing in the wards)' and new regulations were adopted for the continuous revision of each patient's dietary by the supervising medical officer.

At the end of the year, in a further effort to increase subscriptions, the committee issued an appeal to the 'Farmers and Ratepayers of the County of Sussex'. During 1856, the committee stated, 1,039 in-patients were received. Many of these came from the county and a large proportion were agricultural labourers 'whose limbs have been torn and mangled by fearful accidents'. Of these 1,039 patients, 616 were cured, 108 relieved and only 56 died, 'proof of the skill of the Medical Staff and the watchfulness and care by which these sufferers are tended.' Because many of those cured were fathers, which not only 'gladdened the hearts of their sorrowing wives and children', the hospital had also freed the parishes from the burden of maintaining them which had saved the ratepayers '*thousands of pounds*'.

The appeal does not appear to have made an immediate impact on the hospital's finances. The restrictions on the number of patients continued in the following year, which, nevertheless, saw the number rise over the year to 1154, 'with only one exception, considerably in excess of any former year'. 4,687 outpatients were also treated. However, despite the financial difficulties a complete system of drainage was installed, which, the annual report noted, 'in a sanitary point of view, it is difficult to overrate.'

In 1859, however, the restrictions were relaxed (although fewer patients were actually treated) and the financial situation improved with a balance of £816 6s 6d. But it was a sad year for the hospital, which suffered the deaths of many supporters including the Marquis of Bristol and Mr Cazalet.

1860 was an altogether more successful year. Even a wet summer, which affected the harvest leading to higher prices, did not prevent the hospital showing a healthy balance of more than a thousand pounds. The highest ever daily average number of patients was recorded, the number of deaths fell by a third and nearly 900 more outpatients were treated, 4,435 in all.

Because complaints were received from time to time that prescribing to outpatients were subject to delays, two assistant physicians and two assistant surgeons were appointed expressly for the purpose of outpatients. As well as reducing delays, these additional staff enabled outpatients to be seen every day of the week.

All in all, the annual report summed up, 'the experiment of throwing open the doors as widely as possible must be deemed successful'. However, this did not prevent the *Brighton Gazette* from again raising the question of lack of support from the county generally. As with the earlier public appeal by the committee, the newspaper's complaints referred to the working of the Poor Laws: by sending their patients to Brighton the country districts saved on their rates and the town had to bear an unjustifiable expense in return. In the words of the *Gazette*:

> Some of the County subscriptions are made available as a means of relieving the country parishes of poor families at the expense of Brighton. Thus, a village squire subscribes to our Hospital and becomes entitled to orders for admission. He selects for his order some poor man whose complaint will probably take a considerable period for its cure. He is sent to the County Hospital, and shortly after his wife and family are persuaded to remove to Brighton in the hope of obtaining work, and for the sake of being near the poor man in Hospital. A large number

> of families become chargeable to the parish of Brighton in this manner, for it frequently happens that when the patient is discharged, he is from amputation or other causes incapacitated from work – the County parish is thus relieved not only of the expense from doctoring the sick man, but of maintaining his family should he die or become unable to labour, and the parish of Brighton by conferring benefits on the County is made to commit an injury on its own parishioners.

More improvements and a major fire

In 1861 steps were taken to purchase ground in front of the hospital for £3,000. This was intended to secure 'the full enjoyment of the pure air, which forms one of its greatest advantages, free from all annoyances likely to arise from the close proximity of small houses and a dense population.' Four years later, improvements costing £4,500 were approved providing two thirds was first raised by special donations. That this was achieved was due in no small measure to a bazaar held in the Royal Pavilion over three days in November that raised £1,880 after the deduction of expenses. Accordingly, although the committee warned a further £1,500 was needed to complete the proposals, a contract to carry out the works was entered into.

The scheme of improvements was in six parts. First, an improved entrance, which would do without the steep and narrow steps that were painful for some patients to negotiate. A larger kitchen was also needed because of the increased number of patients (the entire cost of this was in fact met by one of the governors). Providing enlarged accommodation in the out-patient department would allow the separation of the sexes. The greater number of patients, the doctors believed, meant there was insufficient space and ventilation. Another staircase was proposed for the west wing where 'inmates [were] exposed to danger in the event of fire'. Finally, improved fireplaces and chimneys were to be constructed in this wing as the rooms were full of smoke in stormy weather or, if the fires were put out, leaving patients to suffer from the cold. Carrying out this work meant there were restrictions on admissions during a large part of the year in 1867

A small surplus, largely the result of legacies, meant it was possible to construct a museum and library outside the walls of the hospital in 1870. Taken together with moving the pupils' day room, this development meant there was more room for patients and also provided facilities for a larger number of pupils.

But all these improvements, indeed the entire hospital, were placed in jeopardy on New Year's Day in 1872, when fire broke out in the Adelaide Wing.

It was a little before five o'clock in the evening that Nurse Plummer heard a crackling noise in the small bathroom in the north west corner of No. 6 Ward on the top floor of the wing. This was soon followed by the sound of an explosion which, the matron said, shook the whole building.

The bathroom contained a tank for hot water supplied by pipes from a furnace in the basement. A gas escape was at first suspected, but it appeared later that the cause was overheating to burning point of an iron bar connecting timbers on either side of the flues.

Normally, perhaps, a few buckets of water would have doused the flames but the seat of the fire was difficult to reach and the decayed wood meant it spread rapidly. There were hydrants on each floor connected to a large water tank at the rear of the building but the force of the water was insufficient to reach the top floor. A high wind was blowing from the south east which fanned the flames and there was a fear that the combination of circumstances, the direction of the wind and the position of the wing in the south east corner, could lead to the destruction of the entire hospital. The view at the time, according to a newspaper report, was that 'nothing less than a miracle could save it.'

At first, patients were moved from the adjacent Fever Ward to the museum library and patients from the eastern wing were moved to the western wing, which was not immediately threatened by the flames. The window blinds were closed so that the patients could not see the falling pieces of fire but by six o'clock the situation appeared so alarming that it was decided to move all the patients out of the building under the direction of the house surgeon, Mr Nicholls, Dr Ormerod and the surgeon E.J. Furner. By this time hundreds of onlookers had arrived, including friends and relatives clamouring to be allowed admission to remove 'those near and dear to them'. According to one report, the decision to remove the patients was not taken a moment too soon 'for scarcely had Mr Kebbell removed an epileptic patient from the ward than the ceiling fell in.'

When news arrived at the town hall, a strong body of police was despatched with hose reels and a fire escape. Hose reels were also despatched from other police stations and the Volunteer Fire Brigade set out from their Russell Street station with their engine and other apparatus. Later a fire engine was also sent from the cavalry barracks at Preston together with a detachment of the 19th Hussars. A party from Lewes Cliffe brigade also attended. During the first hour, the situation looked so desperate that a steam fire engine was summoned by telegraph from London, although this turned back during its journey when better news was received.

By six o'clock the hospital had been cleared of its 'helpless inmates' but flames were pouring from the windows on the north side of Ward 6 and gaining ground on the partition wall. According to local newspaper reports, 'the house surgeon, Mr Keogh, the steward, Mr Percival Boxall, a member of the management committee, a former pupil Mr Kebbell junior, Mr C. Marshall, Mr Willett and a large number of other volunteers climbed on to the roof and formed two rows, one passing full buckets of water, one row returning the empty buckets. An increased supply from the Water Company hydrants at the front of the building then made it possible to pour a stream of water on to the roof and also to flood the ward flooring and the ceilings of the rooms underneath'.

During the next half hour, it was reported, 'the battle was a very close and doubtful [and] one watched with varying emotions by the large and excited crowd'. There were cries of 'the roof must go' and 'nothing can save the building' as large fragments of roof, iron girders and wooden beams fell threatening to break through to the rooms below Ward 6. By then, as the fire fighting continued inside in the corridors and outside on the fire escape ladders at the front and back of the building, the crowds thronging Eastern Road and the surrounding streets were so dense it was difficult to approach the hospital. Fortunately, however, by seven o'clock the fire brigades began to get the upper hand, the flames were totally extinguished and the hospital, with the exception of Ward 6, was spared.

Evacuating the patients had not been easy. Many had to be carried down the long flight of steps leading to the main entrance which were slippery with water 'with a fierce cold wind blowing in their faces' and the only light coming from the burning building. The surgeons 'and other gentlemen' made a road through the dense crowds calling 'make way for the patients' who were taken away in cabs and other vehicles to places of safety including St Mary's Hall, Mohammed's Gymnasium, and St George's Church. Later Miss Elliott offered the use of her Convalescent Home in Sudeley Street and at eight o'clock volunteers carried the patients there from the church, while Dr Ormerod carried one young patient 'pick-a-back' which, according to a newspaper correspondent, was 'a mode of locomotion the little sufferer seemed to enjoy'.

At its meeting held the following Wednesday the board placed on record 'their thankfulness to God for the merciful preservation of the patients'. Special thanks were recorded to the house surgeon, Mr Nicholls and the pupils Kebbell, Miles and Williams 'for the courage, energy and self-devotion with which they laboured for the safety of their patients.' The board also recorded thanks to the matron, Miss Longstaffe, the house steward, Mr Keogh, the carpenter, Mr Gibbs, a former porter, Mr Thomson, the foreman of Messrs. Nell and Tuxford, Mr Warwick Standing and the nurses and servants. A vote of thanks was also made to the families in the neighbourhood 'for their liberal assistance', the Chichester Infirmary and the Sick Children's Hospital for their offer of beds.

According to a later report in the *Brighton Herald* the damage caused by the fire was estimated at £899 13s. A claim for this amount, it continued, 'will be readily met by the Sun Fire office'. The response of the insurance company was more than matched by the generosity of the public following an appeal for funds to reinstate the wing launched by the Earl of Chichester at a meeting in the Royal Pavilion. As a result, the Adelaide Wing was not only restored but improved towards the close of the year which had begun so disastrously at a cost of £2,132 8s 3d.

The Jubilee Fund

As the hospital neared the end of the first fifty years of its existence, it became evident that additional buildings were necessary 'to render the institution equal to its position as the County Hospital.'

In 1874, a small room called the Hankey Ward was furnished for isolation or special treatment but hopes of an additional building for fever and infectious cases the following year were dashed when Mrs Annie Poore of Patcham Place withdrew the offer of £5,000 she had made to erect the building. Her offer had been made subject to a number conditions. These included naming the new building, which was to be built on the site of the hospital, St. John's House. More importantly, it seems, she wanted the privilege of governor to be granted to the vicar of Patcham. Subsequently, however, 'prejudices were aroused by exaggerated statements' against Miss Poore's offer. Through her solicitors, she withdrew her original offer in favour of one giving the hospital £1,500 – subject to the condition that the vicar be granted the privileges of a benefactor of £105 under the existing statutes. The balance of the sum originally offered, it was understood, would be used for the benefit of the poorer inhabitants of Patcham.

In 1876, 1,442 inpatients were treated, the highest number since the hospital opened in 1828. The following year the committee congratulated the governors on the sanitary condition of the hospital, which was 'free from erysipelas, pyrema and other diseases of a similar character'. However, with the same high level of admissions as in the previous year, a sub-committee set up to consider the need for a convalescent home recommended that a separate building should be established for this purpose. With voluntary contributions 'falling off', an appeal was announced for additional funds to erect a number of additional buildings which, according to the annual report, were necessary 'to render the institution equal to its position as the County Hospital.' In particular, the report referred to the insufficient accommodation for pupils and domestic servants, the need for a dining hall for the nurses and servants and a new enlarged linen room and laundry and, finally, to remove the dispensary and drug stores out of the hospital.

Accordingly, in November 1878, in the fiftieth year of the hospital's existence, the Earl of Chichester, as Lord Lieutenant of the County, presided over a public meeting at the Royal Pavilion to inaugurate the Jubilee Fund. This meeting was followed by a banquet with tickets at one guinea 'including wine'. The annual report for the year, published early in 1879, was able to report that already £2,365 2s 8d had been received. In addition more than £500 had been added from the proceeds of a bazaar held in the autumn of 1877 while Lady Grant had offered £1,000 towards the cost of a separate building 'in which such cases as can be more advantageously treated apart from others, may be received.'

The 1880 report was able to record that the hospital's income was the largest on record and that the total amount received for the Jubilee Fund had reached £3,745 8s 1d. The new laundry was opened in January 1882 although plans to alter the museum to provide additional accommodation for six in-pupils and an assistant surgeon had been postponed pending completion of the laundry. Then, because of the cost involved, it was decided that sleeping accommodation for the pupils should be provided 'in the immediate neighbourhood' of the hospital.

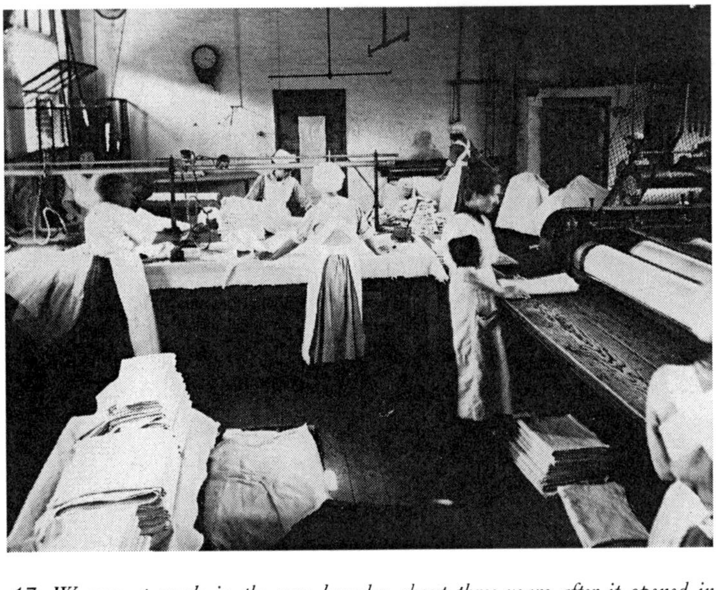

17. Women at work in the new laundry about three years after it opened in 1882.

In 1883, 4 and 5 Clevedon Terrace was rented to provide lodgings where 'for various reasons' it was deemed advisable to have them under one roof. To meet the additional expense to the hospital, the

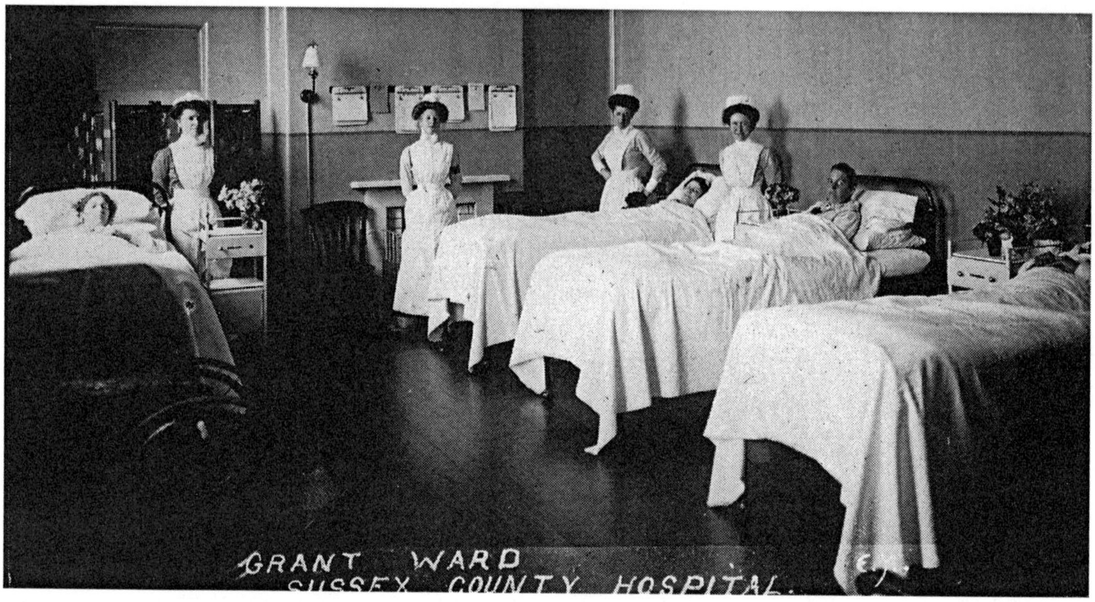

18. Grant Ward in the Jubilee Building named after Lady Grant whose fund raised £1,500 towards the new building.

first year pupils' fees were raised from 80 to 100 guineas and doubled from 30 to 60 guineas for each subsequent year.

In the event, the occupation of the property in Clevedon Terrace was short-lived. In 1886, an alteration to the rules by the examining boards of the Royal College of Physicians of London and the Royal College of Surgeons of England meant that a period of twelve months spent by medical students in provincial hospitals would no longer count so favourably. The lease on Clevedon Terrace was terminated, the in-pupils all left (and the house physician and house surgeon suffered a loss of income).

Thanks to the Jubilee Fund and Lady Grant's Fund (which in 1885 had reached a total of almost £1,500) the building to be named the Jubilee Building was completed in 1887 and one ward was named Grant Ward. The final cost was £5,805 1s 9d. A balance left over was added to a special appeal for the purpose and an isolation block for infectious diseases, for which the medical staff had been pressing, was opened in 1893 and named York Ward in honour of the Duke and Duchess of York whose wedding took place that year.

The Ditchling Convalescent Home

In 1883, the hospital admitted 1591 in-patients, then the largest number on record, and the question of providing a convalescent home was revived. When three gentlemen donated £310 towards the expenses, it was

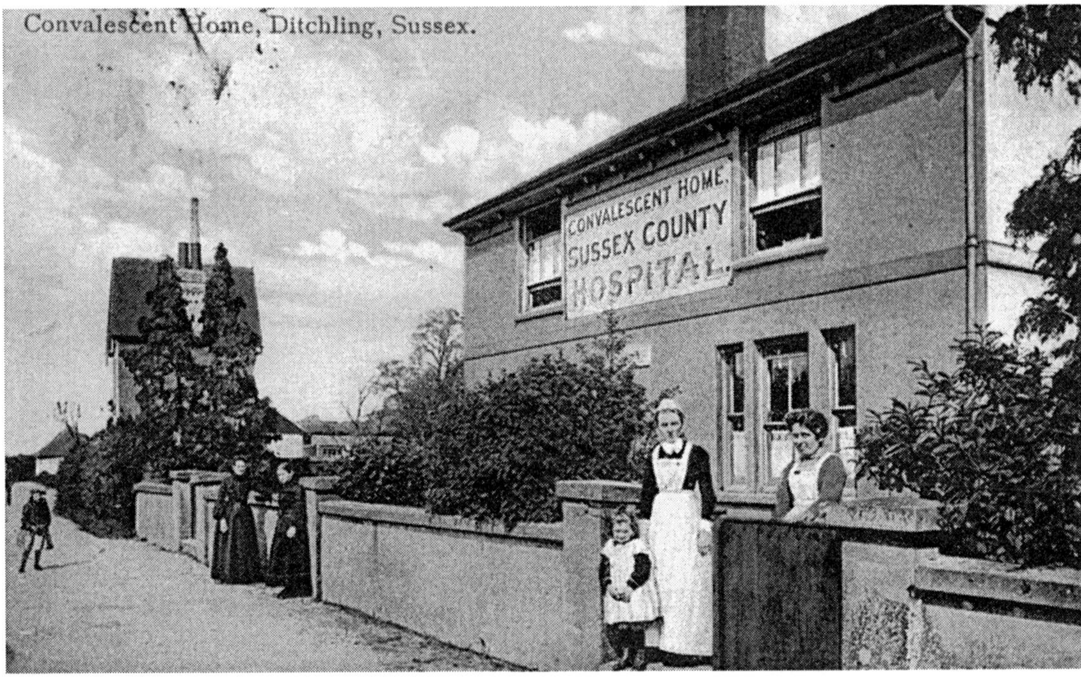

19. The Ditchling Convalescent Home was opened in two semi-detached cottages in East Lane provided through the generosity of Alderman Reeves.

decided to give the plan a trial. Alderman E.J. Reeves, a former mayor of Brighton, offered the use of two semi-detached cottages in Ditchling rent free for three years and the convalescent home opened on the 12th July. As a result, acccording the report for the year, 20 men and 37 women were accommodated for periods ranging from four days to four weeks when they 'benefited from change of air'.

The home came under the threat of closure the following year because of lack of funds but in 1885 it was reported that it had been well supported by special contributions from 'the gentry living in the neighbourhood and the constant supply of vegetables, fruit and other things furnished by them.'

In 1887 Alderman Reeves entered into an agreement to the grant of a lease on the cottages for seven years and fourteen years after the convalescent home opened he used the occasion of the Queen's Diamond Jubilee to make an absolute gift of the cottages to the hospital, which led the *Brighton Herald* to comment:

> To a Hospital a Convalescent Home is an almost indispensable appendage; and during the past fourteen years hundreds of patients have found the change at this pleasant country home after leaving the Hospital an important factor in their restoration to health and strength.

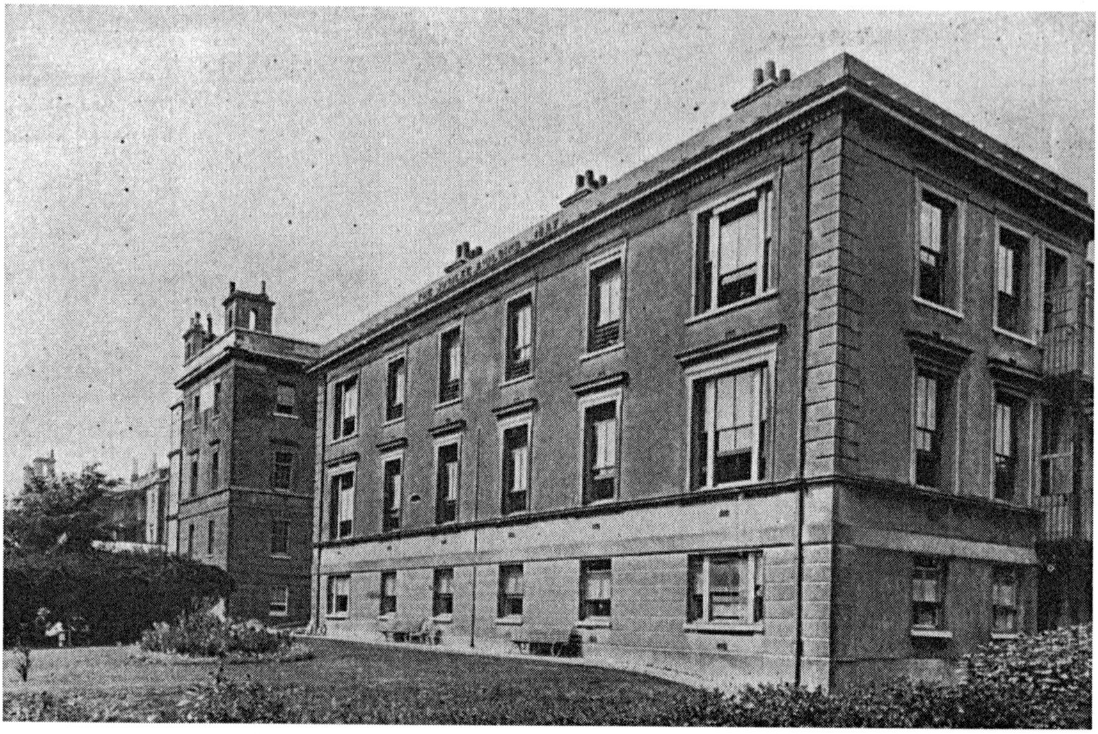

20. The Jubilee building erected in 1887.

Financial problems and the need for improvements

Throughout its history, the Sussex County Hospital was rarely without its financial problems and the final decade of the 19th century was no exception. In 1887, for example, expenditure exceeded income by almost £500 so it is no surprise that the following year the decision was taken to establish a Nursing Institute that would not only meet a demand from local medical men but also provide a source of income for the hospital.

During this first year the Nursing Institute set up in 1888 made a small profit after defraying the costs of setting it up, which the report stated, would not recur in future. The benefit would have been still greater if the matron had been able to recruit sufficient nurses who 'thoroughly commended themselves to her'. The intention had been to recruit sixteen nurses to the institute, but for the first eight months only nine had been engaged. The report noted that demand for the nurses had been 'incessant' and thirty different medical men in thirteen different places had employed them.

In 1890 a number of changes were proposed to meet the demand for additional beds for women; at the time there were only 69 female beds compared with the 88 set aside for men. To achieve this, it was suggested the children should be moved into the upper wards of the Jubilee Block. However, these wards had been set aside for severe cases, which needed to be moved from elsewhere in the hospital who were considered too dangerous to move to the borough sanatorium. The solution proposed was to erect a small building for this purpose costing £2,000 and an appeal was launched to raise the money.

However, there was only a slow response to the appeal and it was not until this reached £2,700, enabling plans for the building to be drawn up.

The new isolation block, York Ward, was completed in 1893 and certain patients from Grant Ward in Jubilee Block were transferred there. Grant was then redecorated and used for general patients, the upper floor being used for children. By using the former children's ward in the main building for women, the number of beds available for them was increased by ten. An anonymous donor, whose name was later revealed when the ward was named 'Overton' as Mrs Jones of Overton House, Brighton, met the cost of fitting and furnishing the new women's ward. Her gift included, according to the annual report, the laying of a new oak floor undertaken 'in the most liberal manner'.

As a result of the changes, the total number of beds in the hospital rose from 173 to 187. Additional nurses' sleeping accommodation was required

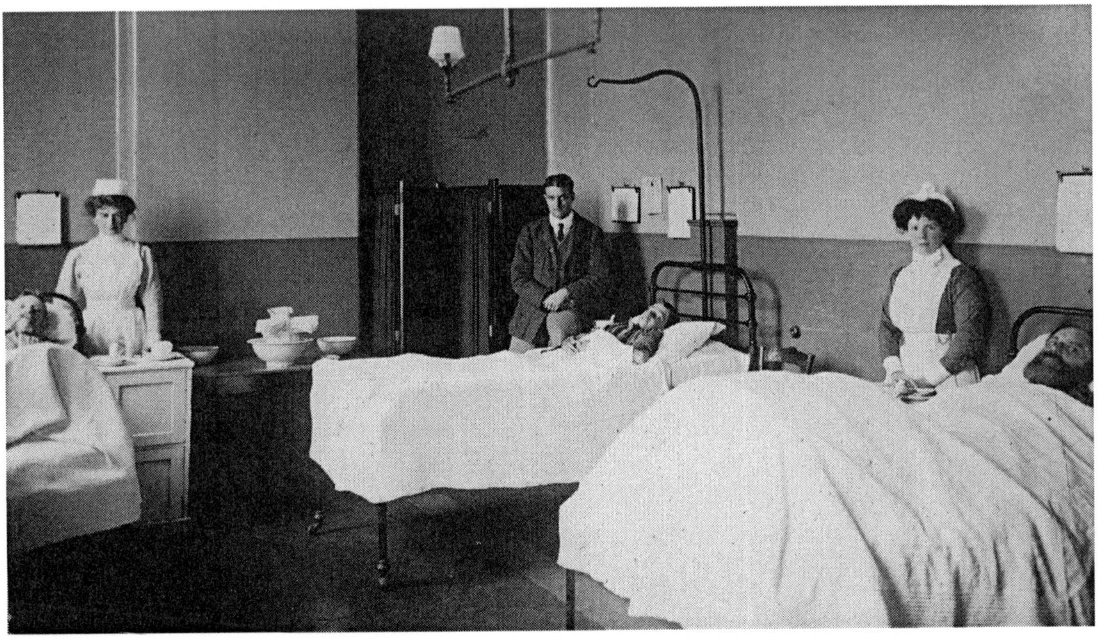

21. York Ward named in honour of the Duke and Duchess of York who were married in 1893.

and this was obtained at 14 Sudeley Place, rented at £50 per annum. By this time, too, the number of surgical operations carried out in the hospital had risen to some 500 a year compared with 208 in 1878.

The annual report includes a breakdown of the 1983 surgical cases which serves to illustrate just how much surgery had developed since the beginning of the century when it was largely limited to fractures and amputations. No details are given of the number of amputations, although from the range of conditions dealt with, it must have been a fairly small one; fractures and dislocations, however, do appear as a separate classification and account for only 71 of the 500 cases. These are far outnumbered by diseases of the skin and subcutaneous tissues (129) and diseases of bones and joints (101). Worthy of particular interest, perhaps, are 39 cases classified as constitutional diseases, which included six rickets and five congenital syphilis; 30 wounds and injuries included 'four cut throat, one bullet wound and one attempted drowning'.

During 1894, it was reported a large sub-committee met 'for many months' to consider the urgent need for alterations and additions to the hospital, which:

> having been built so many years ago, is, in its actual structural state and sanitary condition, in view of the exacting requirements of the present day, a source of never ending worry to the Committee of Management and very heavy drain on the resources of the Institution ...

Once again it was decided to make another appeal to subscribers and the public, the report further noting that since the previous appeal, not only had it been necessary to start work repairing and securing all the ceilings, but 'at the earnest insistence of the Medical Staff', electric light had been installed in the operating theatre, the surgery and the out-patients consulting rooms.

The committee was aware that the time was not favourable for an appeal because of the depressed state of the country, but warned that without considerable support the bank account would be 'largely overdrawn'. To strengthen the case for the hospital's reconstruction, it was pointed out that many older hospitals, including St Bartholomew's and St George's in London, were in a similar position and that totally new hospitals had replaced those in Leeds, Derby and other towns.

Among the suggested improvements were sanitary towers needed to separate lavatories and water closets by cross ventilation from the wards and, 'as in most modern hospitals', an incinerator was required. With many nurses living off the premises and exposed to the weather, a nurses home with a covered approach was needed.

A sub-committee having undertaken a 'searching scrutiny' following allegations of abuse of the outpatient department[1] and concluding that 96 per cent of cases were entirely fit and proper for 'gratuitous treatment', the committee recommended replacing the inadequate, very ill ventilated and dark premises occupied under the wards and making the space available for other purposes including a dining room for nurses and servants.

A hydraulic lift was recommended to avoid jolting patients who were carried up and down by hand and which would enable many to get into the grounds during convalescence. A veranda on the south side would similarly enable patients to enjoy sun and air earlier, while new heating apparatus was needed for the corridors and staircases which were bitterly cold in winter.

Providing a new operating room would bring the cost for all the suggested improvements of £16,550 plus fixtures and fittings and architects' fees, a total cost of £22,360. However, the committee did not leave matters there: the roof of the Barry building needed renewing, four old floors needed relaying and it was desirable to install more electric light for medical and surgical purposes, the report explained, making a gross total of £25,500 excluding the increased cost of maintenance.

The report clearly left no doubt about the extent of the problem the hospital faced. The following year began with a deficit of some £298 and ended with one of more than £2,200. A public meeting in the Pavilion raised £1,000, but most of this was for improvements and little was devoted to maintenance.

Expenditure increased again in 1896, principally because of the price of meat and wages paid to extra nurses employed from outside the hospital needed to attend to patients, and in 1897, the adverse balance was over £4,000. 'If the Hospital is to be maintained in its present state of efficiency and numbers,' the committee warned, 'a large increase of Donations and Subscriptions must be forthcoming. We earnestly commend this fact to the kind consideration of all throughout the County and Town who have the interests of this valuable Institution at heart.'

According to the 1897 annual report, despite the hospital's financial situation, bearing in mind that it existed 'for the reception of the sick and lame poor of every county and nation,' it responded to an 'appalling' outbreak of typhoid in the Kent county town, and offered the use of two beds to the Maidstone Relief Fund for up to six months free of charge apart from the cost of conveying patients from Maidstone.

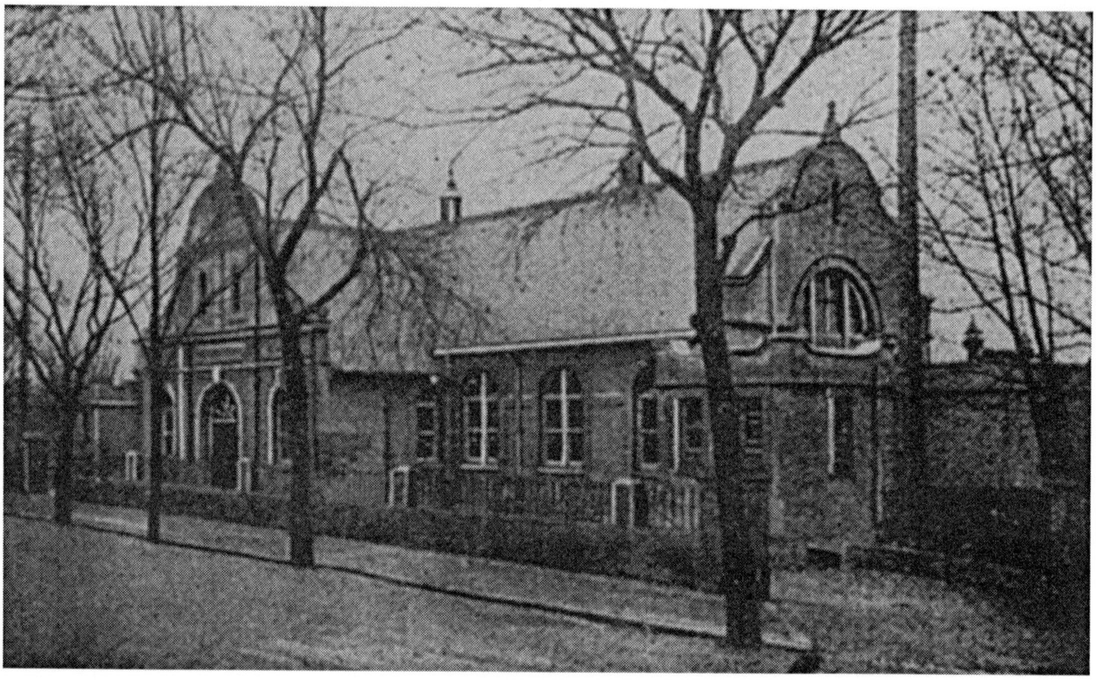

22. An early photo of the Outpatient Department.

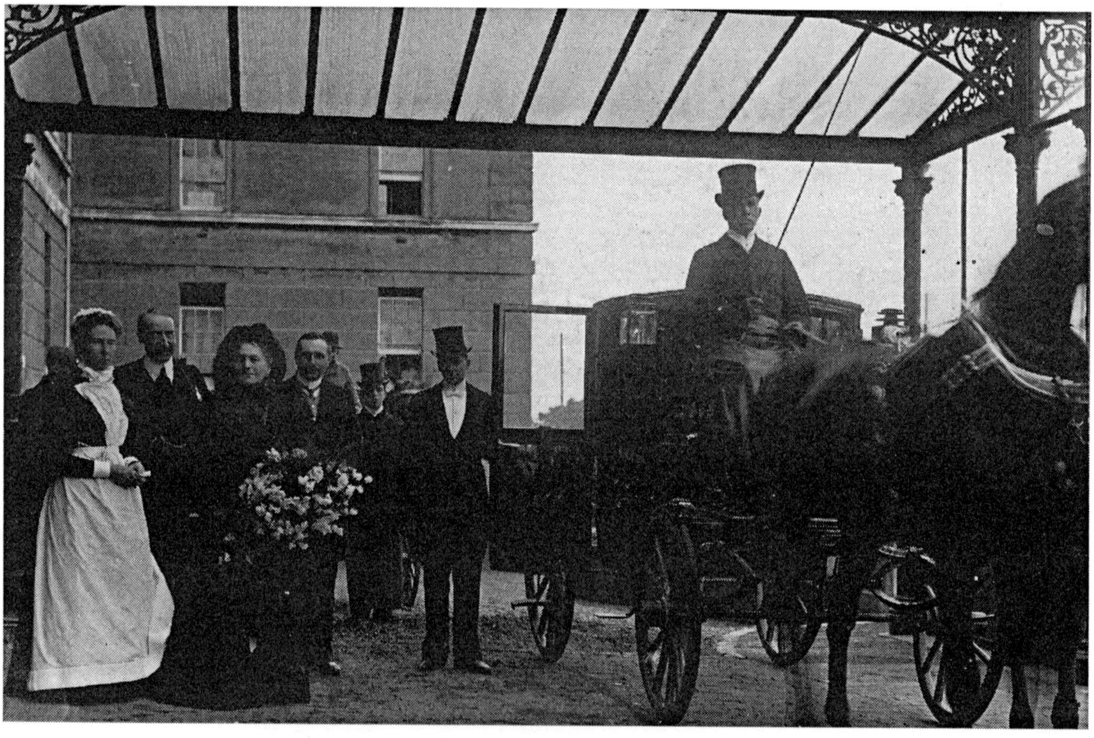

23. The Duchess of Fife arrives at the main entrance of the hospital for the opening of the new Outpatient Department.

Thanks to an exceptionally large number legacies, the committee was able to discharge the 1897 adverse balance the following year but the diminution of ordinary receipts meant that expenditure again exceeded ordinary income by over £3,500.

However, all was not gloom financially. Thanks largely to the 'indefatigable exertions' of the mayor which raised £3,134 8s 7d and £1,690 1s 6d received in purses presented to Princess Louise, the Duchess of Fife, following the laying of the foundation stone for the new outpatients department by the Prince of Wales, almost £5,000 became immediately available for the proposed improvements.

Some historians have questioned the extent of the contribution made by the Royal family to the development of Brighton, but there can be no doubt of the importance of the part they played in the development of the hospital. Throughout the 19th century (and into the 20th) it enjoyed having the reigning monarch as its patron; King William IV donated £800 and subscribed £800 annually; Queen Adelaide subscribed £20 annually and Queen Victoria donated £1,000. The visit of the Prince of Wales to lay the foundation stone of the outpatients department was another example of this. Contemporary accounts leave no doubt as to the welcome he received in the town when despite adverse weather the streets were thronged with people. And although the purpose of the visit was ostensibly to perform the stone laying ceremony, the Prince made it clear he had another important reason for his visit. Replying to the address of welcome, he told the assembled company: 'I come here to assist the cause of charity, and to assist you in your endeavours to place the financial position of your County Hospital' and called for 'a prompt and generous response' to the mayor's appeal.[2]

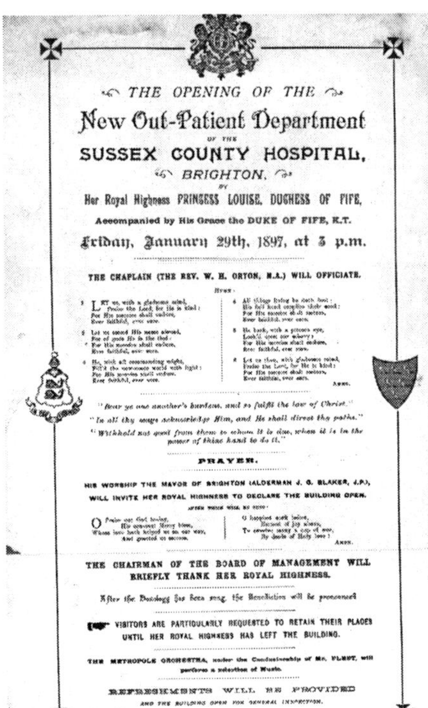
THE OPENING OF THE
New Out-Patient Department
OF THE
SUSSEX COUNTY HOSPITAL,
BRIGHTON,
BY
Her Royal Highness PRINCESS LOUISE, DUCHESS OF FIFE,
Accompanied by His Grace the DUKE OF FIFE, K.T.
Friday, January 29th, 1897, at 3 p.m.

THE CHAPLAIN (THE REV. W. H. ORTON, M.A.) WILL OFFICIATE.

HYMN.

"Bear ye one another's burdens, and so fulfil the law of Christ."
"In all thy ways acknowledge Him, and He shall direct thy paths."
"Withhold not good from them to whom it is due, when it is in the power of thine hand to do it."

PRAYER.

HIS WORSHIP THE MAYOR OF BRIGHTON (ALDERMAN J. G. BLAKER, J.P.), WILL INVITE HER ROYAL HIGHNESS TO DECLARE THE BUILDING OPEN.

AMEN.

THE CHAIRMAN OF THE BOARD OF MANAGEMENT WILL BRIEFLY THANK HER ROYAL HIGHNESS.

After the Doxology has been sung, the Benediction will be pronounced.

VISITORS ARE PARTICULARLY REQUESTED TO RETAIN THEIR PLACES UNTIL HER ROYAL HIGHNESS HAS LEFT THE BUILDING.

THE METROPOLE ORCHESTRA, under the Conductorship of Mr. FLEET, will perform a selection of Music.

REFRESHMENTS WILL BE PROVIDED
AND THE BUILDING OPEN FOR GENERAL INSPECTION.

24 . The official programme for the opening of the Outpatient Department.

Thanks to the efforts of the mayor and the governors, the improvements fund totalled £11,753 17s 8d the following year and although short of the target it was sufficient to erect the new outpatient department and convert part of the old department into a nurses dining hall, to fit up new boilers and heating apparatus, and also to erect two sanitary towers on the western part of the hospital. The

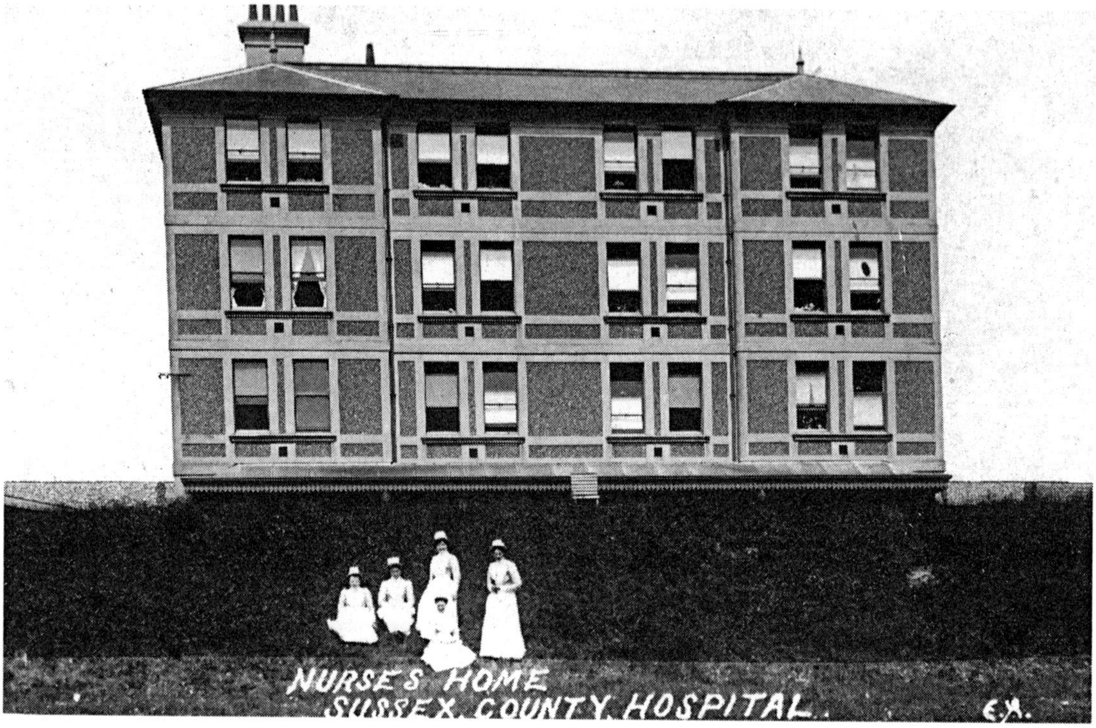

25 . The new nurses' home opened in 1899.

mayor, Alderman Sir John Blaker, donated the unspent balance of the fund for the town's celebrations of Queen Victoria's Diamond Jubilee totalling £822 10s 7d towards the cost of erecting the new nurses' home.[3]

The annual report for 1899 recorded that the nurses' quarters had been completed and opened on the 13th May by Sir Henry Harben, a former president. The new operating room was on the point of completion and the lift had been promised by 'an anonymous friend' (actually Mr C.C. Baily). However, the other improvements called for in the 1894 report, were not likely to be completed until 1900.

6. *Staff and Patients, 1830 – 1900*

Whilst there is adequate documentary evidence concerning the development of the hospital during the nineteenth century, information about life inside the wards is less easy to come by and, in any event, not always completely reliable.

A handbook on Brighton published in 1850[1], for example, described what a visitor might expect to find in 'the principal charitable institution in the town'.

> The patients, although many of them come from the lowest ranks of society, discard their usual habits, and, subdued by suffering and awed by the character of the place, pass their days in a state of repose to which they have been but little accustomed. Enter one of these large wards, in which between twenty and thirty patients are collected – many of them men of the roughest mould – and scarcely a sound is to be heard. Some are reading; others lie motionless on their beds; a few are grouped at the windows; but their conversation is low and all seem to comprehend the sanctity of the sick chamber.

Visitors' reports and the Black Book suggest that the atmosphere on the wards was not always as tranquil as the author of the handbook would have his readers believe. Nevertheless, some of the information the book contains is helpful in building up a reasonably accurate picture of what a visitor to the hospital could expect to see.

> Each patient has a separate bed (iron) furnished with clean bedding and blankets at his entrance, and the sheets of which are changed weekly. He breakfasts at eight and goes to bed at nine, prayers being read morning and evening by the senior patient in the ward. The remainder of the day is passed in reading, talking, or, if the patient's state require it, walking in the grounds by which the Hospital is surrounded; and in which there is one walk for the men, and another for women, with two alcoves for their shelter in wet weather. Above the head of each patient is a shelf for a Bible and a Prayer Book, and another beneath it for his medicine. In front hangs a ticket, stating his name, time of entrance, the name of the surgeon who attends him, and the particular diet prescribed. A piece of wood is also suspended by which he can raise himself.

Although, writing fifty years later, Nathaniel Paine Blaker suggested that the memory of things might not always be relied on, his description of the hospital wards at this time is almost certainly an accurate one.

> The walls of the wards were whitewashed, there was no attempt at ornamentation, the floors were deal boards with wide interspaces, and these were occasionally

> scrubbed. The food was good and stimulants were prescribed freely. The beds were very close, with small cubic space for each. Both nurses and patients conspired to keep the windows closed, especially at night, night air being considered highly injurious. The smell was consequently sickening, and erysipelas and pyæmia were almost always present in a greater or lesser degree.

Nathaniel Blaker's *Reminiscences* also describe the operation on the woman from Pyecombe whose legs had been run over by a railway engine. This took place in a room next to Vallance Ward in which he had been studying when the woman had been brought in. This room, he said, was used for casualties in the morning, for outpatients between 12 and 1, and for casualties (if any) and as a pupil's sitting room for the rest of the day.

> On one side of the fireplace was a washing basin, and above this in the corner, a cupboard containing a skeleton. On the other side of the fireplace was a cupboard with two drawers below, which were used for splints and bandages. In the cupboard above were kept a few cases of casualty instruments, some loose bone and books belonging to the pupils. On that evening, as usual, the pupils' supper, consisting of bread and cheese and beer on a tray, was placed on the table about 9 p.m.

It was on this table that the operation, the first witnessed by Blaker, took place. His book and supper were put into the cupboard, the table was put into the middle of the room and a mattress placed upon it. The instruments were arranged on the windowsill and Mr Vallance operated by the light of three bulls-eye lamps. Following the operation – one leg amputated below the knee and the other above it – the patient was removed, the instruments washed and put away, the table washed down and put in its proper place, and the pupils' supper was brought out and placed back on it.

The Reverend R.B. Matson, writing in 1923, looked back 60 years to the time he was a 12-year-old patient in the hospital.

> There was no separate ward for children. I was mixed-up with men in the men's ward … The patients who could walk about helped to lay the table for meals and also to carry food to the patients in bed. We only had tin pannikins to drink out of. Now it is almost impossible to get the corners inside a pannikin quite clean, so the compound flavours of former liquids all left a sediment which gave its taste to those that came after. I got a friend to bring me in a china mug – which I kept beside my bed for my own use to drink out of and was thought very fastidious and favoured. The hospital only gave patients butter with salt but I could not eat it and a friend brought me some fresh butter every week.

Some ten years later, however, the needs of young children were recognised by the honorary medical staff, who recommended that one of the wards should be equipped as a children's ward. The number of children under ten years of age admitted to the hospital had been steadily increasing from a total of 76 in 1871, 87 in 1872 to 110 in 1873. According to the annual report, when one of the wards was appropriated for children this meant that 'the little patients themselves can be more carefully attended to and amused'. Some of the governors defrayed the cost of cribs and bedding for the ward and through the generosity of the Hon. N.L. Melville a Book, Toys and Games Fund was established. The interest from this fund was used to provide gifts and entertainment for children who had to spend Christmas in hospital.

A former sister in charge of Defflis Ward provided another description of the general wards in the 1880s. Writing fifty years later in the Nurses League magazine, when she herself was a patient on Egremont Ward, she recalled:

> This same place was just a barn with rough floors that had to be scrubbed every Monday, and rolls of coconut matting put down to walk upon. In summer time we had swarms of fleas, which, with other duties, nearly drove us wild.

The Visitors' reports during the 1880s in particular also contain clues to what life was like on the wards. For example, the rule that breakfast for the patients should be served at eight o'clock was not always adhered to.

In 1886, the men on Vallance Ward told the Visitors that breakfast of tea, bread and butter were served at 5.30 instead of 8, as laid down in regulations. They claimed that because of the various ailments patients were restless during the night making it difficult to sleep. Then, when they at last they were 'enjoying a little sleep', they found it hard to be roused at 5.30 when they were unable to eat their breakfasts and considered it too long to fast until dinner time at one o'clock. The matron recommended a compromise. She agreed 5.30 was too early an hour for breakfast, but recommended it should be served between six and seven because delaying until eight meant the wards could not be properly cleaned and the beds made before the arrival of the medical officers.

This situation on Vallance Ward was one that was not peculiar to the nineteenth century. The problem of early breakfasts, in particular, and the organisation of the patient's day in general surfaced from time to time in many hospitals in the twentieth century and even led in 1958 to the setting up of a sub-committee to report on the pattern of the in-patients day which expressed concern at the continued practice of waking patients between 5 and 6 a.m.

The physical conditions on the wards at the Sussex County, on the other hand, should be seen in the context of the time. In her biography of Florence Nightingale, Cecil Woodham Smith wrote: 'In 1845 hospitals were places of wretchedness, degradation and squalor'. She referred to the 'Hospital Smell', which she said was accepted as unavoidable and so overpowering that persons entering the wards for the first time were overcome with nausea, and quoted Florence Nightingale herself from her *Notes on Hospitals* to support this view'.[2]

Many of Florence Nightingale's observations are mirrored in what evidence there is concerning the Sussex County – the smell, wooden floors saturated with organic matter, the lack of sanitary conveniences, inadequate heating and windows closed for warmth 'sometimes months at a time'. However, on the evidence of the official visitors' reports, it seems equally likely that conditions in Brighton may not have been among the worst encountered in hospitals at the time, especially those that began life in unconverted private houses.

Be that as it may, the situation in hospitals was so bad that Sir James Simpson, the Scottish obstetrician who first used chloroform to relieve the pain of women in childbirth, asked, in an address to the Edinburgh Medico-Chirurgical Society in 1847: 'To what extent are hospitals, as in general at present constituted, banes or blessings?' and went on to suggest that permanent buildings should be abandoned in favour of temporary buildings which could be taken down every few years and erected in places where the air was not polluted. Twenty-seven years later the periodic razing of hospitals was still being suggested because, said Sir John Erichsen, they were 'incurably pyaemia stricken. It is impossible to disinfect them.'[3]

Some of the credit for improving conditions during the later part of the century may be due to the change in the quality of nursing staff which occurred following the work of Florence Nightingale and the establishment of the first modern nursing school in 1860.

In 1879, the President of the American Medical Association, Lewis A. Sayre M.D., visited the hospital and reported:

> Its location and construction being all that can be desired in a Hygiene point of view. And in its internal arrangement and management, it appears to be as perfect as our present knowledge of Hygiene permits.

The Case of Sarah Hill

An incident in 1852 serves to throw further light on life inside the hospital at the time, for both patients and staff, and also how press reports then, as more recently, could perhaps unjustifiably cast the hospital in a bad light.

The Case of Sarah Hill was the heading of a paragraph in the *Brighton Gazette* in one of a number of reports during July and August in that newspaper and also in the *Brighton Guardian* and the *Brighton Herald.* One report was headlined 'The Hospital and the Workhouse' as central to the issue was the claim that the hospital, failing to secure admission of patients considered more appropriate to the workhouse, had twice left patients in the street, or to be more accurate, on one occasion on the steps of the town hall.

Late one morning in July, Sarah Hill attended the hospital stating she was subject to fainting fits and Dr King recommended her admission. She was admitted to No. 3 Ward and given some sal volatile by the house surgeon who visited her again during the afternoon. About four o'clock the nurse, Fanny French, sent for help as the patient was becoming violent and unruly and she was unable to control her. She was found to be in a very disorderly state, very abusive and using 'most obscene and disgusting language'. She had frightened all the other patients in the ward into a corner of the room and appeared to be temporarily at least out of her mind.

Henry Hudson the porter was sent for her father who came about five o'clock and tried to quieten her. He said she was a very respectable person but a little given to drink and since her mother's death had not been quite right in her mind. He left after a few minutes. Sarah Hill then became violent again and her language was so obscene that all the eleven or twelve unmarried patients out of the sixteen in the ward were moved to other wards or into the scullery.

By nine o'clock, her screaming could be heard in the grounds and she was taken to the Fever Ward where she was put into a secure room in charge of Nurse Cardiff whose bed was in the room with her. Another nurse, Lower, was in constant attendance during the night. Following more disturbances during the night, one of the porters was sent to bring her friends to the hospital one of whom, apparently her landlady, was told Sarah was not a fit case for the hospital and must be taken away, immediately or a little later. Because she did not want to take her to her own house, the 'landlady' asked for a certificate that the patient was out of her mind and said something about taking it to the town hall. A report placed before the board described in detail the events that followed: apparently the father had left for Portsmouth after passing the certificate to the parish surgeon. He had called at the hospital later on his way to visit a private patient and said he would issue a certificate that the patient was labouring under temporary delusion which, he had no doubt, would secure her admission to the infirmary that night.

What followed, however, was that Hudson, the porter was sent from pillar to post with the certificate trying to obtain an order for her admission to the infirmary. Eventually he obtained an order from the assistant to the workhouse surgeon and took it with the patient to the infirmary where he was refused admission by the governor and returned to the hospital

By this time it was eleven o'clock and there were five or six patients on the ward who had been deprived of sleep the night before and one whose condition had worsened because of Sarah Hill's violent conduct. Hudson was therefore instructed to take her to her father's house, where, after seeking help from a policeman, he finally saw her being taken into the house by one of the women who had been at the hospital in the morning.

This summary of the report to the hospital board scarcely does justice to the various twists and turns of events during the 21st July, but gives some indication of the hospital's dilemma and of what was considered the obstructive behaviour of the various officials connected with the town hall and the workhouse.

The first press reports, however, were an account of a meeting at Brighton Workhouse. These told a rather different story: the request for admission had been made too late. The hospital porter had been told by the assistant overseer the infirmary would probably be closed for the night and an order for her admission would be made in the morning, to which the porter had replied that if the order was not given she would be turned out into the street. He later took the patient to the workhouse where the governor was knocked up but declined to admit her without an order. The patient was then taken to Egremont Street, set down on the pavement and left there. (Cries of 'shame' at the Guardians' meeting.)

Clearly there was ill feeling between the Guardians and the hospital. The chairman said it was not the first time 'the people at the hospital had acted in this way', adding that only a few years before they had brought patients and laid them out on the town hall steps.

At a later meeting it became clear that the Guardians' stance arose from an incident in 1841 with a pauper named Sarah Gable as a result of which the hospital had been informed that no person should be removed from there to the workhouse infirmary without previous notice having been given to the parish authorities.

However, despite the adverse publicity, the affair ended happily for the hospital. Another report of a Guardians' meeting on 19th August related how the chairman had met the hospital governors. After retracting the claim that the woman had been left on the street and accepting the board's version of the way the patient had been taken into a woman's house, he responded to their concern that a remark he had made was 'calculated to injure the institution.'

Referring to his comment that a patient had been left on the steps of the town hall, he admitted that he ought to have said that the person alluded to was left at the office of the assistant overseer at the town hall. The report of this meeting in the *Brighton Guardian* concluded: Here the matter ended.

Surgeons and surgery

In the mid-eighteenth century, surgeons were still operating on conscious patients without anaesthesia and with unboiled, dirty instruments. The introduction of anaesthetics meant more operations were carried out but in the absence of knowledge of bacteriology and antiseptic precautions, the risks were increased by the greater number of operations, and sepsis and gangrene spread throughout the surgical wards.

When Nathaniel Blaker returned to the hospital in 1864 following his appointment as house surgeon, he said the surgeons were still operating in old coats kept for the purpose, which were cleaned by allowing the pus and blood to dry and then simply brushed off. Surgery, he said, had advanced a little since he was first admitted as a pupil, but not very much.

> Diseases of joints which had, during my pupilage, been treated with blisters and cupping, were not put on splints and kept at rest. The first traces of the present aseptic and antiseptic treatment of wounds might be seen in the greater cleanliness, and in the use of such lotions as lead, zinc, and, especially carbolic acid instead of plain water, though it must not be forgotten that Friar's balsam, balsam of Peru, and turpentine in various forms had been used since time immemorial. The three or four sponges, which it had been the custom to use for a whole ward and which were imperfectly washed between each dressing, were superseded by swabs of cotton wool or fine tow, but practically nothing was done to prevent the spread of septic poison.

Cases of erysipelas and gangrene were constantly recurring, according to Blaker, who recorded that in the autumn of 1864 these diseases raged to such an extent that fourteen or fifteen patients, and the head nurse, died in one week in the male accident ward.

To some extent the morbid fear of fresh air was countered by ventilators and blocks placed in the window frames so that the sashes could not be fully closed. Although this produced some improvement, septic cases still occurred.

In 1867, the first ovariotomy was done at the hospital by H.M. Blaker but septic inflammation set in and the patient died. About the same time E,J. Furner tied the subclavian artery on both sides at different times, on the same patient. Both operations were performed without anaesthetic in order to avoid any distension of the veins. According to Nathaniel Blaker, the man scarcely moved during the operation and slept for sixteen or seventeen hours each day until he got well.

Almost certainly Furner's operation took place shortly before Blaker returned to the hospital. The annual report for 1863 referred to two cases 'of a gratifying nature', one of them being an operation which involved 'tying the subclavian artery of a man afflicted with aneurysm, occasioned probably by lifting heavy weights at the railway.' The report continued by describing the operation as 'one of extreme delicacy, the successful performance of which ranks among the triumphs of modern surgery … the man … not only snatched from certain and inevitable death, but restored to active life.'

The nurse caring for him sat up all night for three weeks 'almost literally without taking rest', the report continued. She received a gratuity of two guineas from the board.

The annual reports were well publicised and accounts such as these were clearly designed to enhance the hospital's reputation as well as attracting much-needed funds.

The second case described in the 1863 report concerned the admission of three men with extensive superficial burns sustained following an explosion on a steamboat in Newhaven.

> After remaining within the walls about two months, all three left the Hospital completely cured, owing their recovery mainly to the unceasing attention with which they had been watched and which they could have received nowhere but in an Institution of this nature.

There was more praise for the hospital and its staff in the 1885 report for the way they had responded to an accident in Preston Park. There was an explosion of fireworks during a demonstration by the Ancient Order of Foresters in August, which resulted in many casualties.[4] One 'poor lad' died after admission to hospital from shock following the 'terrible injuries' he had sustained. Fourteen of the 22 others brought to the hospital were seriously wounded, some, in a very precarious state, were detained. Fortunately, according to the report, the staff were equal to the occasion and no further loss of life occurred. Twelve of the fourteen had left hospital by the end of the year, but two remained on the 31st December.

In 1869, Blaker was appointed assistant surgeon and the following year he performed the second ovariotomy done in the hospital, and the first to be successful – despite being told by an elderly retired medical man that the operation was scarcely justifiable. The operation, when first introduced by Sir Thomas Spencer Wells, and those who performed it, had been received with a storm of abuse by the medical profession. Spencer Wells was the first British surgeon to understand the importance of Pasteur's Germ Theory, but despite this, a third of his ovariotomy patients died.

That Furner and Blaker were willing to undertake the admittedly dangerous procedure can probably be considered evidence of the quality of the hospital's surgeons. For a woman, ovarian disease resulted in a year or two of painful illness, relieved only by tapping, in itself a dangerous procedure, and an inevitable fatal termination. Blaker's view was that 'it is not surprising, under these circumstances, that she should take the risk of an operation that would restore her to health, though that risk might be great.'

This view was not universally held. At Hull Royal Infirmary, for example, the first recorded ovariotomy was not performed until 1874, while at the Royal Berkshire Hospital surgeons differed about the point at which the operation should be performed. One view was that it should be delayed until the condition became one of 'grave inconvenience or a serious danger to life'; the other was that early intervention increased the chances of success.[5]

The Rev. Matson provides further evidence of the skill of the hospital's surgeons during this time.

> I was taken to the Sussex County Hospital — it was found that I had diseased bone in my left heel and both my elbows, but the worse was that the whole tibia or big shin bone of the right leg was diseased. The day after Xmas day 1863, two most able and careful doctors Furner and [assistant surgeon Fred W.] Jowers performed a wonderful operation on my leg. It had only been discovered a year before in Paris that such an operation could be done and I think that I was the first case for it to be tried on in England. These two clever doctors removed the whole shaft of the shinbone leaving parts of the healthy periosteum or skin of the bone to form a new bone. The operation was successful but I was 6 months in the hospital 6 months in a Convalescent Home and had to walk 6 years on crutches, and for 60 years that leg has done wonders. The doctors there 60 years ago were in their days equal to any doctors now ...

During the 1870s Lister introduced the antiseptic methods that revolutionised surgical procedures and results. The method was met with incredulity and opposition, one eminent London surgeon even stressing the advantages of the bread poultice compared with the antiseptic treatment of wounds in a professional journal. Many surgeons, while not offering outright opposition, simply waited for undoubted proof that Lister's technique was an advance before they abandoned their own methods. So it was perhaps not surprising that Nathaniel Blaker was subjected to ridicule and difficulty when he first introduced the new antiseptic method at the Sussex County Hospital.

By the 1880s, however, the hospital was enjoying 'the very highest reputation with the [medical] profession,' according to the biographer of Henry Tonks,[6] who added that it was staffed by first-rate physicians and surgeons, who took a great interest in teaching the students all they could. Tonks began his medical career there, in January 1880, as pupil on the advice of his family doctor. At that time, the usual way of entering the profession was to become a student at one of the larger London hospitals, but as well as recommending that Tonks would benefit from the hospital's reputation, it would also appear that the doctor believed that the Brighton air would benefit the young man's health.

In any event, Tonks was well pleased with his year and a half Brighton apprenticeship.

> Every day … Tonks came into contact with new people under new conditions, and watched them being dealt with by cultivated and intelligent men. Had he gone to a London hospital, anatomy and physiology alone would have occupied him for three years; at the Sussex hospital he came at once into contact with medicine.

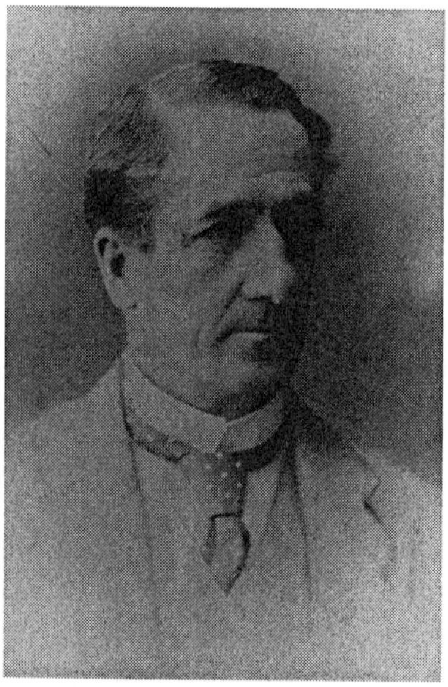

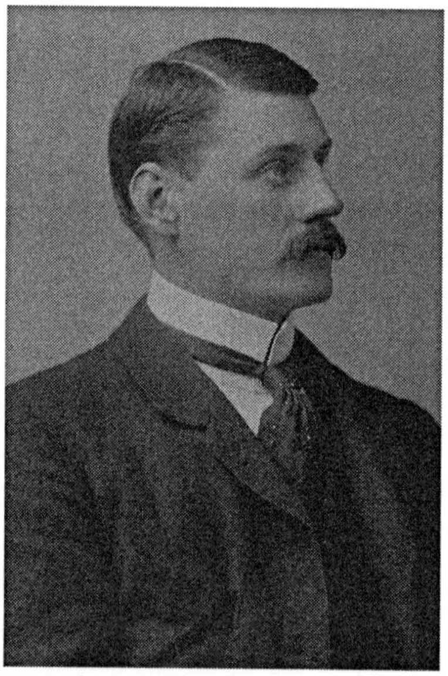

26. Surgeons F.W. Jowers (1869-1889) and R.F. Jowers (1889-1921). Jowers Ward was named in recognition of them and their families for their services to the hospital.

While he was at Brighton, Tonks made what was to turn out to be a lifetime friendship in R.F. Jowers, son of the assistant surgeon. Fred W. Jowers commenced at the hospital as a pupil, later becoming house surgeon, then assistant surgeon and was senior surgeon when he retired in January 1890. Colleagues of the visiting medical staff adopted a resolution, saying, *inter alia*, 'his great surgical skill and administrative firmness during a period exceeding 30 years have combined to elevate the Sussex County Hospital to its present high position.' A similar tribute was paid when sadly he died only a little over three years later.

Fred Jowers brought up his son, Reginald, with the idea that one day he would enjoy the same position as his father. Reginald was appointed honorary assistant surgeon in 1889 and two years later honorary surgeon, a post he occupied for twenty years. During this time he travelled frequently on the Continent and in America, visiting famous clinics and keeping abreast of all the latest developments. Some years later, gratitude for the professional and pecuniary services to the hospital of Reginald Jowers and other members of the family was perpetuated by naming one of the wards the Jowers Ward.

The nurses

When Nathaniel Blaker returned to the hospital in the mid-1860s, he observed there were no sisters, and the head nurse was 'a woman of ordinary intelligence, who had worked her way through the grades of scrubber and under-nurse.' Although they did ordinary nursing fairly well, were very attentive to patients and took much pride in their wards, they could not do dressings, which were usually done by the pupils.

When Henry Tonks came to the hospital in 1880, he arrived as the nurses' Christmas concert was about to begin. Being not quite eighteen and fresh from public school it is perhaps not surprising that he was, in his words,

> overcome by the sight of nurses sitting in rows one above the other, varying in age, some as young as sixteen, for this hospital had a peculiar institution, ward-maids, who were a sort of miniature nurses, and come to the hospital very early in their lives.[7]

The change in nursing attributed to Florence Nightingale brought a different type of woman to work on hospital wards in the latter part of the century. The extent to which this affected the hospital is not clear. For a time the new lady nurses worked alongside the Gamps, who still were still happy to be bribed by relatives to be kind to patients. According the matron Miss E.W. Young[8] 'Patients were still "attended to", not nursed as now [1934], and most of the work was scrubbing and cleaning with occasional instruction in poulticing, bed-making and bandaging. Since thermometers cost 12s 6d (£0.72½) each, they were only touched by doctors and students.'

The establishment of the St. Thomas' training school was later followed by hospitals elsewhere including a well-regarded training school in Brighton.

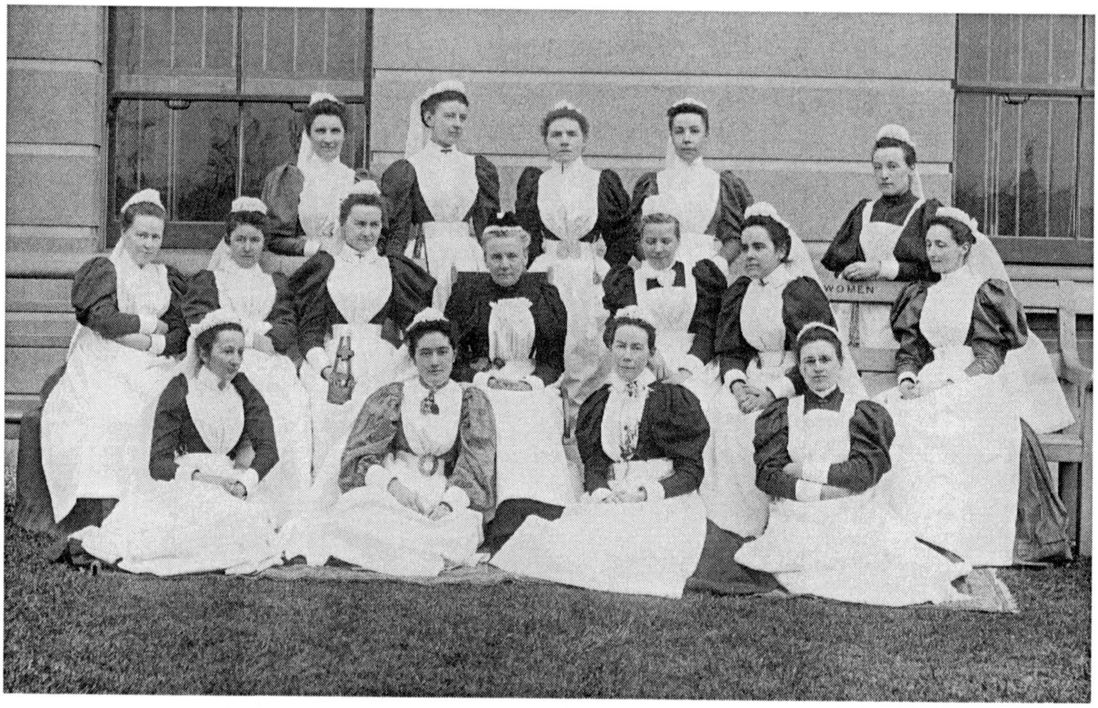

27. Matron Miss Katherine Scott with her sisters at the turn of the century.

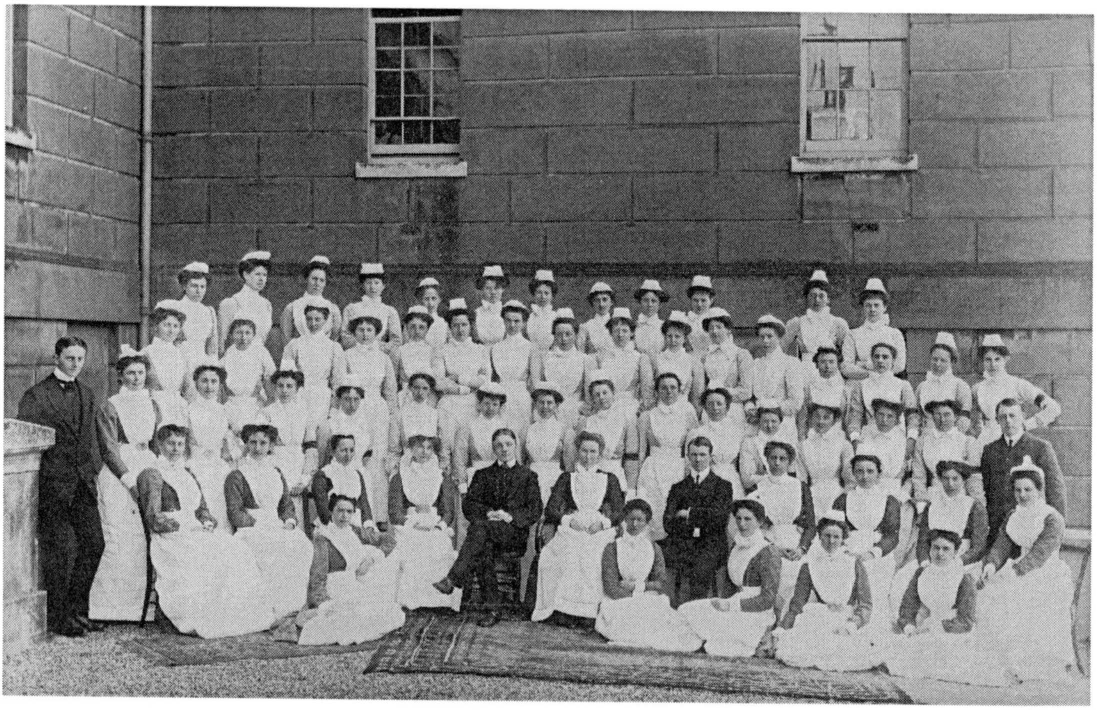

28. A group photograph of the nurses with Matron and doctors

A recommendation that nurses should only work eight hours a day was ridiculed in the first edition of a book on nurse training.

> This committee consisted of men only, and probably did not grasp the fact that it would be bad for patients to be in the hands of three sets of nurses, and that, though eight hours' active work is enough, a woman in good health is easily capable of ten hours of what greatly resembles ordinary household duties.[9]

Nevertheless, applications greatly exceeded the vacancies at hospitals for training as a probationer nurse, despite the long hours and warnings that the work was not simply passive – a mere watching and waiting.

An advertisement for the Sussex County Hospital in 1895 invited applications from young women aged 23 to 30 for three years training for which they had to pay £5. They worked 9½ hours a day with one day off a month and three weeks holiday.

Nurses had to supply their own uniforms. But, as elsewhere, during what was described in the nurse training book as 'the present craze for hospital nursing,' competition for these posts was fierce. Only about twenty applications were accepted, while some 300 were refused every year.

Life for nurses in the new nurses' home, opened towards the end of 1899, was strictly regulated. Staff nurses and probationers had to rise at 6 a.m. when on day duty, make their beds and dust their apartment and be punctual for breakfast at 6.40 a.m. before going on duty at 7 a.m. They were allowed at least two and a half hours off duty each day, one day off a month (staff nurses also had an additional half day each month) and three weeks annual holiday.

Nurses were not allowed to leave the hospital or remain outside for more than two and a half hours without Matron's permission. When off duty they were allowed to receive visitors in the sitting room, subject to Matron's approval. They were also expected to attend family prayers and, of course, Sunday services in the chapel.

Privileges enjoyed by the sisters included an extra week's holiday and, subject to Matron's approval, to receive friends when off duty between 3 and 8.30 p.m. on weekdays and 11 a.m. and nine p.m. on Sundays. However, friends were not allowed to remain during meals without special permission from Matron.

Earlier, in 1888, the hospital had set up the Nursing Institute with the dual objectives, according to the annual report, of proving 'a great public benefit' and becoming 'a source of income to the Hospital'.

The Nursing Institute

Eighteen nurses were employed the following year by forty different medical men and in eighteen places out of Brighton. The hospital profited by £257 16s and in order to maintain the institute in full efficiency and prevent constant changes among the nurses, the board decided to give them a direct interest in its welfare by setting aside one third of the net profits, £25 per annum to go to the matron, the remainder to be divided proportionately among the nurses.

The matron responsible for setting up the institute was Miss G. Scott. Since the retirement of Mrs Comport in 1854, seven other women had held the matron post: Miss Whiteman (1854-1868), Miss S. Longhurst (1868-1870), Miss J. Longstaff (1870), Miss S. Jeans (1871-1879), Miss A.E. Gibson (1879-1880), Miss A.F. MacGregor (1880-1882) and Miss A.K. Robertson (1882-1885). Miss G. Scott held the appointment from 1885-1896 when she was succeeded by Miss Katherine Scott whose appointment was to last some 27 years until 1923.

The Nursing Institute, under the two Miss Scotts, went from strength to strength. In 1890 they served in all parts of the country as well as in Switzerland and the Channel Islands. In 1891, the profits rose to £319 4s 5d and in 1896 23 nurses employed during the year shared a bonus of £214 16s 8d with the matron.

A decade of change

A visitor to the hospital in the mid 1890s would have found a very different situation from the one existing in the earlier part of the century. The plain white washed walls of the wards described in the 1850s and the rough wooden floors covered with coconut matting in the 1880s were largely things of the past.

The writer of the magazine article published in 1896 described the organisation of the wards and some of the work of the hospital and the photographs taken following his visit provide evidence of the changes that had taken place during the preceding ten years or so, not least of the polished oak floors which were replacing the rough wooden floors covered with coconut matting

After visiting various rooms and the surgery 'in which a huge patients' chair, grim and gaunt, was the most prominent feature, he entered the men's accident and surgical Vallance ward and remarked on 'the pleasant aspect of the nurses … the perfect cleanliness and soothing quiet which prevailed, made a strong impression on us.' The writer moved on to the operating theatre then to the women's accident and surgical ward, Peel. On the second floor he visited Bristol and Overton, on the western side, and Egremont on the east, noting they were all for women, the former for surgical cases, the latter for medical.

> On the north side of the corridor leading from the Egremont Ward, we were shown a snug little one bed compartment, such as are used where isolation is necessary. On either side of this corridor are rooms devoted to domestic requirements, the matron's, sisters' and nurses' apartments, dining and boarding rooms, pantry, a large room for the storage of linen, a laboratory for microscopic analysis, the house surgeon's room, and a special room near the Overton Ward for diphtheria.

Following a tour of the third floor wards, Chichester (male surgical) and Defflis (male medical) the writer was taken out of the building to the more recent Jubilee Block.

> The ground floor consists chiefly of isolated departments including a couple of strong padded rooms for victims of delirium tremens and other ailments productive of violence; while the rest are used by the sisters and nurses or are employed as domestic offices. The second floor is entirely devoted to women … ascending the short flight of stairs leading to the third floor, the din and chattering in the rooms above, appraised us that we were approaching the Children's Wards. Despite their ailments they appeared to be thoroughly enjoying themselves.

Numerous though these late nineteenth century changes were, not everything called for in the 1894 programme was made until early in the twentieth when the installation of the lift in the main building, the operating theatre and balconies and fire escape staircases, for example, were brought into use.

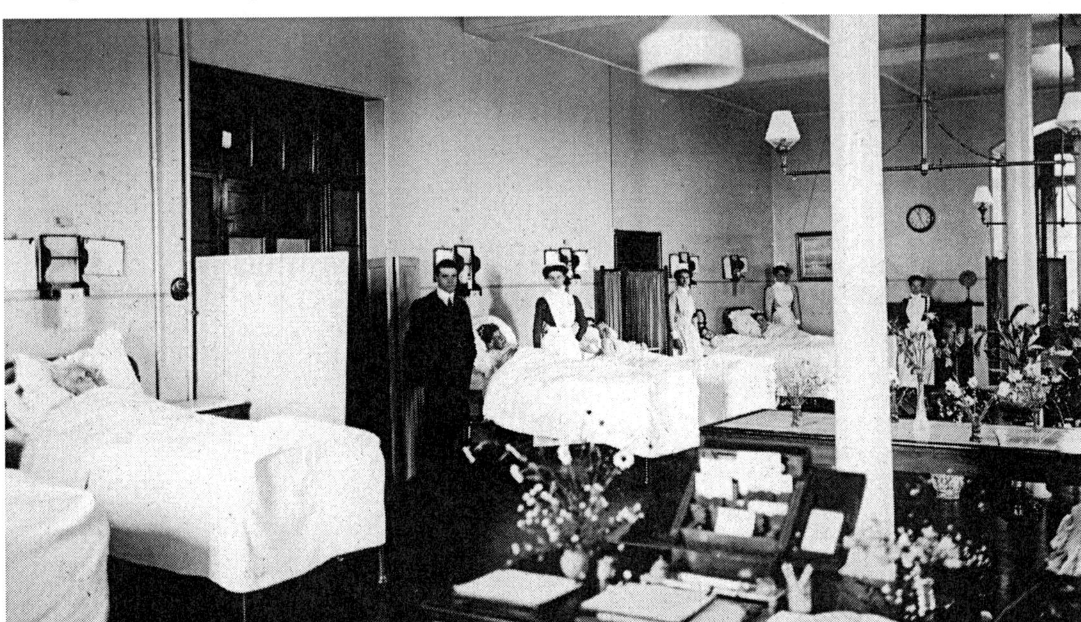

29. A corner of Egremont Ward at the turn of the century.

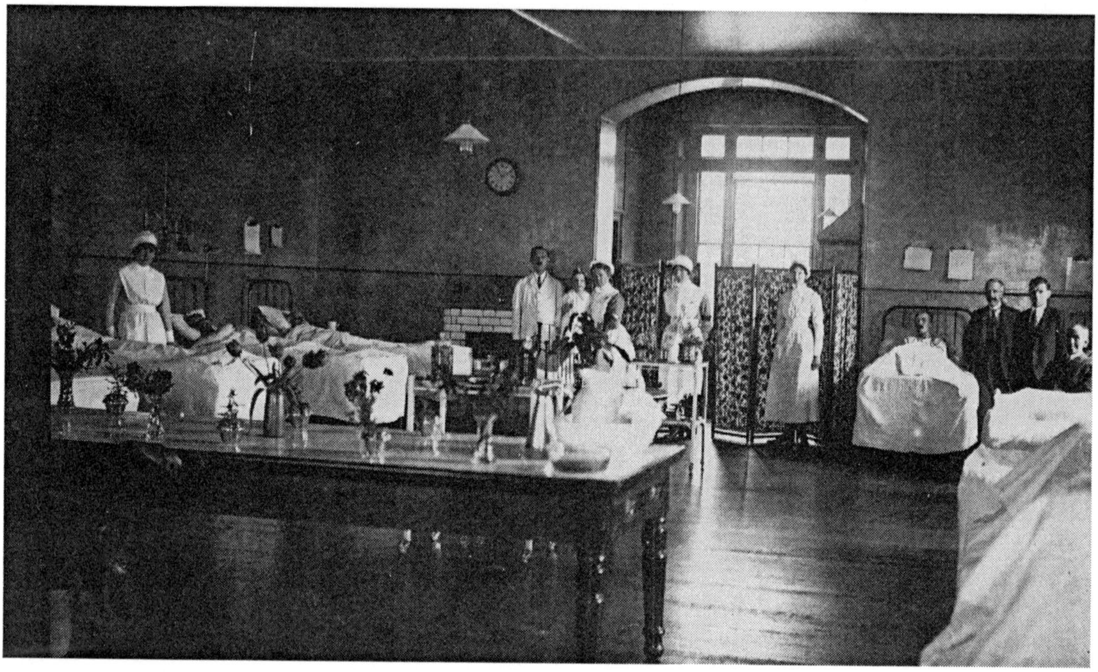

30. Polished oak floors that had replaced the rough wooden boards covered with coconut matting in earlier years were a feature of the wards in the 1890s.

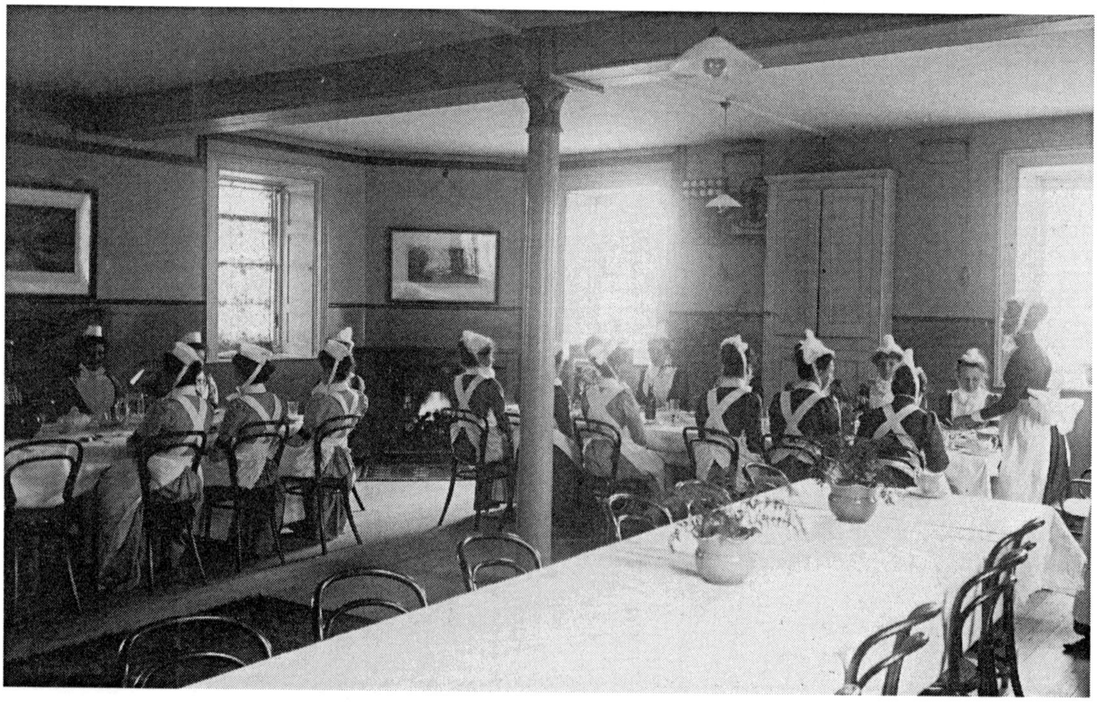

31. The dining room in the new nurses' home.

7. Urgently in Need of Money, 1900 - 1914

From the outset, it became the clear that the financial problems encountered in the 1800s would be even greater in the new century. Nationally, for example, a report in the *Daily Telegraph* on the 27th December 1906 gave details of a number of London hospitals which, 'finding themselves urgently in need of money,' were launching special appeals.

The North Eastern Hospital for Children in Bethnal Green, for example, had a £9,000 debt on a new building and was £4,000 behind in payments to the end of September. If the debts could not be paid off, the hospital was faced with closing half its wards. The Middlesex and King's College hospitals were calling for assistance, Paddington Green Children's Hospital was £2,500 in debt, the Metropolitan Hospital 'suffering a serious falling off of income' was absolutely without funds and needed £5,000 to pay off tradesmen and others.

The long list of hospitals in trouble included, to name just a few, University College Hospital, the London Homeopathic Hospital, the Brompton Hospital and the Cancer Hospital in Fulham Road. Nor was the problem confined to London: Margate's Royal Sea Bathing Hospital, for example, needed £2,000 to settle its account. Hospitals nationally dependent on voluntary donations were in desperate need of funds and the Sussex County Hospital, not surprisingly, was no exception.

A need for prompt action

As early as 1900 it was clear that the hospital was facing serious financial problems. The annual report for that year listed a number of causes: the demand for doctors for the Boer War in South Africa, combined with the exclusion of unqualified men from general practice, for example, meant the hospital had been forced to employ 'temporary substitutes at high salaries'. Fuel costs had increased and there were increased numbers of patients needing special diets. There was also the cost of the triennial cleaning and structural alterations to the wards and outside painting and a 'very serious extra charge' had arisen for putting out washing while rebuilding of the laundry and replacing its obsolete and worn-out machinery.

In 1901, the committee made an urgent appeal for further funds 'to efficiently carry out the work of the Hospital.' During the year, the daily average number of inpatients had risen to 177 compared with 143 in 1900. The number of outpatients and casualties also increased significantly, especially the latter, the number rising by 628 to a total of 4,157 in the year. In the following year, despite 'the utmost efforts of the Committee to economise,' the annual report warned:

> The Institution is now in another financial crisis in its history, and prompt action is needed. It cannot carry on its present work on its present income, and unless timely help is forthcoming the only solution to the difficulty is to close some of the Wards, and the Committee earnestly urge the people of Sussex to avert the necessity for such action.

The situation failed to improve, however, and by 1904 the committee opened its annual report drawing the attention of the governors and the charitable public of the county 'to the extreme gravity of the financial position.'

> The closing of Wards in the largest general hospital in the county, at a time when every bed is urgently required, might well be characterised as a calamity; yet the Committee of Management feel that, unless their appeal for increased support is adequately responded to, they will be forced to recommend the adoption of such a drastic measure in the immediate future.

Coping with the financial challenges

By a stroke of good fortune, the hospital found itself in a much better position at the end of 1906 than the hospitals in the *Daily Telegraph's* report. A number of measures had been undertaken to try to improve the financial position. These included a £10,000 appeal launched by the president, Lord Leconfield, through the local press in October 1902.

In his letter to the press, Lord Leconfield said there was a long list of applicants waiting for admission; expenditure had increased because the hospital was treating more patients and that the increase in the number of cottage hospitals meant that only the more serious cases were being sent to Brighton, in particular surgical cases requiring complicated and expensive operations. He also appealed for support from the country districts, pointing out that at the time of writing 69 out of 193 beds were occupied by patients from outside Brighton. However, the response must have been disappointing, as his Shilling Fund raised a little less than £2,000 in the following year.

On the 14th February 1905, St Valentine's Day, Miss Blanche Fair instituted a Pound Day. Pound Days had already been held very successfully in aid of Brighton's children's hospital and the County's first effort, according to a *Sussex Daily News* report the following day, was 'a huge success.' First reports indicated that £397 had been received in money (the final total was

£426 15s 1d) as well as thousands of articles, for the appeal was also made for pounds of goods in kind. Collections were made at the hospital, at York Place schools and Hove Town Hall.

Enormous quantities of tea were donated at Hove Town Hall and although tea and sugar predominated at the hospital, the range of articles was greater and included fowls, rounds of beef, shoulders of mutton and two huge codfish.

At the boys' school, the 724¼lbs received included 218 lbs of rice, 146 lbs of sugar, 52 lbs of tapioca and 43 lbs of jam and marmalade. Brighton Police sent a 224lbs sackful of sugar. Supplementary efforts were reported in 27 places in the country districts, including 450 parcels at Burgess Hill, Haywards Heath and Shoreham. According to the *Sussex Daily News*, the matron, Miss Scott, was anxious that donors should visit the hospital and hundreds did so, visiting everywhere from 'kitchens to the nurses' home.'

Miss Fair was also a leading light as secretary and organiser of the Ladies' Blanket, Linen and Work Guild. This was established at a meeting of the Ladies Association in 1911 that had organised house-to-house collections in aid of the hospital during the preceding two years.

In 1905, by when a debt of £8,000

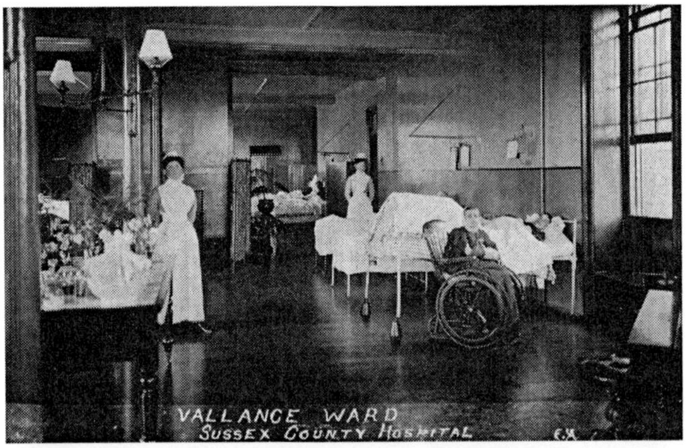

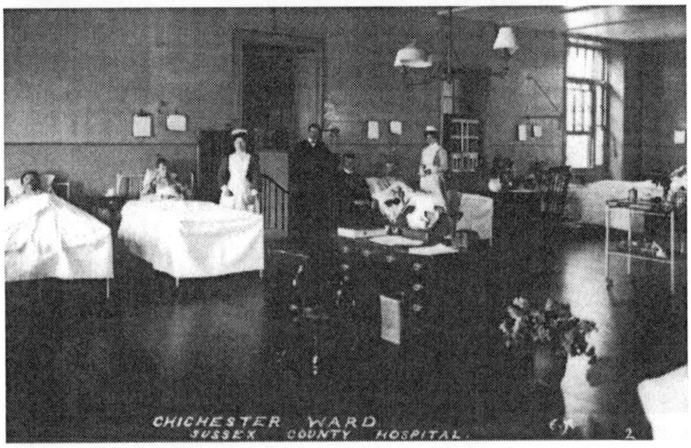

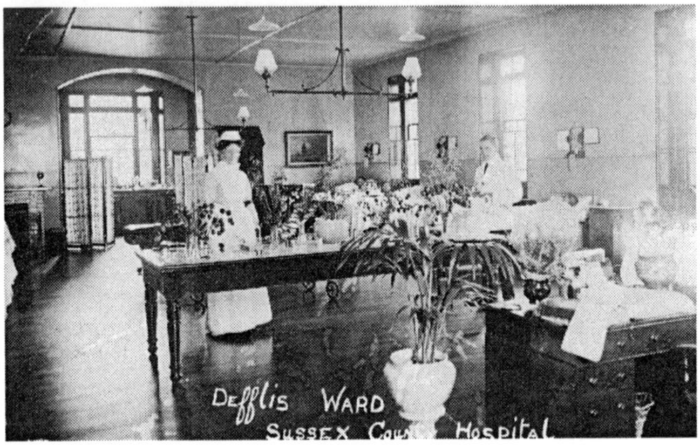

32. The sale of postcards of the hospital's wards was one of the ways by which attempts were made to boost finances. Defflis Ward, then a male medical ward, received its name in 1866 when £10,780 1s 6d. was received under the will of Solomon M. Defflis. More than a hundred years later, the ward was renamed Solomon, many of the patients being admitted apparently mishearing the original name, presumably believing it to be 'deathless' or 'death list'.

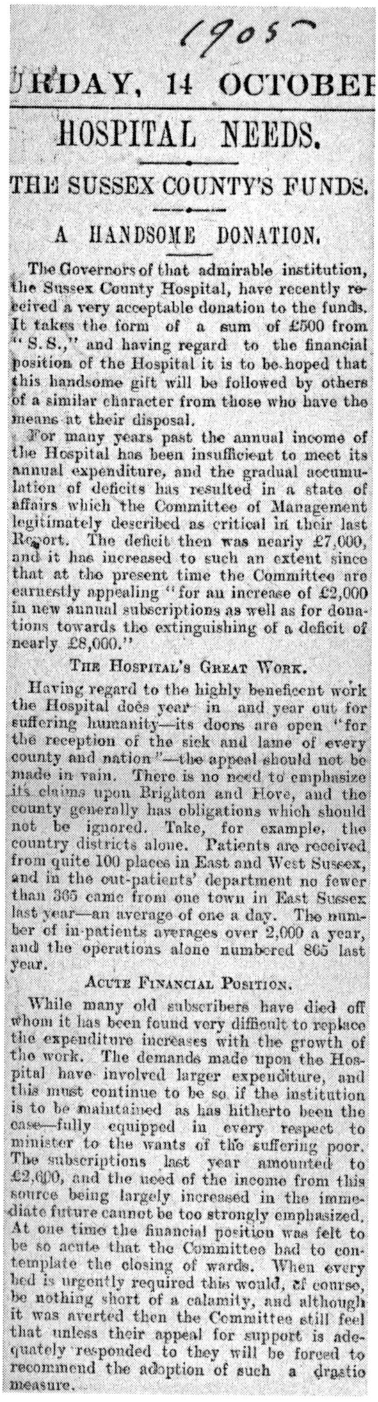

1905

URDAY, 14 OCTOBER

HOSPITAL NEEDS.

THE SUSSEX COUNTY'S FUNDS.

A HANDSOME DONATION.

The Governors of that admirable institution, the Sussex County Hospital, have recently received a very acceptable donation to the funds. It takes the form of a sum of £500 from "S.S.," and having regard to the financial position of the Hospital it is to be hoped that this handsome gift will be followed by others of a similar character from those who have the means at their disposal.

For many years past the annual income of the Hospital has been insufficient to meet its annual expenditure, and the gradual accumulation of deficits has resulted in a state of affairs which the Committee of Management legitimately described as critical in their last Report. The deficit then was nearly £7,000, and it has increased to such an extent since that at the present time the Committee are earnestly appealing "for an increase of £2,000 in new annual subscriptions as well as for donations towards the extinguishing of a deficit of nearly £8,000."

THE HOSPITAL'S GREAT WORK.

Having regard to the highly beneficent work the Hospital does year in and year out for suffering humanity—its doors are open "for the reception of the sick and lame of every county and nation"—the appeal should not be made in vain. There is no need to emphasize its claims upon Brighton and Hove, and the county generally has obligations which should not be ignored. Take, for example, the country districts alone. Patients are received from quite 100 places in East and West Sussex, and in the out-patients' department no fewer than 365 came from one town in East Sussex last year—an average of one a day. The number of in-patients averages over 2,000 a year, and the operations alone numbered 865 last year.

ACUTE FINANCIAL POSITION.

While many old subscribers have died off whom it has been found very difficult to replace the expenditure increases with the growth of the work. The demands made upon the Hospital have involved larger expenditure, and this must continue to be so if the institution is to be maintained as has hitherto been the case—fully equipped in every respect to minister to the wants of the suffering poor. The subscriptions last year amounted to £2,600, and the need of the income from this source being largely increased in the immediate future cannot be too strongly emphasized. At one time the financial position was felt to be so acute that the Committee had to contemplate the closing of wards. When every bed is urgently required this would, of course, be nothing short of a calamity, and although it was averted then the Committee still feel that unless their appeal for support is adequately responded to they will be forced to recommend the adoption of such a drastic measure.

33. A 1905 report in the Sussex Daily News which drew attention to the hospital's financial plight at the time.

had accumulated, a special Committee of Investigation was set up. The committee was charged with investigating the hospital's expenditure in an attempt to avoid or reduce some of its expenses. Much of its work was carried out during the following year with the result that considerable economies were effected, although the committee acknowledged that the result was influenced by savings made on Grant Ward where twenty beds were closed for nearly nine months while it was adapted as a gynaecological ward.

However, at the end of the following year, in reporting 'with great relief and thankfulness [that] the great cloud of debt which had overshadowed the Hospital for some time past has been dispersed,' the committee acknowledged that this was the result of a large legacy over more than £10,000 and so the inadequate level of subscriptions continued to be a problem.

Concluding his report for 1906, the chairman, C. Scrase Dickens appealed for more support:

> The old debt has been got rid of, and it is to the interest of all concerned that a new one should not arise to take its place; all those who take part in the management will do their best if only they are supported by an increased number outside, for surely it is the wish of all that the Hospital should continue to flourish …

The Lady Almoner

At the beginning of March 1904, the hospital's first Lady Almoner began work. The appointment of almoners had gained pace in the London hospitals towards the end of the previous century but their introduction was the subject of some controversy. Their role was seen as necessary to counteract the abuse of voluntary hospitals by patients considered to be 'unsuitable objects for charity.' In particular, these patients were believed to be making unnecessary demands on the hospital outpatient and, to a lesser extent, casualty departments.

Locally, the question of abuse was also raised by members of the public in 1904 in letters to the press. The *Sussex Daily*

News, for example, carried a letter from Mr R.J. Howlett on the 1st February who said he had joined the Ship Street legal firm (Attree and Somers Clarke) 'nearly half a century ago'. The first thing that had struck him was the great abuse of charity by entirely undeserving people. Although this had diminished of late, it still existed, he maintained. Another writer referred to 'the careless way letters of admission to hospitals and dispensaries are distributed by governors.'

The introduction of almoners had been championed largely by the medical profession through the British Medical Association (BMA) and its publica-

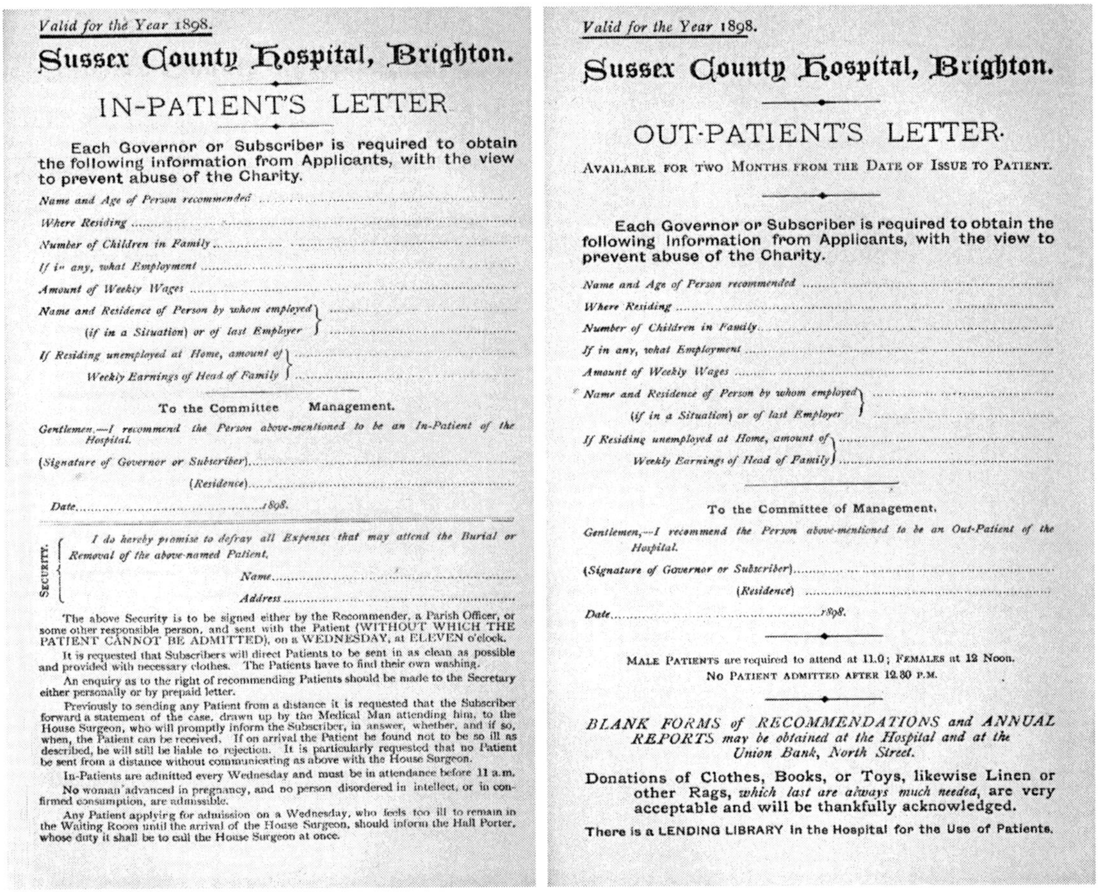

Valid for the Year 1898.

Sussex County Hospital, Brighton.

IN-PATIENT'S LETTER

Each Governor or Subscriber is required to obtain the following information from Applicants, with the view to prevent abuse of the Charity.

Name and Age of Person recommended ....

Where Residing ....

Number of Children in Family ....

If in any, what Employment ....

Amount of Weekly Wages ....

Name and Residence of Person by whom employed (if in a Situation) or of last Employer ....

If Residing unemployed at Home, amount of Weekly Earnings of Head of Family ....

To the Committee Management.

Gentlemen,—I recommend the Person above-mentioned to be an In-Patient of the Hospital.

(Signature of Governor or Subscriber) ....

(Residence) ....

Date ....1898.

SECURITY. *I do hereby promise to defray all Expenses that may attend the Burial or Removal of the above-named Patient.*

Name ....

Address ....

The above Security is to be signed either by the Recommender, a Parish Officer, or some other responsible person, and sent with the Patient (WITHOUT WHICH THE PATIENT CANNOT BE ADMITTED), on a WEDNESDAY, at ELEVEN o'clock.

It is requested that Subscribers will direct Patients to be sent in as clean as possible and provided with necessary clothes. The Patients have to find their own washing.

An enquiry as to the right of recommending Patients should be made to the Secretary either personally or by prepaid letter.

Previously to sending any Patient from a distance it is requested that the Subscriber forward a statement of the case, drawn up by the Medical Man attending him, to the House Surgeon, who will promptly inform the Subscriber, in answer, whether, and if so, when, the Patient can be received. If on arrival the Patient be found not to be so ill as described, he will still be liable to rejection. It is particularly requested that no Patient be sent from a distance without communicating as above with the House Surgeon.

In-Patients are admitted every Wednesday and must be in attendance before 11 a.m.

No woman advanced in pregnancy, and no person disordered in intellect, or in confirmed consumption, are admissible.

Any Patient applying for admission on a Wednesday, who feels too ill to remain in the Waiting Room until the arrival of the House Surgeon, should inform the Hall Porter, whose duty it shall be to call the House Surgeon at once.

Valid for the Year 1898.

Sussex County Hospital, Brighton.

OUT-PATIENT'S LETTER.

AVAILABLE FOR TWO MONTHS FROM THE DATE OF ISSUE TO PATIENT.

Each Governor or Subscriber is required to obtain the following Information from Applicants, with the view to prevent abuse of the Charity.

Name and Age of Person recommended ....

Where Residing ....

Number of Children in Family ....

If in any, what Employment ....

Amount of Weekly Wages ....

Name and Residence of Person by whom employed (if in a Situation) or of last Employer ....

If Residing unemployed at Home, amount of Weekly Earnings of Head of Family ....

To the Committee of Management.

Gentlemen,—I recommend the Person above-mentioned to be an Out-Patient of the Hospital.

(Signature of Governor or Subscriber) ....

(Residence) ....

Date ....1898.

MALE PATIENTS are required to attend at 11.0; FEMALES at 12 Noon.
NO PATIENT ADMITTED AFTER 12.30 P.M.

BLANK FORMS of RECOMMENDATIONS and ANNUAL REPORTS may be obtained at the Hospital and at the Union Bank, North Street.

Donations of Clothes, Books, or Toys, likewise Linen or other Rags, *which last are always much needed*, are very acceptable and will be thankfully acknowledged.

There is a LENDING LIBRARY in the Hospital for the Use of Patients.

34. An 1898 In-patients letter which requested information to prevent the abuse of the charity and a promise by the recommender to pay all burial or removal expenses. Patients were admitted at eleven o'clock on Wednesdays and had to be provided with clean clothes and be responsible for their own washing. Women in advanced pregnancy, disordered in intellect or suffering from consumption were not eligible for admission. Right: Out-Patients Letters in 1898 called for donations of clothes, books, toys, linen or other rags that were 'always very much needed.' Some years earlier, in 1855, there was a special appeal for linen and rags because of a national shortage caused by the need to meet the requirements of the army in the Crimea. This led the local press to report that the hospital needed 'old linen and new subscribers'.

tion, the *British Medical Journal*. In 1897 the Hospital Reform Association had been formed to agitate against abuse. This abuse was seen as misuse of the system by those who were able to pay, which could be dealt with by way of a means test. However, the medical profession, especially the consultants, were also concerned about the use of subscribers' letters. They believed priority for admission should be determined by medical recommendation and not by rules relating to the issue of a letter by a lay person.

The almoner's role involved a rigorous interrogation of new patients about their marital state, their employment and earnings. Patients deemed to be able to afford private treatment were not allowed to attend again. Not surprisingly, there were objections to means testing. This was seen to be against the spirit of voluntary hospitals and by some, such as workmen for example, who made contributions to their workplace collections and believed these entitled them to free treatment. Nevertheless, the committee went ahead and as an experiment accepted the offer of the Charity Organisation Society to pay half the expense of maintaining an almoner in the outpatient department.

In the first full year following the appointment of Mrs Crawford as lady almoner, she reported that she had interviewed 4,846 outpatients of whom 'only 15 have been sent away as judged well able to pay for treatment.' This appeared to satisfy the committee that there was very little, if any, abuse of the charity and that fears that her inquisitional work would drive away deserving persons seeking aid were unfounded.

Much of the almoner's work was concerned with the help she had been able to give to patients, not only by way of grants, but in assisting them 'in obtaining surgical appliances, nourishing food or milk for babies, while in others she has developed the spirit of thrift by encouraging them to saving toward the cost of such necessities.'

Commenting on her work in the annual report for 1906, the chairman noted that with the unqualified support of the outpatient department's medical staff, it had been decided to extend what had been an experimental appointment for a further three years.

Hospital Amalgamation?

More relevant than any possible abuse to the financial situation of the hospital (and others locally) was what Howlett called in his letter to the *Sussex Daily News* 'the mischief of the overlap,' the town's voluntary hospitals all vying with each other for subscribers. Another letter writer, 'A Suffering Householder', suggested there should be only three hospitals in Brighton and Hove, the County, the children's hospital and one in Hove on a site donated for a women's hospital. Moreover, all three should all be under one management and the sites of the other hospitals sold, the proceeds being allocated primarily for building the hospital in Hove. This was probably one of the earliest occasions on which a single hospital for the town had been proposed, something that was to recur throughout the century. If implemented, it would mean either the expansion or, alternatively, possibly the replacement of the County by a new hospital on another site.

What appears to have sparked the debate was a public appeal to build a new women's hospital. Howlett, in his letter, urged the organisers to think again before appealing for many thousands of pounds on bricks and mortar. The mayor of Brighton, Alderman Marx, advocated a possible solution. Writing to the *Sussex Daily News* a month later, he suggested that young patients should be moved from the County to the Royal Alexandra Hospital to make room for women. There would then be no need for a new women's hospital. He entered into negotiations with the committees of the County Hospital and the Women's Lying-In Institution and Hospital at 76 West Street regarding the amalgamation of their gynaecological departments and the borough council donated £2,000 from the Philip Hedgcock Bequest towards the cost of adapting the Jubilee Building. The committee then agreed to proceed with the scheme on the basis that, at a time when every penny was needed for the upkeep of existing hospitals, there was no longer a need for a public appeal for some £10,000 for a new hospital. The work went ahead and an upgraded Grant Ward eventually reopened in August 1906 as a gynaecological ward.

In the meantime, a meeting of the governors and supporters of the local medical charities to promote their amalgamation had been convened by the Brighton mayor and his opposite number in Hove. As a result, the Brighton, Hove and Sussex Joint Hospital Board was set up. Its objects were 'to secure economy in administration (especially with regard to the outlay on buildings) and to prevent overlapping.' The prevention of abuse by 'persons not the proper objects of charity' was another of its objectives.

However, a considerable amount of controversy and acrimonious meetings ensued. There were objections to the membership of the board, especially of the local ministers of religion who, it was said, 'had little knowledge of the intricacies of hospital management'. Also to the membership of the Members of Parliament of Brighton and Lewes, who, it was felt, had enough to do with their parliamentary work. There were fears too of interference in the management of the individual hospitals. Not surprisingly, the opposition, especially by the managing committee of the children's hospital, ensured that amalgamation never took place. The response by the management committee of the County, concerned that 'our cry for help is not lost in the din of conflicting voices' of its competitors throughout Sussex, was to appoint a collector for the country districts in 1908 and a plan to extend his work to Brighton, Hove and Preston during the following year.

More child patients in the County

Moving children to the children's hospital to make room for women in the gynaecological ward did not affect the number of children cared for at the County for very long. The number treated during 1906 fell by 43 to a total of 214. The following year, 229 children were treated and in 1908 the number increased by 54 to 283.

This was largely the result of the Education Act that had come into operation at the beginning of the year. The act introduced the medical examination of children attending elementary schools and placed another burden on the hospital's finances. 'At the lowest estimate it will be a heavy [additional burden], and an expense which, in the present state of our finances, we are ill prepared to meet.'

This may have appeared to be a somewhat gloomy forecast but, in fact, the number of young people admitted continued to rise: The total reached 320 in 1911 and by 1913 had risen to 355, many of whom would presumably have accounted for the 234 tonsils and adenoids operations performed during the year.

Nevertheless, publicity concerning the treatment of children might well have appealed to potential subscribers. This was clearly the view of the writer of an article published in 1896[1] who wrote:

> We saw several instances of the sympathy which is expended upon the little ones, by both doctors and nurses, and the photos we have been able to secure will be welcome not only to subscribers to Hospital funds, but to those unfortunate ones amongst us who may need the benefits which this institution so well affords, yet grieve at the necessity of surrendering their little ones to its care

The care children received in the hospital certainly made good newspaper copy. The *Sussex Daily News* report of Christmas festivities in 1911 told how friends of the institution 'had been specially mindful of the children, sending Christmas cards, toys, bon bons, oranges and other "goodies" to delight the suffering young folk.' After Christmas day, the report continued, the children were entertained and their huge Christmas tree stripped of its toys and distributed among them.

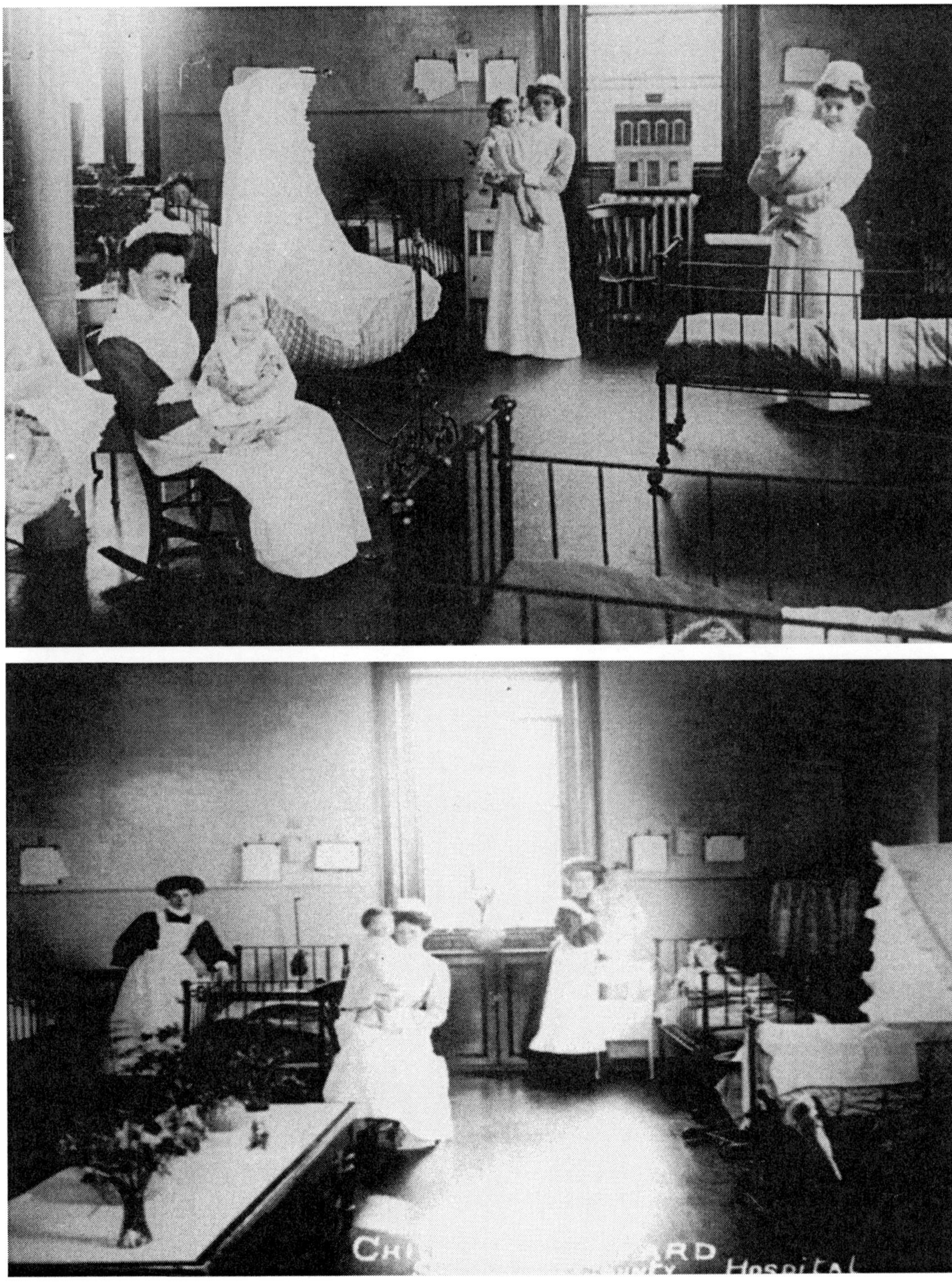

35. The Children's Ward pictured during the early part of the twentieth century.

Many of these toys would have been provided thanks to the Book, Toy and Games Fund set up when the Children's Ward was opened in 1873 for the purpose of providing gifts and recreation for children who had to spend Christmas in hospital.

Doctors in Court

It seems certain, that in the early days of the Sussex County, the physicians were the undisputed leaders medically and the hospital archives contain evidence that rivalry between them and the surgeons still existed in 1908.

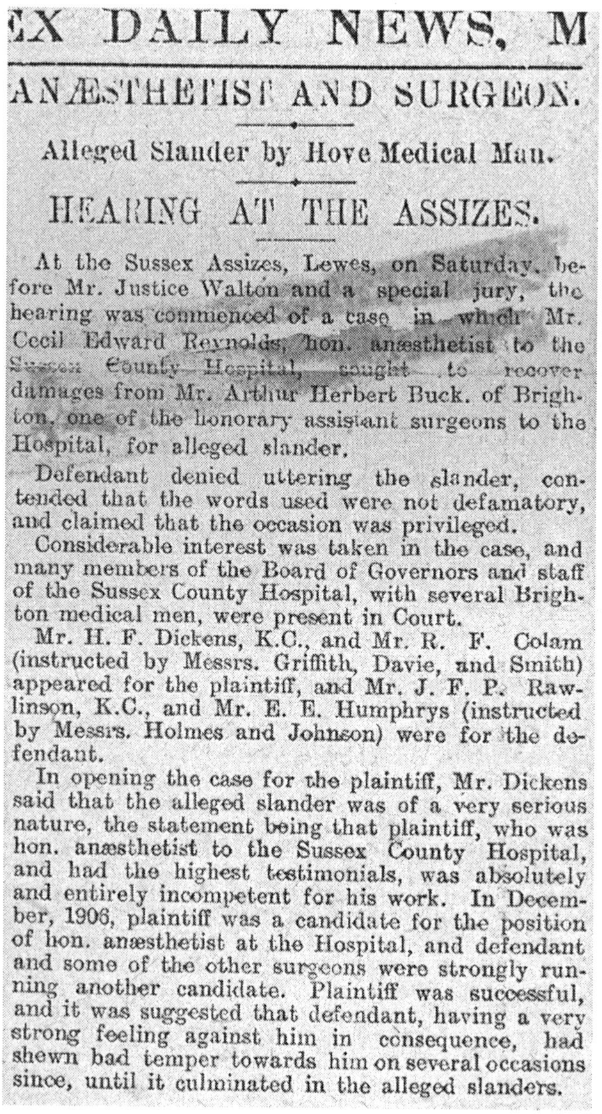

EX DAILY NEWS, M

ANÆSTHETIST AND SURGEON.

Alleged Slander by Hove Medical Man.

HEARING AT THE ASSIZES.

At the Sussex Assizes, Lewes, on Saturday, before Mr. Justice Walton and a special jury, the hearing was commenced of a case in which Mr. Cecil Edward Reynolds, hon. anæsthetist to the Sussex County Hospital, sought to recover damages from Mr. Arthur Herbert Buck, of Brighton, one of the honorary assistant surgeons to the Hospital, for alleged slander.

Defendant denied uttering the slander, contended that the words used were not defamatory, and claimed that the occasion was privileged.

Considerable interest was taken in the case, and many members of the Board of Governors and staff of the Sussex County Hospital, with several Brighton medical men, were present in Court.

Mr. H. F. Dickens, K.C., and Mr. R. F. Colam (instructed by Messrs. Griffith, Davie, and Smith) appeared for the plaintiff, and Mr. J. F. P. Rawlinson, K.C., and Mr. E. E. Humphrys (instructed by Messrs. Holmes and Johnson) were for the defendant.

In opening the case for the plaintiff, Mr. Dickens said that the alleged slander was of a very serious nature, the statement being that plaintiff, who was hon. anæsthetist to the Sussex County Hospital, and had the highest testimonials, was absolutely and entirely incompetent for his work. In December, 1906, plaintiff was a candidate for the position of hon. anæsthetist at the Hospital, and defendant and some of the other surgeons were strongly running another candidate. Plaintiff was successful, and it was suggested that defendant, having a very strong feeling against him in consequence, had shewn bad temper towards him on several occasions since, until it culminated in the alleged slanders.

36. How the Sussex Daily News reported the opening of the three day trial which drew large numbers of doctors and other hospital staff to the Assises at Lewes.

For a period of three days in the spring of that year there must have been a noticeable shortage of medical staff in the hospital. Just how many were absent from the hospital and sitting instead in a courtroom at the Sussex Assizes in Lewes where they were closely following the proceedings in the case of Reynolds v. Buck is not clear. But reports in the *Sussex Daily News* referred to the court 'being crowded with Brighton medical men and members of the Board of Governors and staff of the Sussex County Hospital.'

Ostensibly, it was a case in which Cecil Edward Reynolds, hon. anaesthetist at the hospital, sought to recover damages from Arthur Herbert Buck of Hove, one of the hospital's honorary assistant surgeons, for alleged slander. However, as the trial unfolded it became evident that underlying the alleged slander was the longstanding rivalry between physicians and surgeons.

Opening the case for the plaintiff, Mr H.F. Dickens K.C., said the alleged slander was 'of a very serious nature' that the anaesthetist, who had the highest testimonials, was absolutely and entirely incompetent for his work.

In December 1906 Reynolds was a candidate for the position of hon. anaesthetist and that Buck and some of the other surgeons were strongly running another candidate. 'Plaintiff was successful, and it was suggested that defendant, having a very strong feeling against him in consequence, had shown bad temper towards him on several occasions since, until it culminated in the alleged slander.'

During the trial there were references to operations during which there was friction between the surgeon and the anaesthetist, that on occasions Buck had halted operations because the patient appeared to need air or turned blue and was foaming at the mouth, both allegations being challenged by Reynolds who said he had given anaesthetics in nearly 400 cases at the hospital and not had friction with anybody except Buck.

A senior physician, Dr Dill, told the court that on the day of Reynolds' election, Buck had said to him that the surgical side of the medical staff were in favour of another candidate and hoped Dr Dill would not oppose the unanimous wish of the surgeons and that if the surgeons were disregarded they would not help the physicians in any scheme in which they were particularly interested afterwards.

Another physician, Dr Donald Hall, told the court that on the day of the election, Buck had said to him it was disgraceful that the physicians had set themselves against the surgeons in an election which in the main concerned the surgeons, and that it was enough to break up the entire hospital staff. Another witness told the court that during a motor car journey shared with Mr Buck, the latter had remarked: 'Those d-----d physicians have foisted an anaesthetist upon us. He is quite incompetent …'

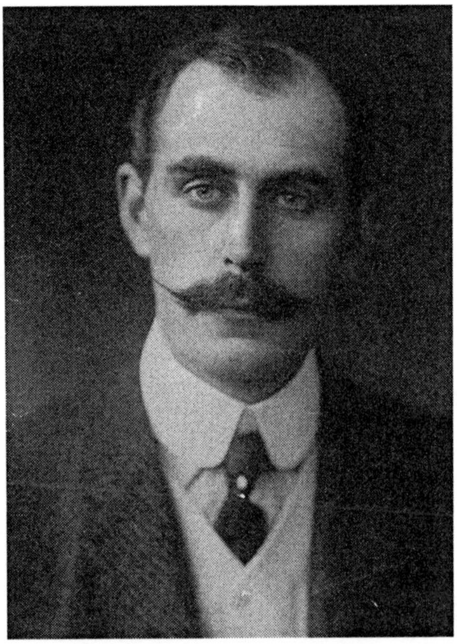

37. Surgeon Arthur Herbert Buck. His actions and statements implied that an anaesthetist was incompetent, the court was told.

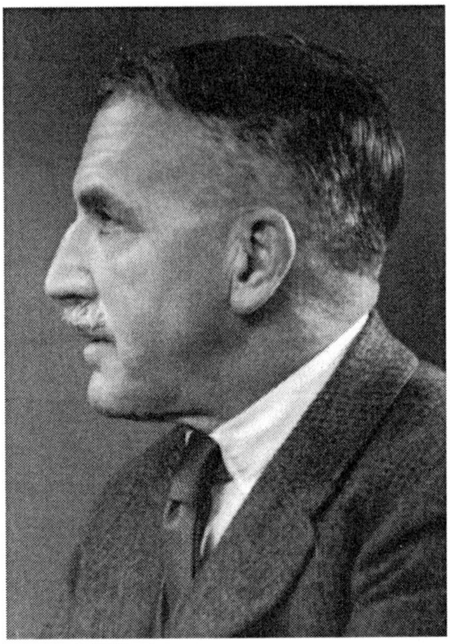

38. Dr Donald Hall, who later gave his name to a ward at the hospital, was one of the eminent physicians who gave evidence against the surgeon at Lewes Assizes.

During the three days of the trial the jury heard at length from several physicians for the plaintiff. A number of surgeons, including Nathaniel Blaker, gave evidence about the relative positions of surgeons and anaesthetists during an operation when the surgeon, they said, must be in command.

However, despite the underlying antagonisms, the trial hinged on whether Buck had used the words alleged by the plaintiff, and if they were, were they spoken maliciously?

Following a lengthy review of the evidence by the judge, the jury found in favour of Reynolds and awarded him, on the advice of the judge, a relatively modest £100 damages.

Developing the Hospital

Thanks largely to a number of generous benefactors, despite all its financial problems, the hospital continued to develop during the years leading up outbreak of war in 1914.

Work on new operating rooms recommended for improvement in 1894, was completed in 1900 costing £3,000. Expenditure of a roughly similar amount had resulted in a completely remodelled laundry. Mr C.C. Baily defrayed the entire cost of the installation of a new electric lift. The following year, the committee used a bank overdraft to provide two sanitary towers at the east end of the building costing £2,500 and a public appeal was made for funds to repay this and defray the cost of a third smaller tower that was still needed.

In 1902 Alderman Brigden paid for an ornamental porch over the main entrance. The third sanitary tower was erected in 1903, paid for by selling an investment. That year, too, Mrs Stephen Ralli made £12,000 available to found and maintain a department for clinical research and bacteriology in memory of her husband. The following year the department known as The Stephen Ralli Memorial was completed in the day room of the museum and library block built in 1870 which had been vacant since the hospital had ceased to accommodate resident medical pupils. Mrs Ralli formally opened the department in June 1905 when she invited guests and the hospital staff to tea and increased her endowment by a further sum of nearly £9,000.

A report on the work of the pathological department was included in the annual report for 1907 and covered the period from July 1904. It recorded that 2,358 examinations had taken place: 894 histological, 138 chemical, 848 bacteriological and 474 microscopical. Diphtheria bacilli were present in 11 of the 61 swabs scrubbed from the throat and nose; tubercle bacilli were present in the 356 sputum samples. The pathologist, Dr F.G. Bushnell, noted in his conclusion to his report: 'Some thirty original contributions have been made to medical literature by research workers in these laboratories since their foundation and publications are being exchanged with other leading laboratories.'

The annual report for 1908 noted that new skin and dental departments were working satisfactorily. The dental department had been established because many patients needed to have old or broken teeth extracted in order to facilitate recovery from other ailments but in sanctioning the new department it had been stressed 'that it is not intended to supply artificial teeth or permanent fillings.' In 1909, fears that houses with their 'smokey chimneys' might surround the hospital were eased by the gift of over five acres of land by Mr Charles Borradaile.

The highlight of 1911 was almost certainly that permission was given to change the name of the hospital. A letter received from the Home Office informed the committee that King George V 'had been graciously pleased to command that the Hospital shall be henceforth known as The Royal Sussex County Hospital.'

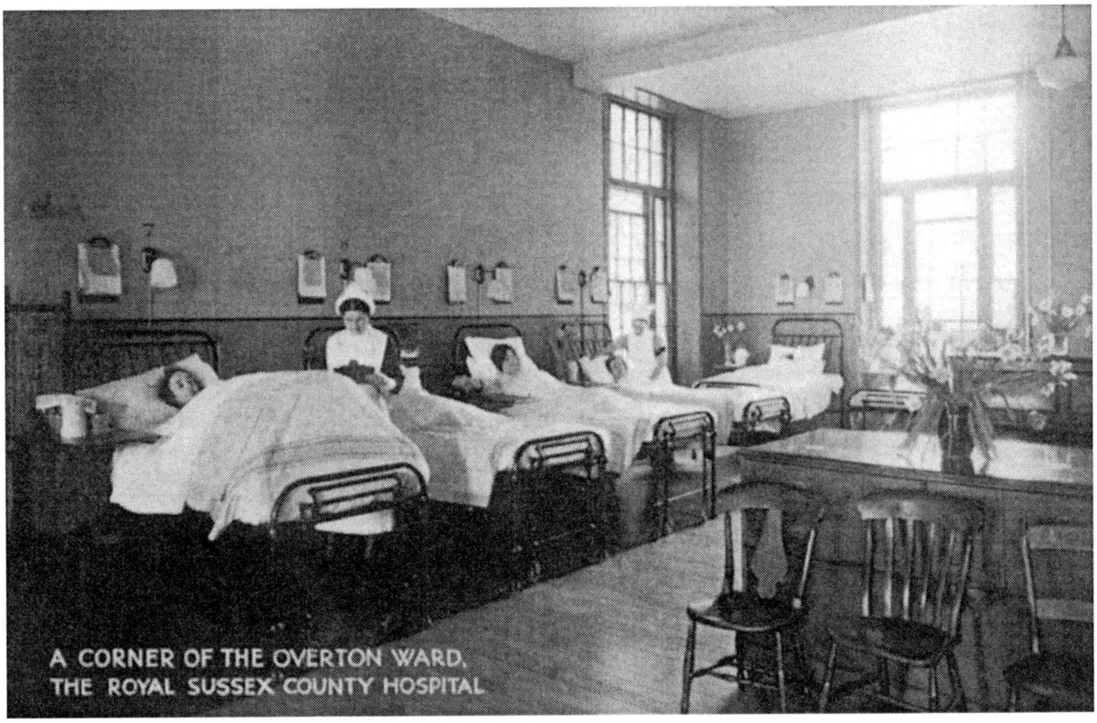

39. Overton Ward: one of a new series of ward postcards on sale in 1912. The women's ward had been named in 1893 after a benefactor, Mrs Jones of Overton House, Patcham, who had wished to remain anonymous

In 1912, balconies were erected over three wards to the west of the building thanks to the generosity of Mrs David Smith. The following year Miss Louise Sassoon met the cost of erecting balconies on the eastern side while the western balconies were extended to Vallance and Chichester wards using a balance in the Mrs David Smith Fund. Mrs Jones of Overton House anonymously defrayed the cost of an extension to a ward, which had been named Overton Ward in her honour. Finally, thanks to the generosity of General Marsland, balconies on York Ward were erected in 1914. The number of beds in the hospital had risen steadily over the years, reaching a total of 201 when the balconies were completed.

In 1913 a central heating system was installed in the hospital but no progress was made in extending the nurses' home. This had been proposed in 1909 by the eminent hospital expert Sir Henry Burdett following his an inspection of the hospital. Burdett believed the extension was essential for the comfort and discipline of staff and that it would help to control expenditure. (Sir Henry also urged the finance committee to look into its financial position and warned that it should not expect its 'unique experience ... of splendid revenue from legacies' to continue.)

There were fears that the National Insurance Act that came into force on 15th July 1912 would have an adverse effect on voluntary hospitals. The committee's belief, that although it would reduce the number of outpatients, there could be an increased demand for admission to hospital for the more serious among the insured, proved correct.

'Shall we be able to receive them all?' the committee had asked in its annual report for 1911. 'That will depend on the answer which the Public may make to our Appeals.'

One effect of providing the extra number of beds and the increasing amount of work meant that more staff were needed and the nurses' home, completed only a few years before, was no longer adequate to accommodate them and a number of nurses and domestic servants had to be accommodated in buildings outside the hospital grounds. The governors therefore issued an appeal for the enlargement of the nurses' home and the erection of a wing for the domestic staff. This had reached a total of £1,112 in 1914 when the outbreak of war meant no further developments in the hospital would be possible until hostilities had ended.

8. *Called to the Colours: The First World War, 1914 – 1918*

In some ways, Brighton appears to have been unaffected by the First World War. Britain entered the war on the 4th August and within a fortnight things had reverted to normal with hotels and shops recovering from the initial shock of the opening of hostilities.

Although the following Easter was quiet, following the first Zeppelin raid on London in May thousands escaped to the relative safety of the town, while the bombardment of Scarborough and West Hartlepool at the same time led many people to take their holidays on the South Coast instead of the north.[1] The Hon. Arthur Stanley M.P., who visited the town in September 1916 to discuss the proposal for state registration of trained nurses, apologised for some little delay in his arrival and said there were still trainloads of people coming down that day to enjoy themselves in Brighton.[2]

The hotels and boarding houses continued to receive fashionable visitors while 1917 was described as a 'year of phenomenal prosperity' with members of the royal families and aristocracy of Britain and Europe among those filling the town.[3] However, the divide between rich and poor that was a major factor in the establishment of the Sussex County Hospital was still in evidence. Towards the end of the war there were demonstrations against profiteering and inequality in food distribution culminating in a march to the Brighton Food Committee offices demanding that the wives and children of servicemen should not want for food.[4]

Because of the war, however, there had been restrictions in entertainment, streets were darkened at night, and women took over many of the jobs previously performed by the men who were away at the front. And perhaps the greatest change could be witnessed in the town's hospitals. War clouds had been threatening for some years and to prepare for the eventuality plans were being made as early as 1903, although its duration and the number of casualties that were eventually suffered were never anticipated. Thus, when the war did break out, there were only 9,000 beds in military hospitals in the UK[5] and far-reaching emergency arrangements had to be made. Brighton General Hospital became known as the Kitchener Hospital providing beds for Indian wounded while the Royal Pavilion and York Place School also functioned as Indian military hospitals.[6] Other schools and even private houses were pressed into military service while the boys' grammar school in Dyke Road was transformed into the 2nd Eastern General Hospital

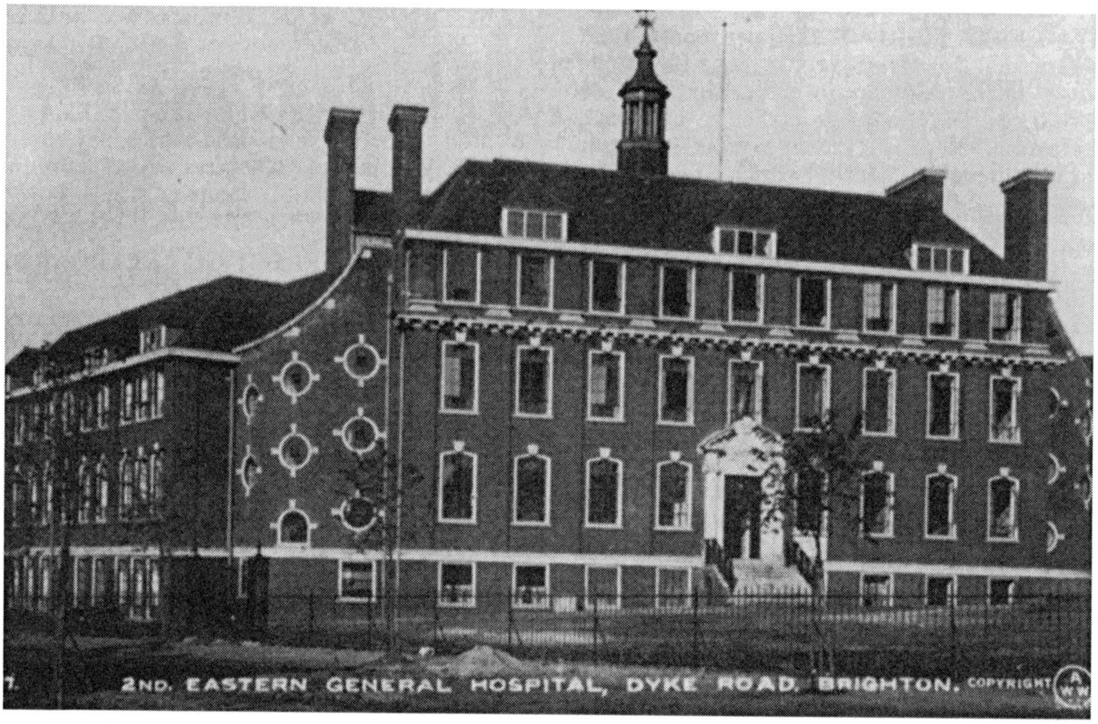

40. A postcard showing the 2nd Eastern General Hospital in Dyke Road, staffed largely by doctors and nurses from the Royal Sussex County Hospital. The postmark was dated 1916.

staffed, largely, by physicians, surgeons, sisters and nurses from the County Hospital.

The Staff

Not surprisingly, the impact upon the Royal Sussex County Hospital was immediate. Six days after the outbreak of war, a letter from the hospital chairman was published in the *Brighton Herald* and the *Sussex Daily News*. Appealing to members of the medical profession to send in only serious cases, he said the board had entered into an agreement several years before to supply a contingent of nurses in the event of war. Several surgeons had already been called to the colours, he added, while many of the honorary staff would be required for the Territorial Medical Service immediately and some wards had been closed temporarily.

The annual report for 1914 was later to record:

> The Royal Sussex County Hospital was among the first to respond to the appeal of the War Office in the matter of Military Nursing, and the Territorial Nursing Association of the South-Eastern District was the first in the Kingdom to have its staff complete. A large number of the Nurses of the Hospital, past and present,

were enrolled on the books of that Association, while many others gave their names for service abroad. All these were mobilized after the outbreak of hostilities, and the Hospital has provided for the service of the Country in its hour of need no less than sixty-five highly qualified certificated nurses, [some] of whom are acting as Matrons and nineteen as Sisters in Military Hospitals.

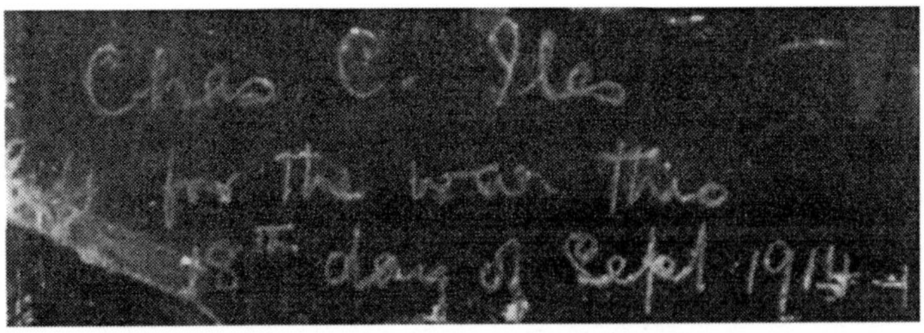

41. The words: 'Chas. C. Iles left for the war this 18th day of September 1914' were inscribed on a glass panel in the Pathology department Dr Iles was killed in action shortly afterwards. Pathology manager Dr Doug Flowers took this photograph in 1993.

The report also referred to others who had been called up: the secretary, Reginald Jay, Dr Gerald Martin, the house physician, who held a commission in the Naval Medical Service and had survived the sinking of H.M.S. Cress, and the resident pathologist, Dr C.C. Iles, who had been killed in France within a few days of joining the forces. In 1915, it was reported that nearly 80 nurses holding the certificate of the Sussex County Training School were or had been doing military nursing and 32 of the private nurses were working in military hospitals or on hospital ships.

According to the report for 1916:

> It is with pride that the Board note the record of Royal Sussex County Hospital Nurses in the Great War, 134 members of staff have joined the Naval, Military, Territorial and Red Cross Services. On these, five have been mentioned in Despatches, and six have been awarded the Decoration of the Royal Red Cross, two of the First Class and four of the Second Class. Several have been appointed Acting Matrons, while many who joined as Nurses have been promoted to Sisters' posts.

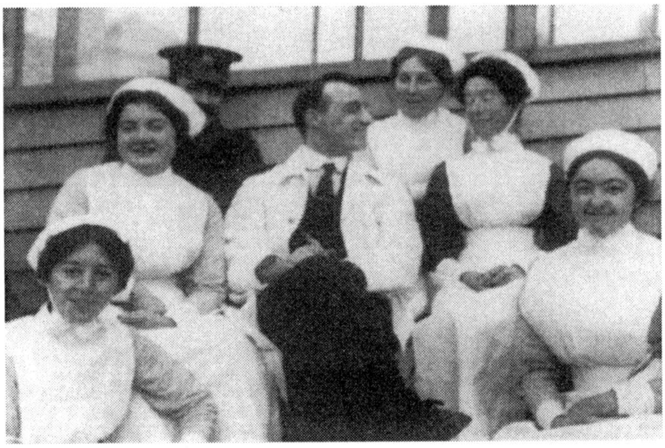

42. In the early days of the war many French and Belgian refugees who had lost their homes during the German advance arrived in Brighton. Among them was a young French doctor, J.D.Deweer, living in Belgium whose nationality prevented him from enlisting in the army. Hearing there was a desperate shortage of doctors in England, he came to Brighton and secured a post as assistant house surgeon at the Royal Sussex County Hospital where he worked from 1914-16. He is seen here with some of the hospital nurses outside the 'chicken run', the covered link corridor leading to the nurses' home.

To help fill the gaps left by these nurses, several others who had left returned to work at the hospital, which was struggling to operate with only a minimal number of staff. For this reason, appeals for exemption from military service were made in some cases. In 1916, for example, an appeal was made for continued exemption of the chief pharmacist, a stoker/sterilising porter aged 28, and a stoker and kitchen porter aged 31. When it was suggested that a man over military age could replace the latter, the hospital's acting secretary, Mr Lionel King, pointed out that several men tried from the labour exchange had proved to be unsatisfactory and that the two porters were also engaged in fire brigade work. However, while a six month conditional exemption was granted to the chief pharmacist and the stoker and sterilising porter, the hospital was given just a month to make arrangements to replace the other man.

The actual acting secretary, Mr Lancaster-Gaye, had been acting as secretary-in-charge during the previous couple of years. A report in the *Sussex Daily News* on the 1st March 1916 noted that on that occasion his appeal for exemption from military service, made because of 'the intricate character of [his] work … that took years to grasp' which involved many military patients, was granted for one month. In view of his delicate health, the board had hoped to retain his services throughout the war. However, in the autumn of 1917, his exemption was finally cancelled and he too was called to the colours.

The report for that year also noted:

> The honours gained by members of the nursing staff engaged in Naval, Military and Red Cross work have been greatly increased. One Nurse has received the Military Medal for gallantry under fire, three have been mentioned in Despatches, one of them for the second time, while no less than seventeen have received the Decoration of the Royal Red Cross, bringing the list for that distinction up to twenty-three, of which four are of First Class. A former Assistant Matron, whose administrative ability is remembered with gratitude by the Board of Management, has also been made an Officer of the British Empire.

During the 1918 summer offensive, three more of the honorary surgeons and physicians were sent abroad and by the time the Armistice was signed in November, 26 Royal Red Cross Decorations had been awarded to the hospital's nurses, four of them First Class.

Wounded Soldiers

Preparations for receiving sick and wounded soldiers from overseas were quickly put in hand and 100 beds were made available to the War Office well before any of the town's temporary hospitals were equipped. However, it was not until September that the first batch of 300 men arrived who were taken to the 2nd Eastern General Hospital in Dyke Road. According to Musgrave: 'Those who saw them arrive were shocked by the terrible wounds caused by modern shells, and by the fact that many of the victims were hardly more than boys.'[7]

The Sussex County received its first detail of 59 wounded soldiers on the night of Thursday the 15th October 1914 and a special Committee on Wounded Soldiers was set up. It met for the first time the following Tuesday, when it was reported that all their kit had been disinfected and labelled and that a tailor was at work repairing the uniforms.

The soldiers' immediate needs were met through the generosity of the mayoress of Brighton and others but the committee decided that a public appeal was necessary for food and extra comforts, in particular:

> Rabbits and game, eggs and bananas;
> Games: easy puzzles, draughts, dominoes
> Tooth powder, hairbrushes;
> Shag in half ounce or one ounce packets, pipes, Woodbine cigarettes;
> Writing paper, stamped envelopes;
> Handkerchiefs.

The appeal sent to local newspapers the following day also added:

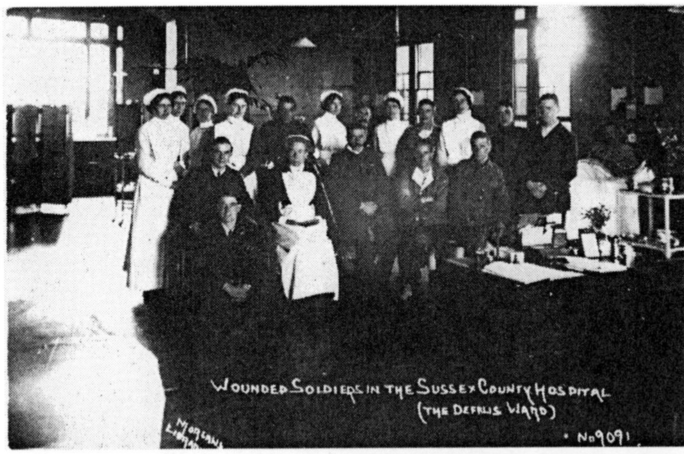

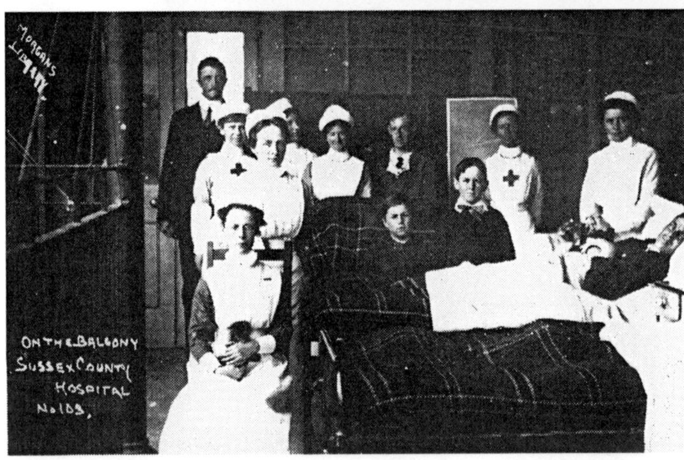

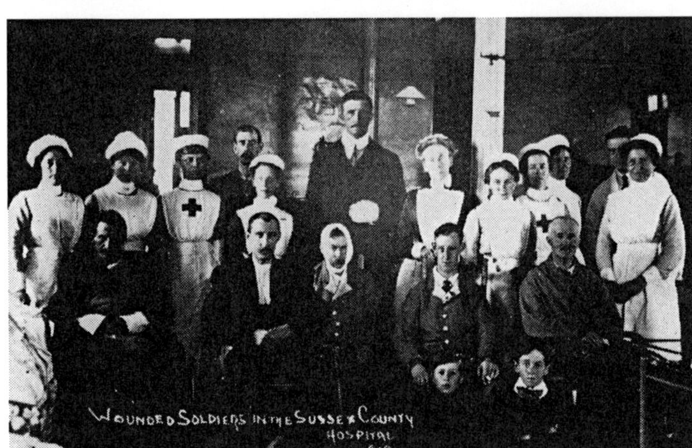

43. Three examples of a series of postcards that were produced during the First World War showing wounded soldiers and members of the medical and nursing staff at the hospital.

> Though most of the cases received were serious ones, they are making good progress, and soon some of them we hope, will be able to go out for motor drives, but the weather is growing colder, and they cannot be sent out without proper clothing, and we shall therefore be grateful if readers having them spare will send us some warm overcoats, and others will supply is with money to purchase some. Several contributions in money have already been received.

At a later meeting of the committee, it was reported that in December some of the soldiers had enjoyed visits to the Grand Theatre and that they had enjoyed a 'huge dinner' that included pheasants from Sandringham that had been distributed among the hospitals.

The first public appeal was successful but a year later a second appeal was made for renewed support. This called for stamped envelopes, which were 'in much demand, while game, rabbits, fruit, sweets and jam and cakes etc provide a much appreciated change in diet.' Contributions of money were also welcomed. Another appeal appeared in the *Brighton Herald* in December:

> Sir, At the opening of the pheasant season you were good enough to insert a letter from me asking for game, rabbits etc for the wounded in this hospital, and the response made to that appeal has afforded from time to time a pleasant variety to the diet of the Soldiers.
>
> We are now approaching the holiday season, and much game will be shot this week and next, so I again venture to ask those who are having shoots not to forget the sick and wounded in this hospital.
>
> Pheasants and rabbits make splendid Christmas fare, and, with nearly four hundred people to provide for, gifts of the kind are of great financial assistance as well in these days of war prices.

Interestingly, unlike the original appeal, there was no reference to the need for tobacco or cigarettes. Perhaps it was a coincidence that in May Mr Ball Dodson, chairman of the Board of Management, wrote to the Wounded Soldiers committee suggesting that wounded soldiers were allowed to smoke too much. Whether this was on the grounds of cost

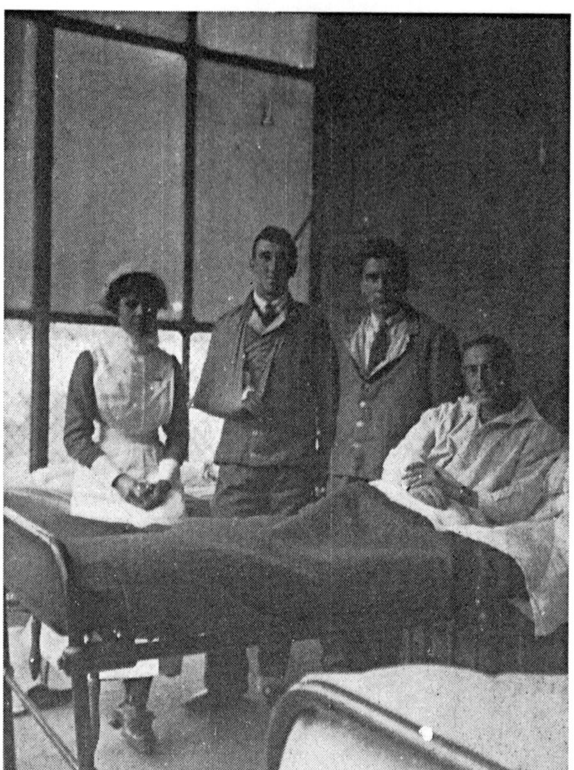

44. Two of the wounded soldiers pictured on this corner of one of the balconies wearing the hospital blues uniform that were to be seen around Brighton during the First World War.

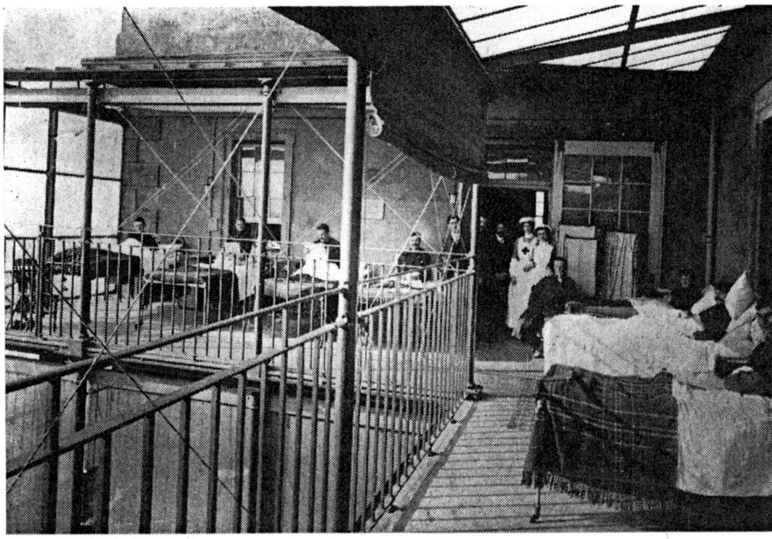
45. Wounded soldiers in beds arranged round one of the hospital balconies.

or their health is not clear, although it was decided that the honorary surgeons should be consulted on the matter. However a minute of a meeting later in the year would suggest that cost was the real concern, for this noted that although cigarettes were given to the soldiers on admission, they were to pay for future cigarettes from their pay book accounts. (A year later, however, it was reported to the committee that the matron had been authorised to purchase 20 cigarettes a week for soldiers who were unable to go for walks.)

The annual report for 1915 noted that ten more military beds had been added and there were 71 wounded soldiers on the wards at the end of December. Following the admission of 191 military cases the previous year, 642 more were admitted during 1915, eleven of which were military nurses 'who had broken down in their work' while the report for 1919 reported that by the end of the war, a total of 3,328 members of the British Expeditionary Force had passed through the wards.

Civilian Patients – and the Role of Women

While soldiers were allowed to smoke in the hospital, this was not always allowed in the case of civilian patients. There had been a relaxation of the rules and regulations concerning patients since the hospital opened in 1828 and by 1914 this had extended to smoking. Smoking was then allowed in the wards or on the balconies with the permission of the sister, but then only between four and six in the afternoon. Smoking at other times was allowed in the grounds.

By 1914 there was no longer a requirement to read the rules to patients regarding their behaviour every Friday morning in every ward. They were, however, expected to behave with 'propriety and civility' at all times and to 'refrain from any undue familiarity with the Nursing Staff and Servants.'

They were still not allowed to bring cards and dice into hospital although the rules regarding religious observation now required only attendance at chapel service on Sundays 'when able'. Violation of the hospital rules still rendered patients liable to expulsion and readmission was possible only with special permission of the board of management.

While life on the wards was therefore somewhat easier by 1914, the possibility of admission became somewhat harder during the war years. During 1915 it was reported that the majority of beds were filled with the very old and the very ill who recovered only slowly: as a result patients were staying in hospital longer and there were serious problems with the waiting list. The following year it was reported that 'the demands of all male civilians were met' although these must have been lessened to a large extent because vast numbers of men were now away on military service.

For women, however, it was a different matter, and Miss Blanche Fair wrote to Mr Ball Dodson asking that the thirteen women's beds 'rightly taken over for the treatment of wounded soldiers' should revert to their original use 'as a great deal of suffering was being caused by the shortage [of women's beds] and the women's waiting list was very long'.

With the demand for male beds down, the committee was able to respond by transferring some male beds to female. Things later improved, however, and, presenting the report for 1917, Mr Ball Dodson was able to announce, that with practically all men of military age in the army, 'the complete obliteration of the waiting list for civilians'.

Miss Fair's campaign for women patients was accompanied by a call for a change in the management of the hospital. She wrote:

> Women, although they provide a great part of the funds of the hospital, and are at least as generous as men in post-mortem gifts, are without any voice in the management of this institution, which concerns their welfare so closely. The whole governing body is male and even when suggestions are put forward for change in administration or information sought by a woman, a meeting composed entirely of men thinks it compatible of right to ignore such a communication. Should a man be treated in the same way there is ample opportunity for him to seek a remedy.

A special general court was called to discuss the question of the ineligibility of women to sit on the Board of Management. During a legnthy debate, the view that women have certain special qualities' for the work of hospital managememt prevailed. The statutes were amended deleting the word 'male' and, according to the 1917 annual report, 'the disabilities of women were removed, and subsequently four were co-opted as members of the board.'

War and Medical Progress

Throughout recent history, developments in medicine have followed as a result of wartime experiences, and one example of this during the Great War is evidenced by events at the Royal Sussex County Hospital.

The treatment of wounds brought about developments in the electrotherapeutic and massage departments and the experience gained was applied in general orthopaedic practice. Receipts from a legacy made it possible to provide and equip a new X-ray treatment room while another room was added to the massage department and during 1918, it was reported, both rooms were 'taxed to their full capacity'.

The war also contributed to a development at the hospital of a rather different kind. The growing prevalence of venereal disease was seen as a threat to both the military and civilians and in 1914 a Royal Commission was appointed which was expected to issue a report in 1916. In fact, some 40,000 military cases were treated in Britain and France between 1914 and 1918. The Royal Commission duly reported in 1916 when it was estimated that ten per cent of the population in large cities were infected with acquired or congenital syphilis and considerably more with gonorrhea.

Free diagnosis and treatment was recommended in the report, as well as instruction of medical students and the education of special groups of the general public. Public Health (Venereal Diseases) Regulations gave immediate effect to some of the recommendations, including a requirement for county and county borough councils to establish services for free diagnosis and treatment, with 75 per cent of the cost being paid for by central government.

There was a problem with the proposed provision of these services at the County Hospital with its remit to provide treatment for the necessitous poor. The chairman dealt with this saying that as they wanted to stamp out the disease, for the time being they would not ask if the person was poor. Moreover, he added, one reason the scheme should be taken up by general hospitals was that in a very large number of cases the disease was contracted quite innocently, therefor 'they must learn to look upon the matter in a more generous and charitable way than hitherto.'

The hospital then entered into contracts with the corporation and both county councils and a special clinic was opened in the outpatients department on 31st July 1917. A progress report on the work of the clinic during its first eight months revealed that it had made a considerable impact on the outpatients' department. Several patients attended on the opening day and the number increased week by week.

> Up to the 1st of May 1918 no less than 375 cases had been treated, 1164 intravenous injections given, 357 blood extractions for Wasserman tests made, all without a single mishap, thanks to the skill and care with which the Medical Officer, Mr Lawson, has conducted the Clinic loyally supported by other members of the Staff.

The report made it clear that a fourth clinic was desirable immediately but that enlarged facilities would be needed at some future date. In 1918 plans were drawn up to provide these in a building behind the department, although no further progress would be made until after the end of the war.

The Rising Cost of the War

The problem of financing the work of the hospital again came to the fore in 1915. 'Only by the curtailment of many legitimate items of expenditure in maintenance and repairs has total expenditure been kept within reasonable limits' it was noted in the annual report. One reason for this was a great increase in the cost of living: meats, groceries, provisions and coals, the report pointed out, had 'risen enormously in price'.

Even more serious, it seems, were the rises in the 'costs of those special supplies which are the very essence of hospital treatment' caused by the demands of the military hospitals and by the monopoly Germany had secured in many drugs.

The following year the financial position was giving the board 'cause for the gravest anxiety'. Prices had risen by 87 per cent since July 1914 and were still rising. Despite postponing practically all work on renewals and on the upkeep of the building and exercising strict economies in every department, the year ended with a deficiency of £2,703 6s 4d. Moreover, this was after spending every penny of the £5,000 received in legacies during the year and selling £1,766 of shares held by the hospital. 'A veritable wartime Budget for 1917,' was predicted.

Legacies received in 1917 amounted to only £2,356 and although there had been a generous response following the issue of the previous year's annual report, the financial position continued to give serious concern. Not surprisingly, an emergency appeal for £10,000 for necessaries was made to the general public towards the end of 1917.

There was strong support for the appeal from the hospital's senior physicians and surgeons. In a letter published in the *Sussex Daily News* they pointed out:

> The institution of many small medical charities, while diverting money from the Royal Sussex County Hospital, has not lightened its labours, as the more serious, and therefore more costly, cases of illness continued to be sent there for treatment, and

> for some years before the war the work was only made possible by the receipt of several generous legacies …In our opinion an enforced limitation of the activities of the Royal Sussex County Hospital, especially at this crisis of our affairs, would be a calamity to the country.[8]

Fortunately, the appeal was successful and by the end of 1918 £10,554 10s 10d had been received and expenses amounted to only £300 as no commissions had been made. The 1917 deficit was wiped out and 1918 ended free of debt. However, this was not achieved as the result of the successful emergency appeal alone. The cost of hospital commodities had continued to rise and with coal and milk now three times their pre-war price, for example, the year might well have ended in deficit but for what the board described as 'exceptional receipts falling within the year.' Contributing to these were the continuing successful Pound Days and efforts of the ladies of the Linen, Blanket and Work Guild.

In 1917, the guild had supplied 1,278 yards of sheeting and all the requirements such as linen and blankets for all the hospital, including the wards, staff and household and the convalescent home, according to Miss Fair in a letter to the *Sussex Daily News*.[9] Two years earlier, according to another report in the same paper, members had also donated the doctors' and nurses' operating caps as well as patients' garments and towels used in the operating theatre.[10]

One fundraising event not specifically mentioned by the board was nevertheless of special interest. A charity concert at the Brighton Hippodrome in 1918 raised £1,400 that was divided equally between the Music Hall Artiste's Benevolent Institution and the Royal Sussex County Hospital.[11] The manager of the Hippodrome, Mr W.H.Boardman, and Mr Harry Preston, owner of the Royal York Hotel, organised the concert. Mr Preston also made a personal donation of £30, a relatively modest one in the light of what he was eventually to contribute to the hospital, particularly in the gravest financial crisis that it was ever to face in the immediate post-war years.

9. An Uneasy Peace, 1919 - 1929

The end of the war did not mean life returned to normal during the next decade. The years were marked at times by industrial unrest, an outbreak of deadly influenza and rising inflation. Each, in different ways, impacted on the hospital.

Brighton was greatly affected by the general strike in 1926 when there were no trains, buses or newspapers, and to a lesser extent by a strike by railwaymen in 1919, which led to accusations of unfair treatment of local strikers. According to the *Brighton Herald*[1] many railwaymen were in fact treated at the hospital and the rumour arose because a doctor had refused treatment in Outpatients to the wife of a striker. Although the reason for refusal was not known, she apparently suffered from a only a trifling disability, a skin infection, the paper explained. The main impact of the strike at the hospital, however, according to the *Herald,* was on the relatives who were prevented from coming to see sick, and possibly dying, friends on visiting day. It seems likely that this was also the situation during the general strike when whole-time volunteers ensured that there was no interruption to the hospital's activities and the main impact appears to have been on its finances. The prolonged stoppage of work in the coalfields, for example, raised expenditure on fuel by nearly a thousand pounds.

The hospital also escaped the worst effects of the Spanish flu pandemic in 1918 and 1919, but it was not so fortunate in the influenza epidemic of 1922. That outbreak was so severe that the *London Evening News* reported on the 3rd January that the hospital had been closed to all but urgent cases, one third of the nursing staff being affected. The *Sussex Daily News* reported on the 14th January that 62 patients and staff were affected: two resident medical officers, five sisters, a large percentage of the nurses, 29 in all, seven maids and two porters had been 'stricken since Christmas'. The result, according to the annual report for 1922, was that for some months two of the largest wards were closed because of the lack of nurses. In a way, this was a foretaste of what was to come: bed closures were again to hit the headlines later in the year when the critical condition of the hospital's finances became the subject of newspaper reports, nationally as well as locally.

However, it was not all gloom in the months leading up to the 1922 crisis. In April 1919, the building ceased to be a military hospital. All members of the medical and surgical staff who had been called up were demobilised; so too were the majority of the nursing staff who had volunteered for war service. Finance was a problem because of the enhanced cost of maintaining the hospital, largely the result of depreciation and the reduced purchasing power of money. Despite the generosity of the public there was 'a heavy debt on the year's working' but this 'black cloud' hanging over the hospital was dispersed the following year, thanks largely to generous public support.

On the 1st January 1921, following the lead set by London voluntary hospitals, patients were asked to contribute towards the cost of their maintenance 'according to their means' and in their report for the year the board acknowledged the 'ready and willing spirit' by the 53 per cent of patients who had contributed. The total received from them together with the small payments made by outpatients was well over £4,000.

During the early part of the 1920s, the number of those awaiting admission grew to 'an abnormally high figure'. A number of convalescing patients were sent to the Sunshine Home at Hurstpierpoint and extra beds were erected in the wards. Extra beds, however, meant extra nurses and thanks to a large legacy from Miss A.E. Walker, a start was made on the addition to the nurses' home, which had been delayed by the outbreak of war in 1914. Regarded by the committee in the 1921 annual report as 'the most important event of the past twelve months', the addition was completed and formally opened by Her Royal Highness the Princess Mary in November.

In his address, the president told the Princess that the extra accommodation comprised 45 bedrooms, a large sitting room for sisters, a large sitting room and writing room for nurses, a small kitchen and box room. 'We trust that the building will commend itself to your Royal Highness as suitable, sufficient and satisfactory,' he concluded.

Other developments in the aftermath of the war included the provision of additional facilities for massage and electric treatment, and with somewhat less fanfare, the building of a 'temporary' wooden building behind the outpatient department to cope with the increasing demand for the treatment of venereal diseases.

A Great Blow to the Sussex Poor

The desperate financial situation faced by the hospital in 1922 dominated the annual report and the columns of the local press and was even featured in many national newspapers. 'Critical Condition of the Royal Sussex County Hospital. An Appeal to Readers of the *Sportsman*' were the headlines of an advertisement that was published in August. The hospital's press cuttings

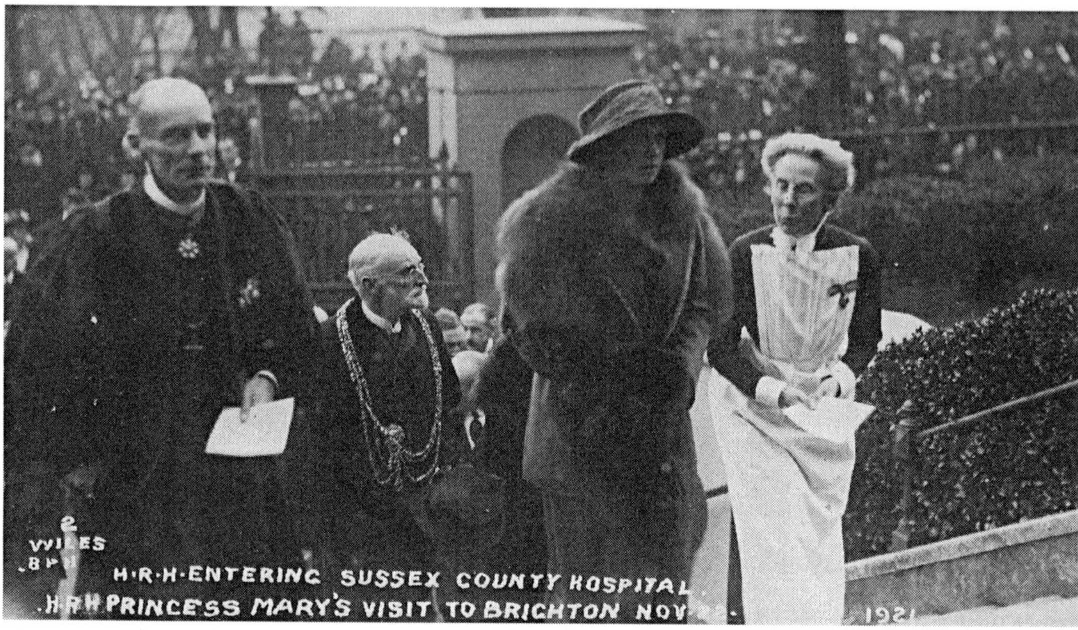
H·R·H·ENTERING SUSSEX COUNTY HOSPITAL
H.R.H. PRINCESS MARY'S VISIT TO BRIGHTON NOV
1921

46. The Matron, Miss Katherine Scott, with Princess Mary entering the hospital when she visited Brighton to open the additions to the nurses' home in November 1921.

include a similar appeal to readers not only of Sussex newspapers but also to readers of the *Daily Express,* while reports on the hospital's plight also appeared in the pages of the *Daily Mail* and the *Daily Chronicle.*

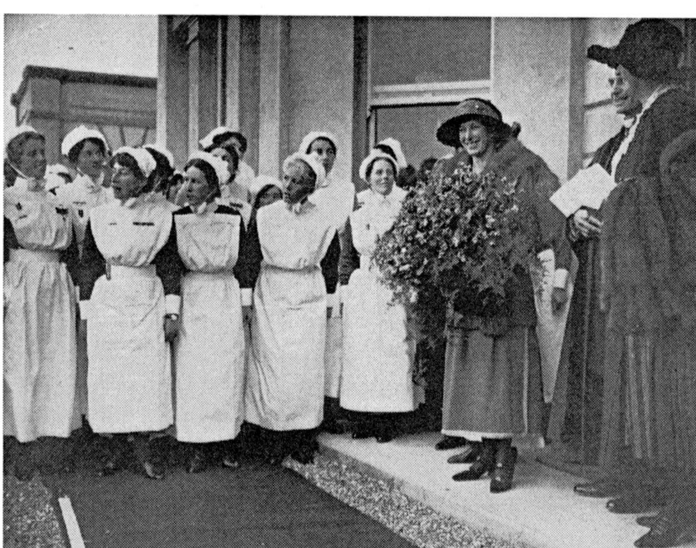

47. *Princess Mary pictured outside the nurses' home at the end of her visit during which she also presented badges to 25 nurses who since the war had joined the Territorial Army Nursing Service of the 2nd Eastern General Hospital.*

The annual report for 1921 had referred to financial anxieties but there were high hopes that a generous response to an appeal for 250,000 half crowns in the autumn (at eight to the pound this would have raised over £30,000) would see the hospital through. The report for 1922, however, conceded that the general tone of the previous year's report was 'undoubtedly sanguine'. The first three months of 1922 showed that the target would not be realised and in March, when the 1921 report was made public, a leaflet was enclosed

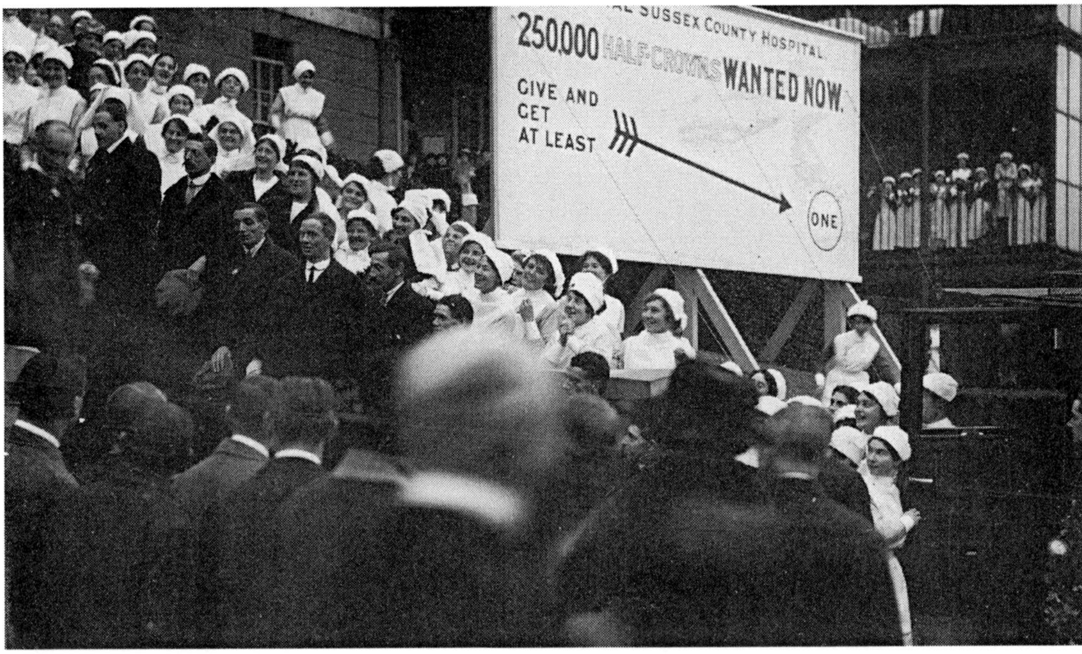

48. Faced with a financial crisis, a Half Crown Appeal was launched in 1921 hoping to raise £33,000. This photo was probably taken before the opening of the nurses' home extensions in November 1921.

with each copy containing the words 'in all the 96 years of its history, [the hospital's] financial state has never been so serious as it is today.' A further public appeal was made in May but the half yearly accounts revealed a situation so serious that a further appeal was made in the summer. This stated that the general funds were completely exhausted and that 'the Board have two courses open to them at this critical juncture, the one to carry on and incur further debts, the other to close down beds and restrict work generally.'

A letter in the *Brighton Herald*[2] signed by the president and chairman made it clear they would not be justified in incurring further debt and beds would have to be closed unless they were provided with the means to carry on.

> Expenses are still high and fresh sources of revenue will have to be developed.
> Meanwhile the hospital cannot wait: help is urgently needed and needed now.
> You are earnestly begged to assist.
> The bank account is overdrawn £2,000.
> There are bills due: last month still unpaid in the amount of £3,500.
> To get square at the end of the year there is needed £10,000.
> Total sum required, £13,500.

The response, according to the annual report, 'was practically nil'. A special general court was ordered on the 7th September and the board was directed to close all but 100 beds 'until such time as they saw their way to re-opening the Wards with a fair prospect of fully supporting them.' The proposal to close the beds was moved by the chairman of the honorary staff. He said:

> There was nothing the staff would regret more than the curtailment of their hospital work, and it must be realised that the closing of beds would mean a great hardship especially in the coming winter, to the poor of Brighton and the neighbourhood … [but] the deficit was so enormous that nothing they could think of would obviate the measures they now suggested.[3]

If the public had failed to react in response to earlier appeals, this was not the case when the press reported the decision to close half the hospital's beds. Not surprisingly perhaps, most of their subsequent anger was directed at the way the hospital was managed by what one newspaper described as 'the somewhat aristocratic rule we have known in the past,'[4] while a detailed criticism of the committee occupied a column in another edition of the *Sussex Daily News*.[5]

The criticisms of what it called 'a panic decision' included failure to set aside money from the good years to form a nest egg for the lean as some other institutions had done; a claim that they had not taken advantage of the sum of £275,000 that was available for distribution to voluntary hospitals; the establishment of new departments, such as throat and ear, dental, eye and children, which led to extra expense although other hospitals in the town already provided these facilities; the unnecessary expense of employing four resident medical officers; and the payment of a salaries to probationer nurses.

In conclusion, a public meeting was called for with the object of setting up a committee of inquiry. Whether or not these criticisms were justified, they seemed to catch the prevailing mood that all was not well with the management of the hospital, that businessmen should be brought in to sort things out and that a committee of inquiry should be set up.

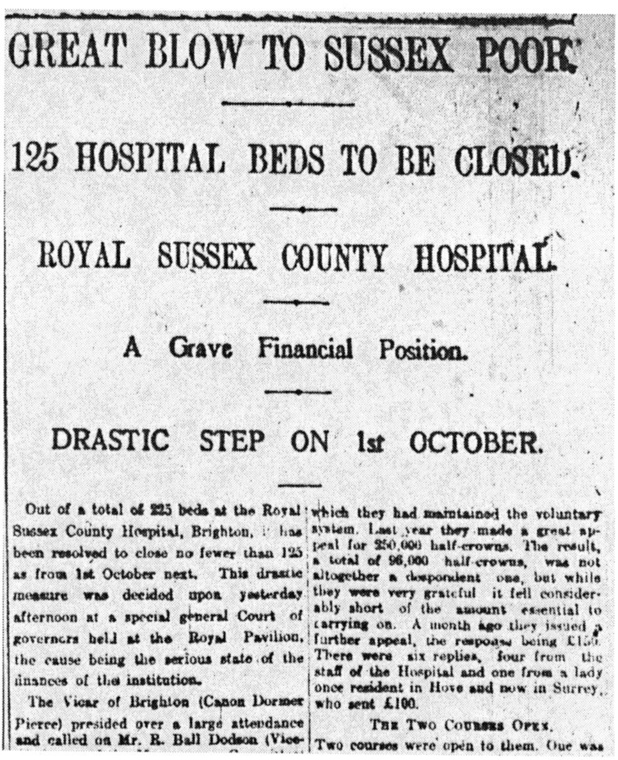

GREAT BLOW TO SUSSEX POOR.

125 HOSPITAL BEDS TO BE CLOSED.

ROYAL SUSSEX COUNTY HOSPITAL.

A Grave Financial Position.

DRASTIC STEP ON 1st OCTOBER.

Out of a total of 225 beds at the Royal Sussex County Hospital, Brighton, it has been resolved to close no fewer than 125 as from 1st October next. This drastic measure was decided upon yesterday afternoon at a special general Court of governors held at the Royal Pavilion, the cause being the serious state of the finances of the institution.

The Vicar of Brighton (Canon Dormer Pierce) presided over a large attendance and called on Mr. R. Ball Dodson (Vice-

which they had maintained the voluntary system. Last year they made a great appeal for 250,000 half-crowns. The result, a total of 96,000 half-crowns, was not altogether a despondent one, but while they were very grateful it fell considerably short of the amount essential to carrying on. A month ago they issued a further appeal, the response being £150. There were six replies, four from the staff of the Hospital and one from a lady once resident in Hove and now in Surrey, who sent £100.

THE TWO COURSES OPEN.

Two courses were open to them. One was

49. How on the 8th September 1922 the Sussex Daily News reported the decision to close 125 beds at the hospital.

The crisis persuaded the chairman of the management board, Mr Ball Dodson, to postpone a visit to America 'in order to be at the helm,' reported the *Sussex Daily News,* which had secured an interview with him.[6] Ball Dodson responded to a number of the criticisms; the new departments, he said, were intended for the patients already admitted primarily for other illnesses; the children's ward was being closed, but without it nurses would be unable to complete their training; paying probationers, as other hospitals did, had become necessary because the small professional class who provided most of the nurses had been hardest hit by the war and could no longer afford to maintain their daughters while they were training. As for the proposed committee of inquiry, he believed it was urgent action that was necessary; there was no time to wait for a committee to deliberate and report.

The original newspaper criticism, however, included something much more fundamental. It was the voluntary system of hospital management, it maintained, that was on trial.

> The older constituency, which has hitherto largely provided the funds, has no longer in its power to continue the help it has rendered in past years, because of altered circumstances; and the new holders of wealth have not yet fully realised their responsibilities to lend their help. But the whole community is in one mind of recognising the advantages of that system, which brings a humane sympathy to bear upon the sufferers who cannot help themselves; provides an outlet for Christian charity; and breeds so much nobler a spirit than could by any possible stretch of imagination be expected in an institution governed by officialdom, which is the only alternative.

What the hospital's records do not make clear, but which the newspaper's readers will have been aware of, is that since the war the question of the way in which the country's hospitals should be organised and administered was the subject of impassioned debate. The war had revealed (as the Second War World War was again to do) that the eighteen and nineteenth century hospital system, comprised principally of poor law hospitals on the one hand and voluntary hospitals on the other, was no longer appropriate in the new century. 'The case for an integrated approach to the nation's health which had been canvassed by a minority of "experts" before the war became widely accepted in the national crisis.'[7]

The Ministry of Health was established and various suggestions were put forward proceeding from there. The Labour Party, for example, envisaged the establishment under the Ministry of a National Health Service under democratic control centrally and locally, although, recognising the fears of the medical profession regarding the establishment of a whole-time state salaried medical service, offered an olive branch in the form other possibilities.

However, there were also others who wanted to learn the lessons of the war, principally Dr Bernard Dawson, a major general in the army, who was convinced there must be some form of state aid and central control.[8] Sir Bernard Dawson became chairman of the Council on Medical and Administrative Services established under the Act which had set up the Ministry of Health. He gave his name to the report in 1920 which made what were considered revolutionary proposals for the way medical services should be provided. This led, however, only to the setting up of a committee to consider the financial problems of voluntary hospitals in the realisation that voluntary contributions could no longer be their principal source of income and that a system of patients' payments had to be extended or substantial aid had to come from central or local government.[9]

This, then, explains much of what lay behind the situation in Brighton (and elsewhere) in 1922. The voluntary hospitals did not favour state control: they firmly believed the voluntary system was the right one. Moreover, despite their precarious financial position, some were not prepared to accept grants-in-aid from public authorities. It was to this attitude that the *Sussex Daily News* referred in its criticisms: the board's failure to take advantage of a possible government grant was rumoured to have been the reason for the resignation of the chairman of the management committee who preceded Mr Ball Dodson.[10]

Replying to the suggested need for a committee of inquiry and for seeking the advice of businessmen, Mr Ball Dodson asserted that running a hospital was not something for 'benevolent amateurs'[11] and announced that the hospital would hold its own commission of inquiry. An open meeting was called at the Royal Pavilion on the 16th October. A specially invited guest, the superintendent and secretary of Manchester Royal Infirmary, spoke about 'The Post-War Problems of County Hospitals.'[12] He told the meeting that he was impressed with the hospital, that it was efficiently run and that its great weakness was the lack of dependable income which he attributed largely to a lack of publicity.

Mr Ball Dodson clearly accepted the need to increase the number of annual subscriptions and he announced that a Hospital Week would be held in December. The programme, he said, would include appeals from church pulpits explaining that house to house visitations would be made during the week by authorised collectors armed with bankers orders, promise slips for annual subscription payments and receipt books for cheques and cash. In rented houses and flats of more than £50 per annum, he suggested, people would be asked to subscribe one per cent of their rent annually.

Collections would be made on both Sundays at the churches while shops, cinemas, theatres and the railway company would be asked to arrange a collection on one day in aid of the hospital. The week would be inaugurated, he explained, by a great boxing tournament at the Regent Cinema organised by that 'great little wonder man, Mr Harry Preston.'

Despite the earlier reluctance to set up an inquiry, at the conclusion of the meeting a motion to set up a committee of governors and supporters 'with power to inspect all books and accounts … to advise on increased sources of income and increased economy of administration' was accepted. But the mover, Mr Jennings did not leave it there. Whether or not the criticisms were justified, he believed that the committee had to command the confidence of the public and suggested, and had accepted, an additional list of names, including a member of the Voluntary Hospitals Commission, to serve on it.[13]

Nevertheless, the annual report for 1923 was to note, the year 'commenced in the deepest gloom in the history of the Hospital.' The first gleam of hope came in the offer of a grant from the Voluntary Hospital Commission. There was no reluctance to accept government help on this occasion, which was conditional on 50 beds being re-opened in March and the remainder in September, with the proviso that all the beds should be kept open throughout 1924.

'Such a mark of confidence, coming from a body acting under the Ministry of Health, could not be refused,' the annual report continued, 'and the Board accepted the responsibility thrown upon them in the belief that their faith in public support would be justified.'

Facing the Challenge

The hospital's dependence on legacies and subscriptions necessary for its financial survival was supplemented by the efforts of fundraisers, not least of whom was Mr (later Sir) Harry Preston. The tribute paid to him at the public meeting when Hospital Week was announced was well deserved.

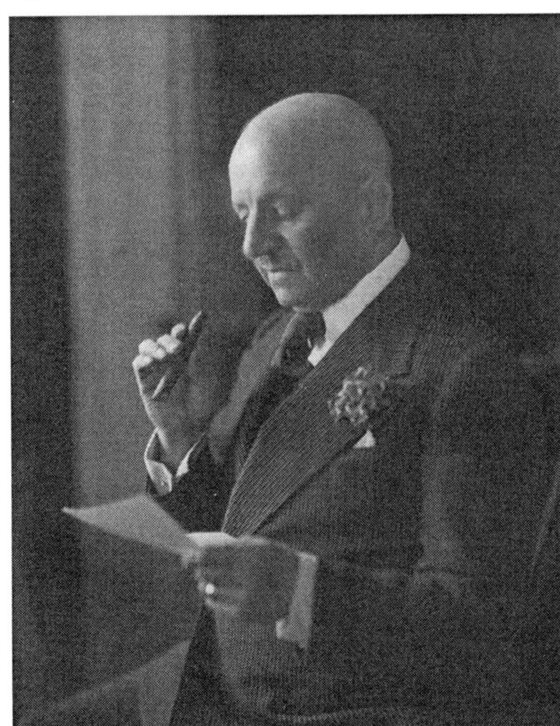

50. Mr Harry Preston's presidential portrait taken in 1923.

Harry Preston, who became president of the hospital in 1921, was well known locally as the owner of the Royal York and Royal Albion hotels. The boxing tournaments he organised in aid of the hospital raised thousands of pounds. To achieve such success the tournament included exhibition bouts by some of the most famous names in the world of boxing – Jack Dempsey, Bombardier Billy Wells, Billy Wilde and Georges Carpentier, to name but a few – and Preston himself took part in an exhibition match.[14] The tournament in 1920 raised over £3000 for the hospital. This was in addition to his annual Christmas time effort, a sale of dolls, that produced a further £1,200.[15] According to the annual report for 1922, Harry Preston had raised nearly £15,000 including £3,000 from his personal pocket, while the 1925 report noted he had 'contributed well over £22,000 to the coffers' since 1918.

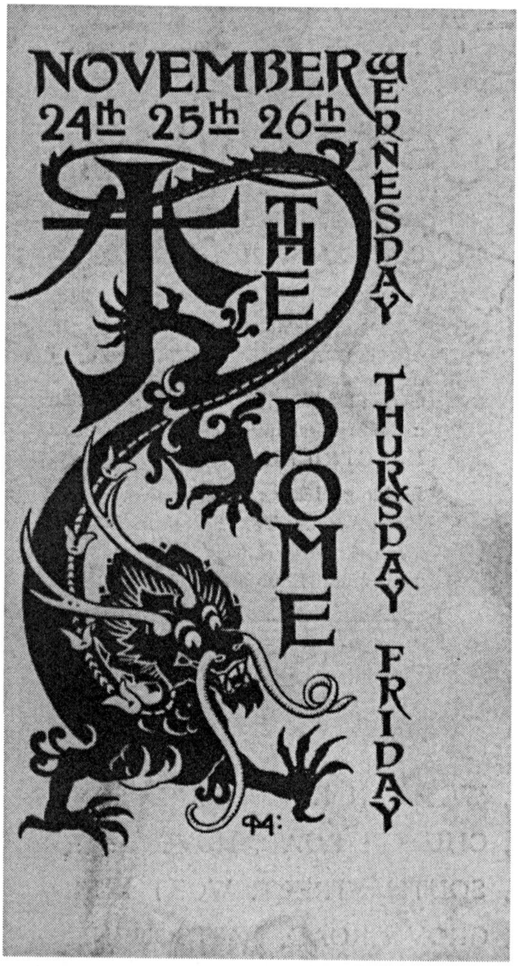

51. The cover of the souvenir programme for the Chinese Fair in November 1920.

To help meet the desperate financial situation in 1922, Preston launched his Shilling Fund. With twenty shillings to the pound, this was a significantly lower amount than the somewhat disappointing Half Crown Appeal (two shillings and sixpence) launched earlier, but as the *Sussex Daily News* reported on the 23rd September, it would appeal to all 'because people of the humblest resources can contribute as well as those of more affluent means.'

There were many other donors, of course, including individuals and organisations the length and breadth of the county. One of these, a nurse from the Private Nursing Institute, set up a doll fund to help re-open the children's ward following its closure in 1922.

Fundraising fairs, a feature of the previous century, continued in the peacetime years of the twentieth. The Chinese Ambassador opened a Chinese Fair at the Dome in November, 1920. Held over three days, it raised £2,600 in the first two days.[16] Events organised in 1925 included a two-day Regency Fair and a Dickens Fair and Pickwick Pageant in 1926, both held in December at the Dome.

The programme of the Chinese Fair concluded with a paragraph that summed up the desire of its supporters to safeguard the voluntary hospitals system:

> It is proposed that Hospitals should be rate-aided; if we can but keep this – the Sussex Hospital – off the rates for just eight more years, it will attain its century as a Voluntary Institution, and many of the abnormal conditions under which we live at present will, by then, have passed away.

One fundraising event in 1922 was so unusual it was widely reported in the national press. Evening papers on the 1st June reported that the public were to be allowed to visit a mystery tower at Shoreham Harbour by Major E.F. Sexton who was bearing all the expenses and giving the proceeds to the Royal Sussex County Hospital. The necessary scaffolding and gangways set up for the safety of the public had employed 27,000 feet of timber at an approximate cost of £1,000.[17] Admission to the tower, which had taken eighteen months to build and had been the subject of questions in Parliament, was to be one shilling and it was the only opportunity to view it before it was demolished.[18]

The following morning more reports appeared, one, 'from our special correspondent from Brighton', was headlined: Mystery Secret Tower Room Which Nobody Must Enter[19] and spoke of 'a secret chamber which is zealously guarded and nobody, not even the sentry who stands over the barred door may enter'. According to the report, the Admiralty kept the key of the room and only the highest officials were allowed to use it. Another newspaper[20] reported that 'the Admiralty still retain the utmost reticence concerning the uses to which this unwieldy [nearly

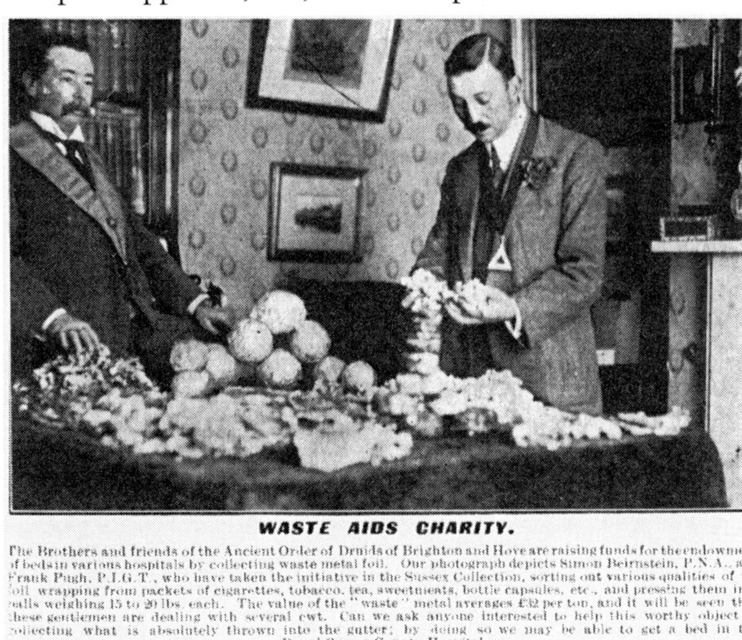

52. This postcard illustrates one of the many ways money was raised to support the hospital. The proceeds of the collection of tinfoil by local masons that realised the considerable amount of £32 a ton were used to endow a bed in 1918. In the 1930s, silver paper was collected to raise more funds.

1,000 ton] structure was to be put' and predicted, correctly that no doubt many thousands of holidaymakers would take the opportunity of visiting it. According to a later report, 12,200 people turned up on the day[21] and, according to the annual report, the event yielded £750.

An unusual feature of the hospital that attracted interest many years later, was a niche in the pillar on the west side of the hospital entrance Until 1927, the niche contained a post box and below it there was believed to be a box for the deposit of the half crowns donated for the special appeal. What is certain is that the niche later housed a milk churn to collect two pence pieces to help meet the annual milk bill while a former nurse recalled that in the 1930s when she was a small child it was used to house donations of silver paper.[22]

New Developments

Following the crises of the previous year, 1923 was considered to be not merely one of 'recovery and recuperation' but also one of progress, two of the most noteworthy developments being the opening of the John Howard Wards and the completion of a new orthopaedic department and reconstruction of the massage department.

Twenty beds in the John Howard Wards in the Jubilee Block were officially opened in March. They were intended for patients who were ineligible for treatment in the ordinary wards but whose means were insufficient to pay for a private nursing home. They were charged not more than £4 a week, the sum being made up where necessary by a contribution from the Howard Estate.

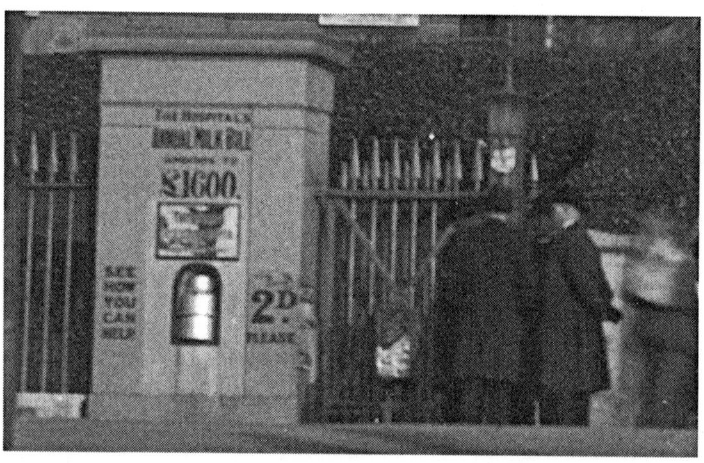

53. The pillar in front of the hospital that may have contained a box to collect half crowns in a 1920s appeal and later to collect donations to help meet the cost of the annual milk bill.

The new orthopaedic department, formally opened in December, was made possible thanks to a £2,000 grant made in 1920 by the Joint War Committee of the British Red Cross and Order of St John. It was conditional on work being started no later than April 1st 1923 and also a similar sum being raised locally to cover the cost and building and equipment. The committee of the Lady George Nevill

Hospital, who transferred their entire orthopaedic equipment to the new department, also announced their willingness to equip and endow a new electro-cardiographic department.

A Miss Poulter, who twelve years earlier had created the School of Massage, 'contributed lavishly' to the creation of the new massage department, which was transferred to the hospital. However, it was found it needed more students if it was to meet modern requirements and to be run economically and as this would have required a considerable increase in accommodation, the board reluctantly decided to close it five years later.

The Ditchling Convalescent Home, which was no longer considered to be suitable for its purpose and had been out of use since 1920, was finally sold in 1924. The interest on the invested proceeds was allocated to the Christmas Fund.

During the year, a special committee had been considering the need for isolation quarters for nurses 'for the many cases of slight infection so often contracted in a General hospital' and the provision of a wing for the maids. It was agreed this had become a 'matter of first importance' and £2,000 was earmarked for new buildings. Plans and estimates for an annexe to the nurses' home were completed in 1925 when the question of further expansion of hospital came to the forefront. 'The whole matter is fraught with difficulty,' the board warned in its annual report. 'Our main building is a hundred years old, and the site does not easily lend itself to expansion. Our accommodation is taxed to breaking point and a very great amount will have to be done if the Hospital is to be made worthy of the County.'

Faced with this problem (one to emerge again later in the hospital's history) the board engaged a hospital design expert, Colonel J.D. Mackintosh, to advise on future expansion.

The result was an ambitious programme estimated to cost £100,000: an additional 50 to 60 beds; more bedrooms and a lecture room for the nurses; an annexe to accommodate the domestic staff; remodelling and updating the operating theatres; the expansion of the X-ray and massage departments; and the enlargement of the casualty and emergency departments.

1926 marked the centenary of the laying of the hospital's foundation stone and to help fund the developments it was decided to launch a Centenary Appeal in October for the £100,000 needed and also for £10,000 in increased subscriptions. By the end of 1927, £41,843 had been reached, including £10,000 from Mr Bernhard Baron that was earmarked for a new casualty department. Meanwhile, work had begun and was nearing completion

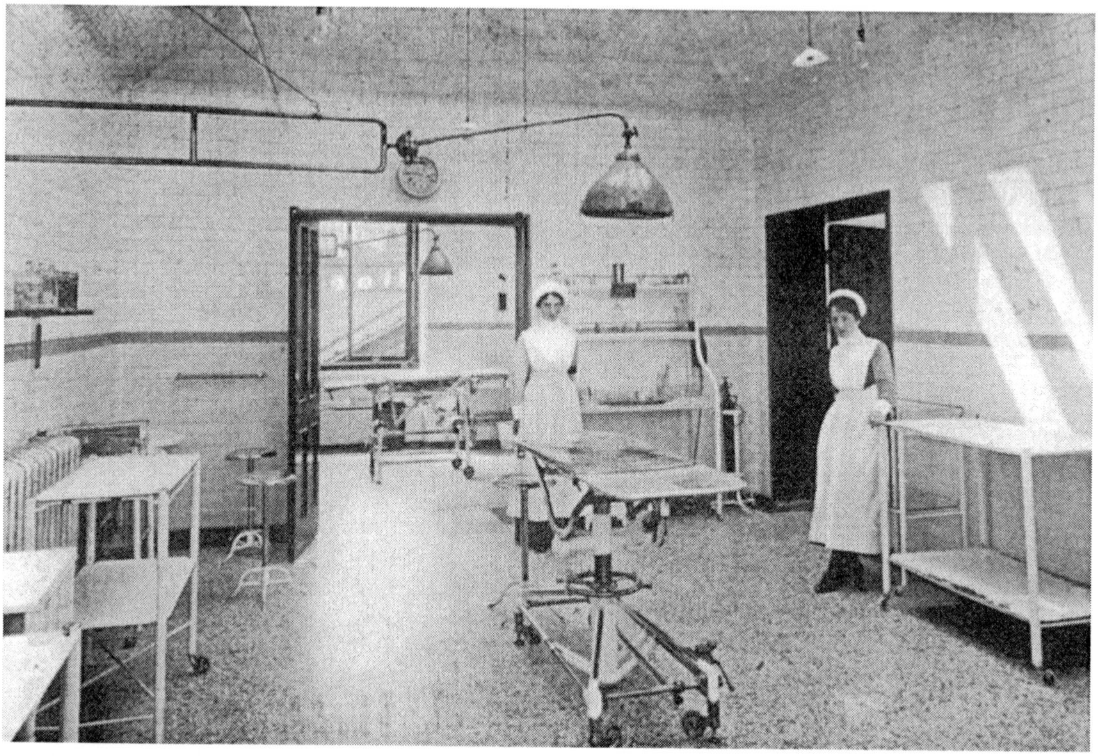

54. An operating theatre in the main building pictured in the annual report for 1927.

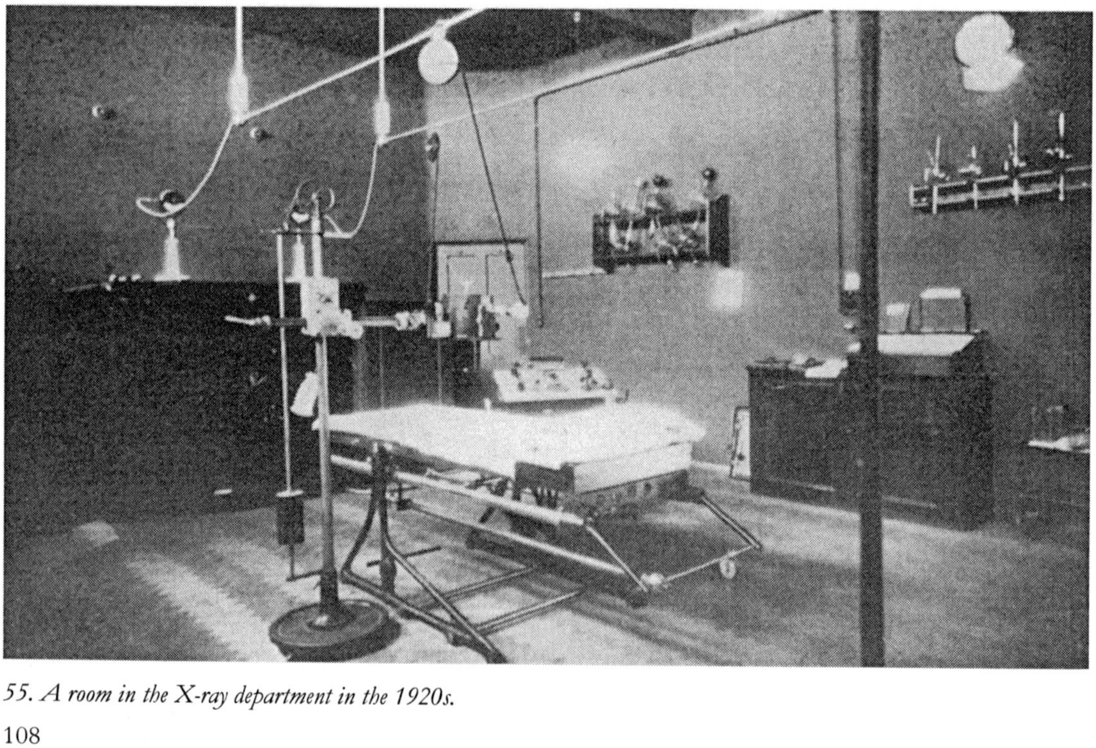

55. A room in the X-ray department in the 1920s.

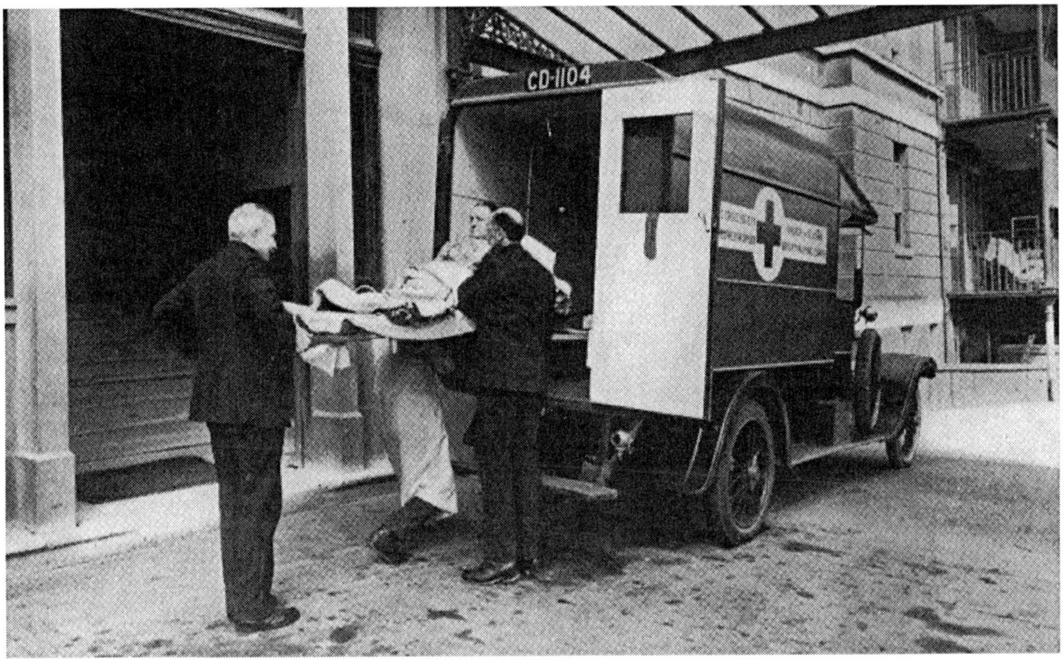

55. Porters Joe Kenyon and Joe Large receiving a casualty at the main entrance to the hospital, probably in about 1927. 10,000 casualties attended the hospital during 1928 when the need for a new department was established.

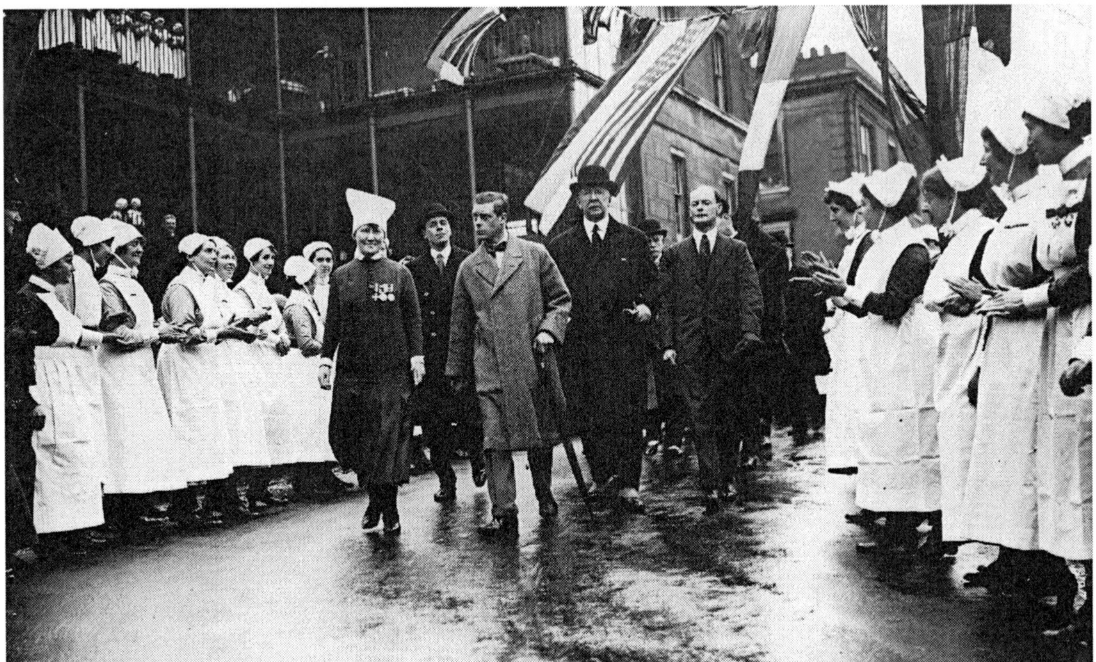

57. Sisters and nurses formed a guard of honour for the Prince of Wales who inspected Overton and Bristol wards during a brief informal visit on the 23rd March 1927.

on the additional accommodation and lecture hall for the nurses and the home for the domestic servants and these were opened on 31st July 1928 by Dame Ann Beadsmore Smith.

In spite of the encouraging start, the final total reached by the Centenary Appeal in 1928 was only £45,000. This meant that many necessary and urgent improvements could not be undertaken. Thanks to the donation by Bernhard Baron, however, work was able to go ahead on the new casualty department. The original plans for the new department envisaged this as being at the front of the hospital.

The plans eventually drawn up utilised a site under Vallance ward that was accepted at first by representatives of the medical staff. This was a cheaper option and would have left some of Bernhard Baron's gift available for other purposes. However, the medical staff were not entirely happy with this. On reflection, they felt the new site proposed would be 'deficient in height, light and ventilation', that access would be poor and that the noise of ambulances would affect the ward. A staff meeting was called which urged that the original site at the front of the hospital should be adhered to. The feeling was that it would be 'poor propaganda' not to use the gift in a way that would visibly improve the hospital.

At the meeting this view eventually prevailed with the new department officially opened on 30th April 1929 by Prince Arthur of Connaught prominently occupying the space formerly filled by the two exterior flights of steps leading up to the hospital.

Staff in the Post-War Period

One of the causes of increases in expenditure that had to be met after the war was that many more staff now had to be paid. This reflected not so much an increase in the number employed but the fact that during the war years many of the gaps left by those who were serving in the armed forces or nursing services had been replaced by unpaid volunteers 'doing their bit' for the war effort. Also, since working in hospital often offered the prospect of a reserved occupation, it had been possible to employ men on much lower wages than normal.

The payment of probationers, which had been questioned by those critical of the way the hospital was managed, also added to the problem. The matron, in an interview published in *The Nursing Mirror*[23] dealt with this at some length.

Until the spring of 1919, she said, probationers came not only without remuneration, but they used at one time to pay a premium. Three years before, when the cost of clothing had become a serious problem, they were given their uniform, which previously they had paid for themselves. In April 1919, it was decided also to make a payment of £12 for the first year, £16 for the second and £20 for the third.

She also explained that although she would prefer one, there was then no preliminary training school. Probationers had to be between the ages of 21 and 34. For the first three months they were on probation and if suitable had to agree to serve the hospital for at least three years, including the trial period. During the final six months, they had to pass a final examination to qualify for their certificate.

Miss Scott admitted that at the time they had been unable to introduce a 56 or 58-hour week. However, every nurse had two and a half hours off duty in the day, or three hours in the evening, a half day once a week and a day once a month. Because the first year was 'particularly trying', probationers were granted a week's leave after the first six months. Sisters were allowed a weekend once a month from 2.30 on Saturday to noon on Monday in addition to their weekly half day. Nurses had a three week annual holiday and sisters a month.

During the visit, the writer of the article was taken to the nurses' home, which could be approached in bad weather, it was explained, by a covered subway popularly known as the 'Chicken Run.' The description of the accommodation left no doubt about the need for the postponed improvements. The off duty arrangements for the nurses, on the other hand, appeared to leave little to be desired: no meals were served in the home with the exception of breakfast in bed for nurses on their days off when they could, if they wished, remain in bed all day and have their meals brought from the hospital.

The article concluded:

> If the interior of the Nurses' Home is not at present all the authorities would like it to be, the outside surroundings are delightful. In the gardens sloping down to the road are tennis courts, and plenty of seats for outdoor life. At the back of the Home are the downs; and here, in their off-duty time, the nurses take full advantage of the privilege they are allowed of using a private gate and getting away in a few minutes from the hospital atmosphere, straight to the delight of green sward, wild flowers, and the glitter of the sun on the sea below.

The effect on the hospital's often precarious finances of having to pay probationers was a prelude to similar difficulties throughout the Twenties. In

1918 and 1919, there were fears that as they returned in increasing numbers from war service there would be a surplus of nurses. However, these fears were short lived and it soon became apparent there would be a national shortage, not helped by the introduction of state registration. This was to persist throughout the Twenties and into the Thirties when there were two major inquiries into the reasons for the shortage.[24]

The effect on the Sussex County was compounded by the need to employ more nurses, for example because the probationers now spent more time at lectures instead of attending to patients on the wards; the introduction of private beds was another factor, as more individual attention was necessarily given to private patients.

Recruitment difficulties in 1925 resulted in increased salaries of £20, £25 and £30 to first, second and third year nurses and consideration was given to instituting a pension scheme. From the 1st January 1927 the salary scales of senior nurses were also increased: the ward sisters' scale rose to £65 to £85 per annum from £60-£70. In order to extend off duty hours, the number of nurses was increased from 100 to 108. To meet the current training and examination requirements, a full-time sister tutor was appointed, the post having previously been combined with the home sister post. Because of the financial situation, however, the board felt unable to introduce the proposed pension scheme.

Earlier, in 1923, the hospital had said farewell to Miss Katharine Scott, who had reached retirement age in July after 27 years service as Matron. Some idea of her reputation locally can be gained from the rumours spreading wildly during the 1922 influenza epidemic that she had died and her funeral had been arranged. The truth was she had suffered a minor accident and sprained her ankle.[25] A tribute to her was paid in the annual report:

> It is hard to express adequately the debt which the Hospital owes to Miss Scott. During the War, her services were invaluable and her sympathetic personality did much to attract the support which all who came into contact with her were only too pleased to offer. But it will be as a trainer of nurses that she will probably be best remembered, for it is mainly due to her noble qualities and her special gifts in the development of character that the Royal Sussex County Hospital Nurses have attained a reputation unsurpassed in the profession.

Miss E.F. Spencer from St Thomas's Hospital was appointed to succeed Miss Scott. She retired in 1924 when her health broke down and was succeeded by Miss S. Williams, then in 1927, Miss E.W. Young, assistant matron at the West London, who had trained at the County, returned to take over as Matron.

The Private Nursing Institute went from strength to strength during the Twenties. In 1920 the board bought the freehold of St George's Vicarage and, now renamed 1 Chapel Terrace, the nurses moved there the following year from the three small houses from which they had worked in Eastern Road. This enabled more nurses to be maintained on the staff (by 1922, 50 had been enrolled) and it was hoped the profits of the Institute would eventually cover the cost of the building and the adaptations that were necessary.

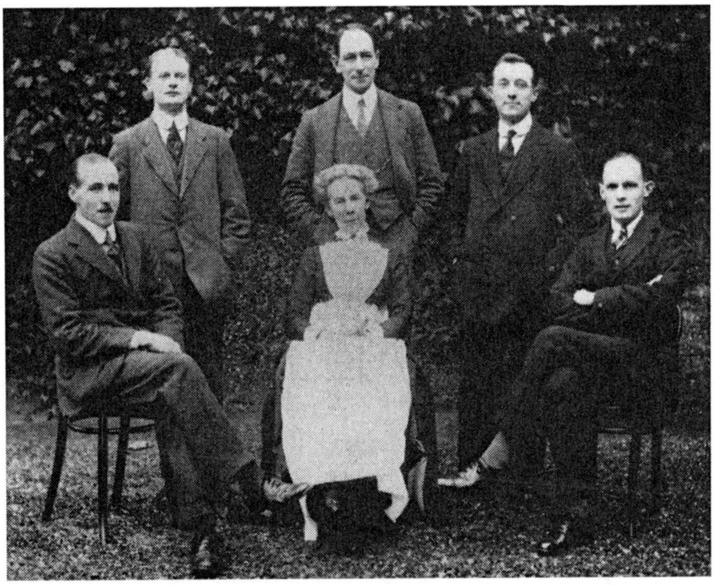

58. Matron Katherine Scott with (standing) A.F. Cowan and E.F. Crabtree (1st and 2nd house surgeons) and house physician Dr P.C. Fenwick and (sitting) the secretary, Mr Lancaster Gaye, and J.D. Deveer (3rd house surgeon), probably taken c.1914-16.

This was achieved in 1926 when the success of the Institute meant that there was sufficient profit made during the year for wireless to be installed and for another sum of £192 8s to be transferred to the hospital's general funds. A successful year in 1927 led to a further transfer of £881 to general funds and £746 6s 5d the following year. In 1929, despite an increase in the number of nurses, a number of applications for the nurses' services had to be refused.

The opening of the extensions to the nurses' home in 1928 brought a number of benefits to the hospital. The eastern annexe provided additional bedrooms for the nurses and a larger lecture theatre than the one previously situated over the pathological laboratory. By 1929 this had enabled the hospital to become one of the centres for the nurses' state registration examinations.

The annexe on the west provided new accommodation for the domestic staff. Previously they had been accommodated in three houses in Eastern Road, which were 'inadequate, insufficient, poor and sunless'. As a result, only 31 members of the staff were resident. The remaining 24 were employed uneconomically by the day. They were paid 3s daily exclusive of food at an annual total cost of £1,200 compared with £770 for the larger number of resident staff. With the new accommodation, the board hoped to achieve better control of the hospital's domestic services and to achieve 'a definite reduction in the number of Maids employed'.

The annual report for 1926 was unusual in that it paid a tribute to a member of the engineering staff, sadly following his death. Ernest Albert Malpass had been resident engineer for 25 years when he died from severe scalds suffered during an accident while he was on duty. A tablet was erected to his memory in the hospital chapel. Mr Malpass had also been hon. secretary of the local 'Men's Effort' that had set out to raise £200 for the Half Crown Appeal[26] and eventually raised £840 12s 1d. He was succeeded by his son, popularly known as Frank, who had been born in the engineer's cottage. Frank eventually retired at the end of December 1967, bringing to a close a family association with the hospital extending over 66½ years.

10. The Thirties

The ten years from 1930 to 1939 began in a depression and ended with the beginning of the Second World War, both of which, in their different ways, made their mark on the running of the hospital. In 1930, for example, the depression was in part responsible for a deficit on the running costs of over £4,000.

In the event, however, financially this proved to be a relatively good year, only marginally worse than 1934. Throughout the rest of the decade, the day to day running costs of the hospital exceeded income by amounts ranging from £5,350 in 1931 to £13,118 in 1938.

In common with most of the nation's voluntary hospitals, there was a never-ending struggle throughout the Thirties to meet the cost of maintaining the institution, which, despite appeals for more subscribers and supporters, always seemed doomed to failure. Rising costs, at one time of bed linen, coal and rates, were one problem. Another was the effect of medical advances that led to the need for expensive replacements of old and worn out apparatus, in X-ray for example, and the general need for more and newer medical and other equipment generally.

The growing use of the motor car, like the previous century's growth of the railway, also put pressure on the casualty department and contributed to increased financial pressure. In 1930, 294 motor accident cases received treatment in casualty and 79 of these were subsequently treated as inpatients. In 1934, 440 were treated in casualty, 120 in the wards. A new Road Traffic Act, promised to ease the burden on voluntary hospitals by raising the maximum that could be claimed for treating any one case from £25 to £50. Nevertheless, the financial burden remained: the following year the board reported that the cost of treating 171 such patients was approximately £1,830 but the hospital received only £988

To keep abreast of rising costs, the hospital was forced to rely on legacies of large and small amounts, which generally brought in several thousand pounds a year. Among these was a total of £18,000 bequeathed by the Misses Eugenie, Elizabeth and Florence Stewart in 1937 and 1938. In gratitude for their bequests, it was decided in 1939 to name the children's ward Stewart to perpetuate their memory.

There was one occasion in 1935, however, when the board had to correct the widespread belief that the hospital was about to receive a large legacy from Sir Francis Montefiori, believed erroneously to be in the region of £160,000, and as a result was no longer in need of funds. The adverse effect of this on the hospital's financial situation led the board to remind subscribers that its anxiety 'with regard to the maintenances and future progress of the Hospital remains and is desperately real.'

This situation would have been even worse without the continuing efforts of many organisations and individuals to raise funds for the hospital. The Sussex Provident Fund, an insurance scheme inaugurated by consultant physician Dr Gordon Dill in 1922, prospered to such an extent that in 1933, for example, it was able to reimburse the hospital for the treatment of its members during the previous fifteen months with a sum of just over £9,900. In 1938, £9,856 was received for the treatment provided in just twelve months.

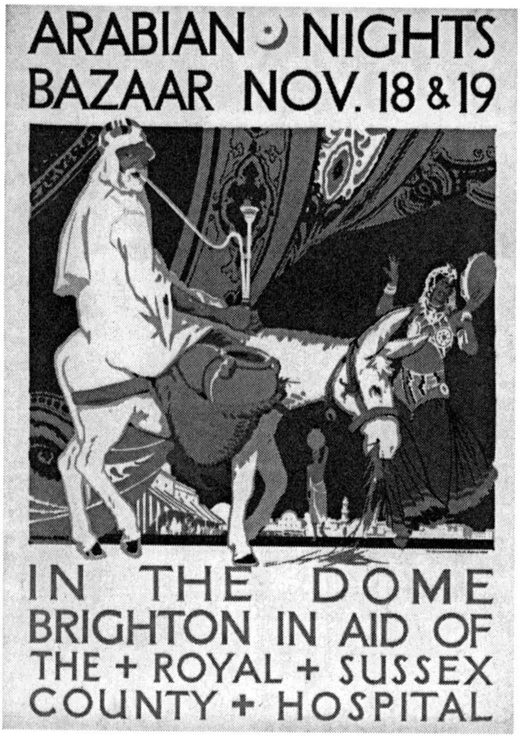

59. The Arabian Nights Bazaar was held in 1931 during the economic depression. In the programme's foreword, the chairman, Brig. Gen. D'A. C, Brownlow urged that while everyone had to make drastic economies, subscribers should not discontinue a subscription to a hospital or charitable institution, but 'leave this cut to the very last.'

The annual bazaars normally held over two or three days in the Dome usually raised between two and three thousand pounds. The Hospital Sunday Fund similarly contributed amounts in the region of £500. In 1934, Sir Harry Preston's Hospital Fund contributed £1,176. Some idea of the range of organisations working for the hospital can be gained from that year's list of contributors. This included the Alexandra Day Committee, Seaford Village Fayre, Cowfold Ball, Burgess Hill Hospitals Fete Committee, Steyning Hospital Week Collection, Seaford Flag Day, Uckfield and Hurstpierpoint carnivals and Brighton Students' Association

Two new associations established in 1934 widened the ways in which funds were raised. The Old Patients Association recruited 660 members in its first six months and the following year subscribed over £100 for the upkeep of 'Grateful Remembrance' beds. The Golden Penny League established in April recruited 2,000 members to hold their special collecting boxes. By the end of 1936, membership had increased to 5,372 who subscribed over £1,200. Annual subscribers of 2s 6d to the Birthday League, whose Birthday League Book was kept in the main entrance of the hospital for signatures, also contributed to the general funds. The Blue Bird Club set up in 1937 with a subscription of one shilling presented a cheque for £232 9s 10d at the end of 1938. In April 1939, a scheme to encourage children to take an interest in the work of the hospital was inaugurated, with the Duchess of Norfolk as president. Called the Sussex Shrimps, 170 children were enrolled by the end of the year.

The annual reports also paid tribute to the continuing work of the Blanket, Linen and Work Guild, the Ladies Association, who maintained the library as well as making other gifts, and the Brighton and Hove Centre of the League of Remembrance. The Clothing and Household Bureau raised funds towards the purchase of 4 Paston Place which was to house the Appeals Department.

Supplementing these efforts, the hospital continued to receive the proceeds of box collections at schools and public houses throughout the county, congregation collections and staff and working men's collections.

Developments

A hospital's financial matters can be considered under two headings: firstly, expenditure on maintenance, where rising costs could lead to calls for economies and even to bed closures like those in 1922. Then there is capital expenditure on new buildings and major equipment that necessitate special appeals or rely upon the generosity of benefactors like Bernhard Baron whose gift resulted in the building of the new casualty department.

The first noteworthy development of the Thirties, a new operating theatre block, also owed a great deal to Bernhard Baron. He promised £5,000 towards the cost of the new facilities (estimated to cost £15,000) shortly before his death in 1929 at his home in The Drive.[1] Construction work began early in 1930, although an estimated £6,000 was needed for completion. Determined to ease the pressures on the surgeons and remove the 'many difficulties

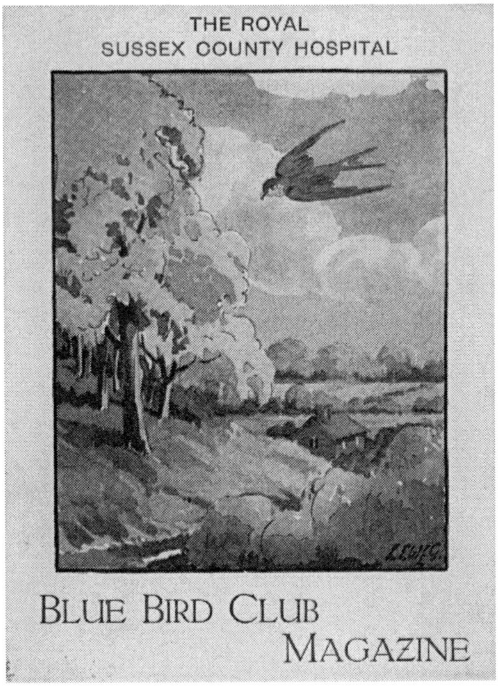

60. The first issue of the Blue Bird Club Magazine, issued free to members who paid a shilling a year, was intended to form a close bond between patients and staff of the hospital.

under which they have so patiently carried on their work,' the board hoped for a generous response to an appeal for funds made by the president. However, when the block was officially opened on the 16th April 1931 by Lord Moynihan, the president of the Royal College of Surgeons, the cost had risen to over £17,000 and a debt of nearly £7,000 remained. As a result, the board had to sell some of the hospital's investments to reduce the overdraft at the bank.

The opening ceremony was described in some detail in the *Nursing Mirror and Midwives' Journal:*

> ... sisters and nurses formed an attractive guard of honour as they lined both sides of the long corridor leading to the entrance to the new theatre block ... A broad line of white ribbon stretched across the archway in front of them, and close by a sister waited, holding a case containing a shining pair of surgical scissors with which Lord Moynihan would presently cut the ribbon while declaring the new block open. Matron – Miss C.W. Young – flitted up and down the corridor to see that all was ready for the ceremony, and at the far end appeared for a moment 'Absolom', the hospital cat, aloof, indifferent yet vaguely inquisitive concerning the unusual stir ... Lord Moynihan came to the archway, where he was presented with the scissors, and in return smilingly tendered sixpence to the sister for the theatre fund, in traditional exchange for what might otherwise prove an unlucky 'gift'.[2]

The value of the new theatre block to the hospital quickly became apparent. According to the 1931 annual report, 3,160 operations were performed during the year, 625 more than in 1930. The average length of stay decreased by 1.6 days and there was an appreciable reduction in the time patients had to wait for a vacant bed. The theatre in the Jubilee Block, now used for eye and ear, nose and throat cases, was also renovated and altered at a more modest cost of £255 14s 6d, while York ward was extended at a cost of £235.

These were only the first of a number of developments that took place in the years leading up to the war. Alterations were made to the X-ray department and new equipment installed in 1933, although the cost of more than £3,000 had to be met from general funds.

In 1934 more adequate accommodation for Matron and an additional nurse's bedroom were added in the nurses' home, while a chapel was added to the mortuary. Further replacement of diagnostic equipment costing almost £2,000 took place in 1936 but more space was required if X-ray therapy services were to be extended to meet the needs of cancer patients. Radium treatment had been available at the hospital on a limited basis during the Twenties and was made more available from 1929; now there was also a need for special equipment to be installed and maintained in X-ray. This included the expensive Chaoul apparatus for low voltage contact X-ray therapy, possessed by only a few hospitals in the country, donated to the hospital by the Sussex branch of the British Empire Campaign. The solution to the X-ray department's problems was eventually provided by another major development, the provision of a new massage department.

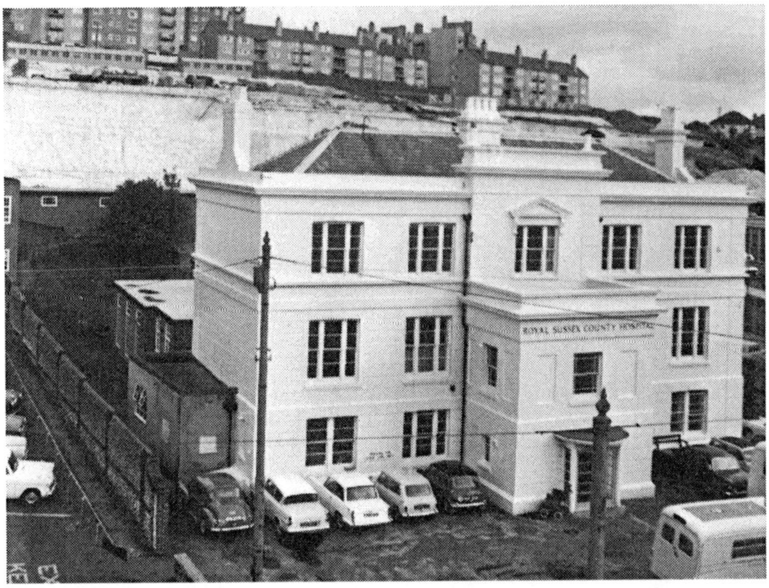

61. The Girls' Orphanage at 177 Eastern Road, a Regency style building with an unusual staircase in the porch of the building, was bought and extended to become the Latilla Department of Physical Medicine.

For many years, the board had cast envious eyes on the adjacent Brighton Girls Orphanage in Eastern Road, which prevented further expansion of the hospital to the east. In 1936, they were able to purchase the property for £5,000, which gave access to the land already owned fronting Bristol Gate.

Thanks to donations from Mrs H.G. Latilla of nearly £5,000, the building was extended to provide a new massage department, known as the Latilla Department of Physical Medicine. Dr R.W. Windle, who became honorary consultant in 1937, advised on the planning of the department with the sister in charge, Miss Ward. When finally completed, he later recalled, the Latilla was looked upon as one of the eight foremost departments in the country and the Ministry of Health sent various groups to see it.[3] It certainly impressed a writer from *The Nursing Times:*

> In a newly reconditioned and extended house next door the hospital has an immensely busy department of physical medicine fitted with plaster room, ultra-violet ray therapy department, wax and foam bathrooms, a gymnasium, and a special diathermy room with an ultra short-wave diathermy apparatus that treats patients through their dressings, e.g., in chest and sinus cases. A Paevex machine for gangrene, the only one on the South Coast, was operating in one of the cubicles. The department has evening clinics for village patients as well as daytime ones, and altogether does about 1,300 treatments a week.[4]

One of the benefits of the new department was that it accelerated the early return to normal activities of patients suffering fractures – the hospital dealt with 184 fracture cases as inpatients and 600 outpatients at the time and earlier in 1937 a special fracture clinic had been set up with three sessions weekly in casualty.

On the 19th April 1938, Sister Ward and her six physiotherapists transferred to the new accommodation, which contained all the electrical and mechanical apparatus for up-to-date massage treatment. With the additional accommodation now available in the main building, the way was open for an extension of the work of the X-ray department and a special committee was set up to consider a suggestion by the Sussex Branch Council of the British Empire Cancer Campaign to install additional deep X-ray apparatus to be used by all the hospitals in Brighton and Hove and to establish a centre fully equipped for diagnosis and X-ray and radium treatment of cancer cases. Unfortunately the outbreak of war in 1939 meant the proposal was put into abeyance.

In 1929, following a change in the law that meant patients could receive psychiatric treatment without being certified as insane, a new departure had been proposed: the establishment of an outpatient department for cases of early nervous disorders referred from other departments of the hospital. On the 1st October 1930, the new department was established in close co-operation with the Lady Chichester Hospital under the charge of Dr A. Helen Boyle and Dr. G.H. Harper-Smith. Under the scheme, it was agreed that the Lady Chichester would allot twelve beds for cases recommended from the County Hospital's outpatient department, an agreement that meant 'crossing a Rubicon' for the Lady Chichester. As six of the beds were to be for borderline male patients, not only would it have to bear the cost of the necessary alterations, it would also cease to be purely a women and children's hospital.[5]

More new departments were established in 1939. An orthopaedic department was established in the early part of the year under the charge of Mr R. Brooke and in May, a gynaecological department was established to take over the whole of the gynaecological work of the Sussex Maternity Hospital. The existing eleven beds were allotted to the new department under two honorary gynaecologists, the County's honorary assistant surgeon, Mr H.J. McCurrich, and Mr K.F. Mackenzie, honorary surgeon to the maternity hospital and the governors were offered land for a new maternity hospital to the west of the new Sussex Eye Hospital.

The new eye hospital had been erected in 1935 on the south side of Eastern

Road on what was part of the large hospital vegetable garden and had been offered to the hospital on a lease for 999 years at a peppercorn rent.

Early in July, the County Hospital's eye departments closed and eight probationers were transferred to the new hospital to obtain three months' experience in nursing eye cases. This arrangement was essential in order that the Sussex County would continue to be recognised by the General Nursing Council for England and Wales as a first class general nurse training school.

This was not the first occasion that the hospital had emphasised that a full range of services was essential to meet the requirements for nurse education. The value of the children's wards in this respect had been explained in answer to criticisms of the local duplication of services in the 1920s and it was referred to again in the annual report for 1932. Describing the extent and nature of the accommodation provided, the report reiterated the need 'for adequate facilities for the treatment of both adults and children, suffering from medical or surgical diseases' without which it 'could not continue to hold its present proud position as an efficient Training School for Nurses.'

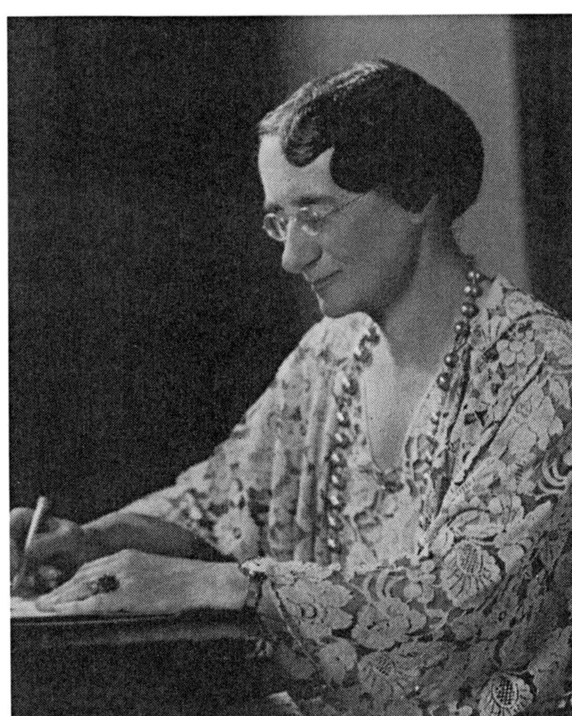

62. Dr Helen Boyle was one of the two medical officers in charge of the hospital's new department for early nervous diseases. She was appointed consultant in nervous diseases in 1937 'in recognition of valuable services rendered'.

In 1932, according to the report, there were 246 beds, including 62 allotted for medical cases, and provision for the treatment of eye, ear, nose and throat, skin and dental cases, and for those suffering from early nervous disorders.

22 beds were allotted for children, 13 of the cots (the majority of which were either 'named' or 'endowed') were accommodated in a separate children's ward. Altogether, 374 children under the age of 15 had been treated in the wards during the year.

The number of beds increased on several occasions during the 1930s. Thirteen extra beds were provided in 1930 when Chichester Ward was divided into two self-contained wards, each in charge of a sister The additional ward,

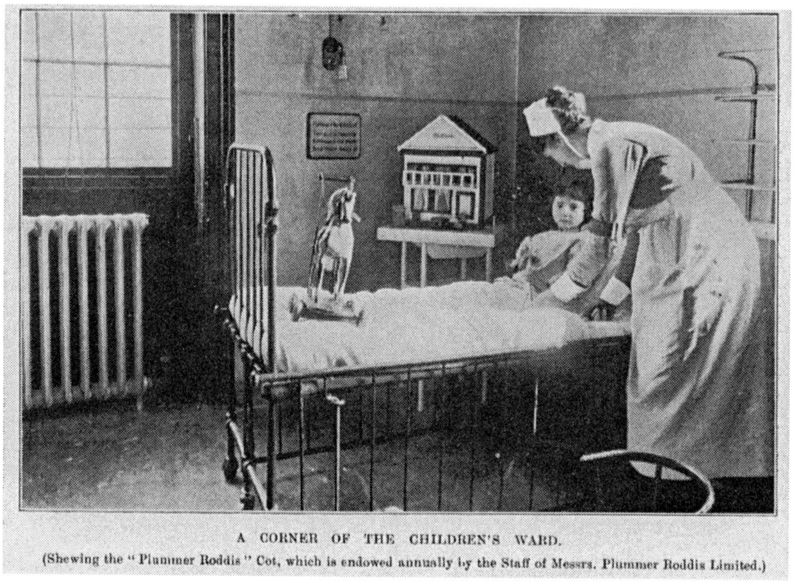

63. The Plummer Roddis cot, one of the majority of cots that were named or endowed in the children's ward.

opened on the 31st August, was named 'Baily' in recognition of the generous support of Mr C.C. Baily and his family. Eight more beds installed in 1931 brought the total to 246.

In 1934, the board reported that the number of beds had risen to 250 but that 100 more were needed and that it believed that an appreciable number could be added with further division of some of the wards. To bring this need before the general public, a Festival Dinner was held at the Royal Pavilion on the 14th July 1935 followed by a postal appeal for £60,000 towards the 'Special Building and Extension Fund' and for an additional £8,000 maintenance income.

During the year, 22 additional beds were made available, again as the result of dividing three wards, Bristol, Overton and Vallance, into two separately administered units. The eastern end of Vallance became Jowers Ward, to perpetuate 'an expression of gratitude to Mr R.F. Jowers and members of his Family for the valuable professional and pecuniary services they have rendered to the Hospital.'

These changes brought the total number of beds to 272, not including the 12 beds maintained at the Lady Chichester Hospital. However, these increases and the other developments not only necessitated the employment of more nurses, but also made demands that had to be met, for example, on staff accommodation, the engineering services, kitchen and laundry. Because a number of the domestic staff had become non-resident, accommodation for the nurses was found in the maids' quarters. Approximately £1,500 was spent in 1933 on the first part of a £3,000 scheme submitted by the hospital's consulting engineer that involved increasing the efficiency of the boilers and installing electrical generating plant.

Lack of finance restricted laundry improvements to the replacement of a forty-year old hydro extractor in the laundry. Eventually, in 1937, when it became clear that there was not sufficient space to install additional equipment, some of the work was placed with an outside contractor. At the same time, although some additional equipment was installed in the kitchen, no more was possible because of the shortage of space.

The need for a third operating theatre was acknowledged in 1939 because of the establishment of the gynaecological department and increased surgical work generally, but this was not proceeded with because of the national emergency.

Publicity in the national press and elsewhere in 1933 stressed the advantages that could be gained by voluntary hospitals from providing facilities for paying patients. The Royal Sussex County had taken a step in this direction by establishing the John Howard wards in 1923 for patients of moderate means who were unable to pay the full cost. Lack of funds for the capital outlay involved, however, prevented the board from making provision for patients able to pay higher fees including, unlike the patients in John Howard, payment to the medical staff.

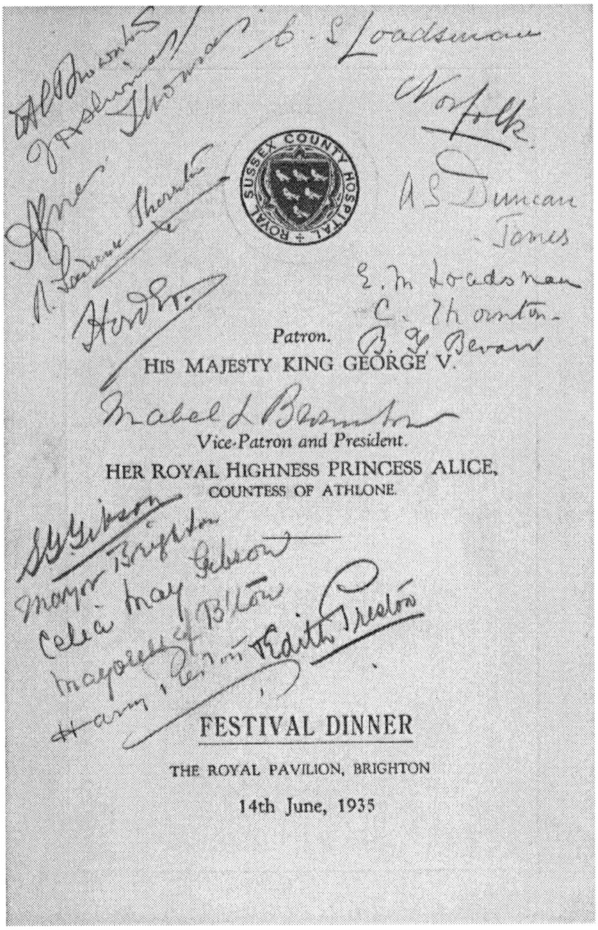
ROYAL SUSSEX COUNTY HOSPITAL

Patron.

HIS MAJESTY KING GEORGE V.

Vice-Patron and President.

HER ROYAL HIGHNESS PRINCESS ALICE,

COUNTESS OF ATHLONE.

FESTIVAL DINNER

THE ROYAL PAVILION, BRIGHTON

14th June, 1935

64. The programme of the Festival Dinner held in 1935 to launch a fund for new buildings and extensions to the hospital.

The situation promised to change, however, following the death of Sir Harry Preston in 1936. An appeal was launched to build a paying patients' block in his memory and the amount raised, nearly £4,000, was earmarked as the nucleus of a fund to proceed with the proposal that was expected to cost £45,000. Land to the east of York Block was identified as a suitable site for the block which was to be connected to the third operating theatre and X-ray department by a covered corridor. Direct tunnel communication to the Latilla department was also planned.

According to Dr Windle[6], who had sat on the sub-committee planning

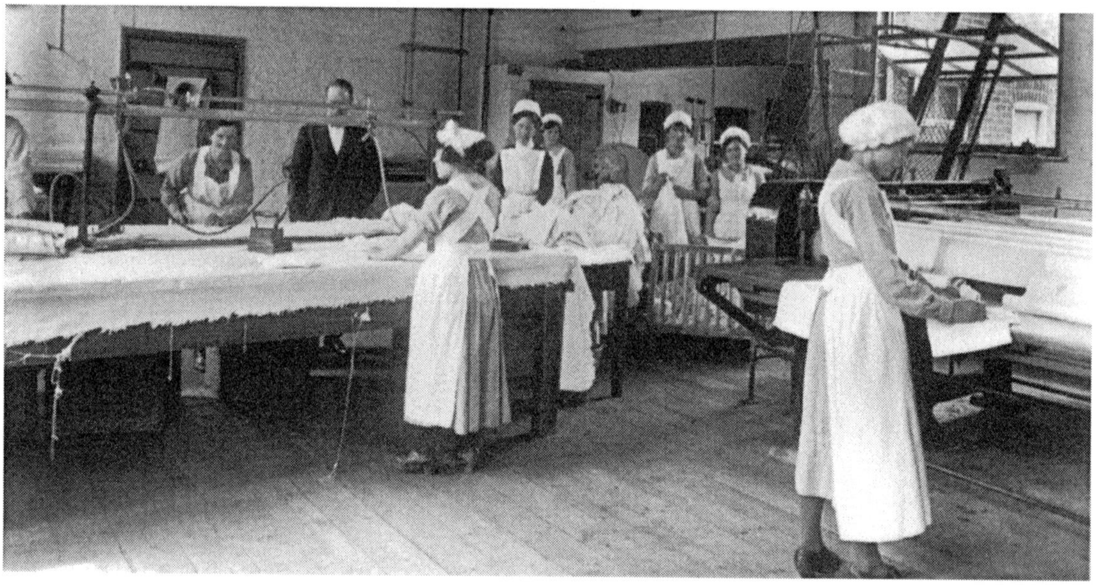

65. The hospital laundry c.1931. Mrs Sarah Mitchell (centre, back to camera) told the Brighton Hospitals Bulletin (August 1969, shortly after her retirement) that there were 8 women in the laundry when she first worked there. 'Hours were from 7am to 7pm. all for 12/- per week including food which was really good. We had to wear black shoes and stockings with our uniform or else get out!'

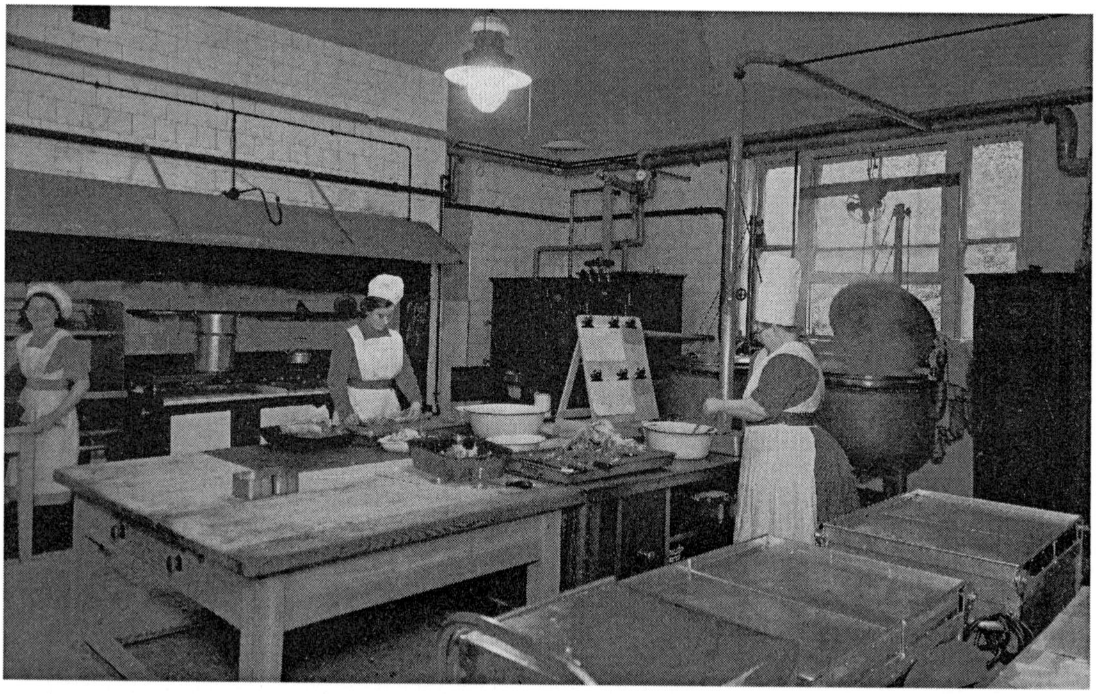

66. Kitchen staff preparing vegetables that were grown on hospital land on the opposite side of Eastern Road, part of which was used to build the new Sussex Eye Hospital in 1935.

the block, patients were to have been charged from five to nine guineas a week. The beds were to have been open to any general practitioner to have charge of his own patients and who had to select a member of the honorary staff if he required a consultation, while operations could only be performed by a member of the staff.

33 beds for inpatients and accommodation for 26 nurses were also to be included in the scheme, which, however, like the operating scheme, was held in abeyance because of the outbreak of war.

The Nursing Staff

A shortage of nurses was a major problem for hospitals in the 1920s and 1930s, although voluntary hospitals appear to have fared better than the municipal hospitals. The depression brought some improvement as girls who could not afford the expensive outlay needed to qualify in other professions turned to the nurse training schools. The situation deteriorated as the economic situation improved and in 1937 the Athlone Committee found that the shortage was worse for trained nurses than probationers.[7]

A nurse at the Sussex County in the early part of the Thirties worked a 56-hour week with three hours off duty during the day and a day off each

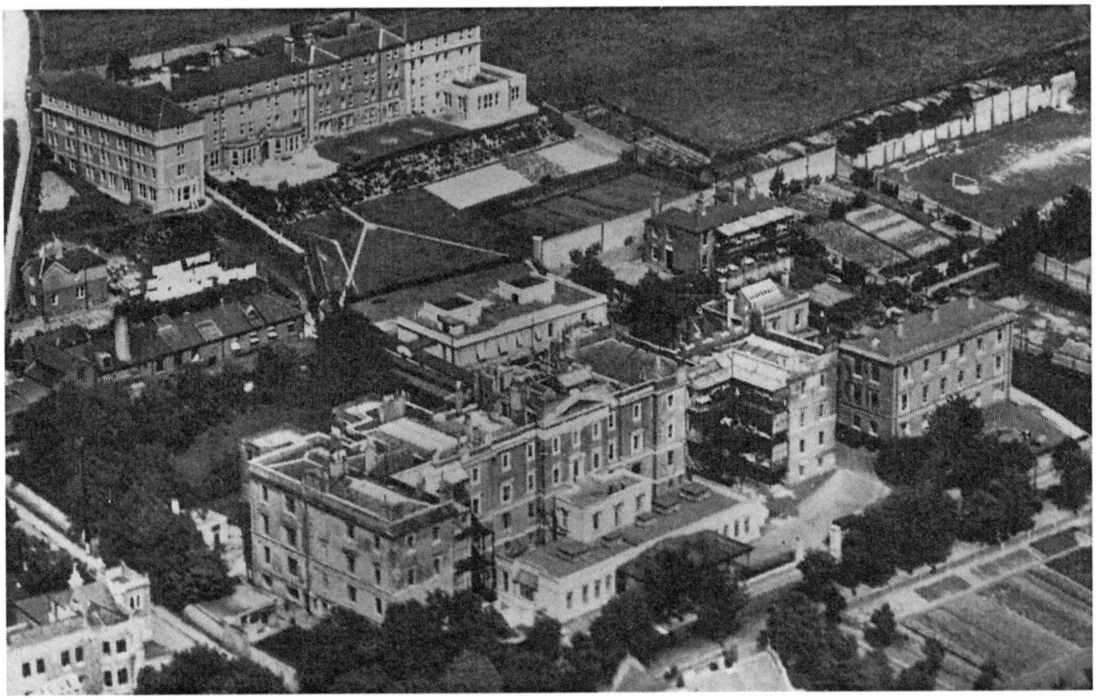

67. A picture postcard showing an aerial view of the hospital in the 1930s.

week. Night duty was longer and harder: eleven hours on duty with meals eaten in the ward kitchen.

> When on day duty, we should be called at 6am. Beds had to be stripped and the mattress turned before re-making. Our bedrooms had to be neat and tidy at all times. We had to be in our own rooms by 10pm and lights out by 10.30pm. While on duty we were not allowed to wear any make up or nail varnish. Nails had to be short. As little hair as possible should be shown. No fancy pins or slides should be worn.[8]

The conditions under which the nurses at the hospital worked were, as a result of the Athlone report and the consequent press publicity, 'much in the minds of the Governors,' according to the 1937 annual report. Although there had never been any shortage of suitable candidates for training, recommendations during the preceding years had been approved by the board to help ease the lot of the nurses. According to the report, duties had been reorganised, more nurses allocated to night duty, inpatient beds had been grouped into smaller nursing units, the superannuation scheme had been introduced in 1935, sisters had been given an additional week's holiday in the spring, off-duty hours had been extended and night domestic staff had been employed so that night nurses could take their midnight meals away from the wards.

Further improvements were reported in 1938 when the board stated its intention to work towards implementing a 96-hour working fortnight. A large number of nurses' bedrooms had been redecorated and complete

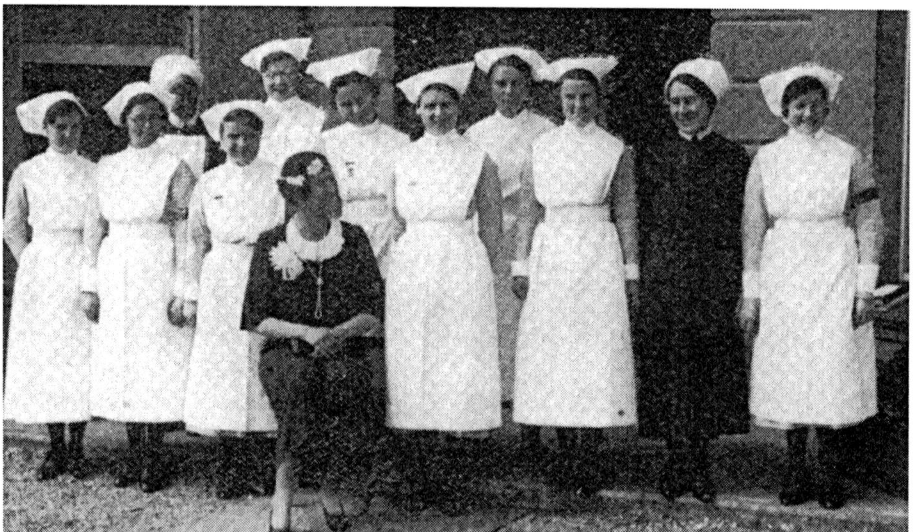

68. Prizewinners and medallists with Lady Leconsfield, president of the hospital, at the nurses' annual reunion in July 1937

new suites of 'durable bedroom furniture' purchased and plans for a new £7,000 sanitary wing had been approved. This extension would allow 13 additional bedrooms to be provided. 'A slight but practical change in the design of uniform,' suggested by Matron had been made. According to the *The Nursing Times,* dress reform was gradually changing their uniform to short sleeves and brown shoes and stockings[9], which would have replaced the black woollen stockings and black flat-heeled shoes worn earlier.[10]

Although earlier reports suggested there was no problem at the hospital with the recruitment of probationers, during 1937 the minimum age of entry for student nurses was lowered from 19 to 18 years. At the same time, young women of 17 pending acceptance for training were allowed to attend lectures 'and to do such practical work as can be conveniently arranged in their interests.'

According to the *Nursing Times:*

> Life is good for the nurses here ... they have a most comfortable home perched up behind the hospital... There is an air of comfort and solidarity about everything in the nurses' home. Outside summer tea parties use the terrace, and tennis players have a hard court at their disposal. Down on the beach is a chalet with electric plug where student nurses make tea for themselves and their elders after bathing. [11]

The article went on to describe the Sussex County as 'a happy, lively, very busy hospital'. But within a few months the idyllic scene it painted of life for the nurses was to change dramatically with the outbreak of the Second World War.

11. The Second World War

The impact of the Second World War on the hospital was even greater than that experienced during the earlier conflict in 1914: preparations prior to the outbreak of hostilities in September 1939 reflected the knowledge that hospitals had to be ready to receive not only military casualties, but civilian ones as well.

Twentieth century technological advances, especially the development of the aeroplane, meant that aerial attack became a very real threat. There was, for example, the evidence of China, where Japanese bombing had caused heavy casualties and spread panic in the cities; in Ethiopia, the Italians had added to their bombing raids the spreading of mustard gas from the air; and, finally, and probably of greatest importance, was the effect of air attacks during the Spanish Civil War in the late 1930s, especially the tragedy inflicted on Guernica in 1937 by German airplanes. This air attack on market day, Monday the 26th April, destroyed over seventy per cent of the houses and caused large numbers of casualties, a catastrophic event that is recalled in Pablo Picasso's celebrated painting bearing the name of the devastated small Basque town.

The result, in Britain, was that the fear of large numbers of casualties led to the setting up of the Emergency Medical Service (EMS) in order that a sufficient number of hospital beds could be made available for their treatment. The EMS was also expected to cope with military casualties, but it was the sheer scale of anticipated air raid casualties that was largely responsible for setting a target of beds that it was believed would be needed, 300,000 in all.

On the 31st August 1939, Hitler ordered an attack on Poland. On that day, although Britain was not yet at war with Germany, the evacuation of women and children from London began, a large number coming to Sussex. To make room for the evacuation of the most serious patients from central London, including Guy's and St Thomas's hospitals, the County was immediately faced with the task of discharging a number of patients to their homes where possible or alternatively to other institutions. 120 beds were set up in the wards bringing the total available to 395, of which 250 were designated as 'casualty beds' under the EMS scheme, and 164 patients from London were received on Friday the 1st September. According to a reporter who visited the new arrivals a few days later, the patients on Sister

Ainsworth's men's medical ward ' lay back in their comfortable beds and breathed the invigorating air. One, a little fellow with a shock of grey hair grinned cheerfully when I asked whether he was contented. He said: "Lady, it's almost worth a war to be ill in such a grand place." '[1]

This was not the end of the matter, however. Precautions had to be taken against the possibility of enemy air attack. These included the need to black out 1,496 windows, an expense for which the hospital was to be responsible just like ordinary citizens living in their homes. 865 of the hospital windows were not normally fitted with blinds: in any event, to be really effective the blinds had not only to stop light escaping, they also had to allow for ventilation and for the use of the powerful lights needed to carry out surgical procedures. The outside of the building had to be protected with blast walls and sandbags. 750 tons of sand was delivered to the hospital and staff and volunteers, who included some of the children evacuated from London, filled the bags. The National Radium Commission advised that a bore hole 50 feet deep for the safe storage of radium was essential and 'the unheralded and unwelcome addition to the hospital's costs,' was fortunately avoided when a board member presented a cheque for £100 as a 'thank you' offering for the maintenance of his health by members of the medical staff.[2] A first aid post with a mobile unit attached, managed by the town's medical officer of health, was set up in the outpatients department. and the old physiotherapy department was turned into a gas decontamination unit in charge of Dr Windle.

The fear of gas attacks had led to the distribution of gas masks to the entire population, including special masks for babies, but there remained the threat of mustard gas and the decontamination unit was established to meet this eventuality. Practices carried out under instruction from the War Department were described by Dr Windle:[3]

> 'Casualties' were brought in to the Unit by ambulance. The entrance ... was on the south side of the existing X-ray department and the stretchers were taken through a light lock. The 'casualties' had to be undressed by workers wearing heavy mackintosh clothing, gum boots and thick rubber gauntlets. This was extremely difficult. They were then wheeled into the Unit itself where they were thoroughly hosed down by physiotherapists, who wore bathing dresses and mackintosh aprons.

Ironically, it was not until about a year later, Dr Windle recalled, that it was found these precautions were entirely unnecessary. All that was required was the use of anti-mustard ointment.

Another problem was posed by patients confined to wards on the upper floors. Most hospitals attempted to deal with this by treating seriously ill

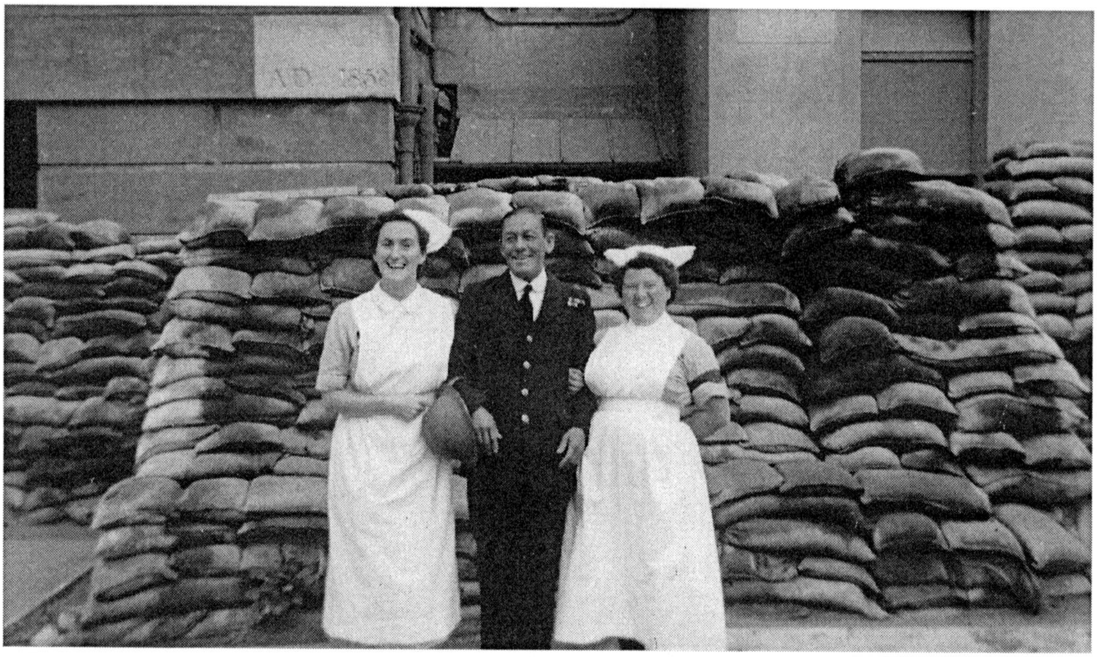

69. Thousands of sandbags were placed around the hospital as part of the air raid precautions undertaken when war broke out.

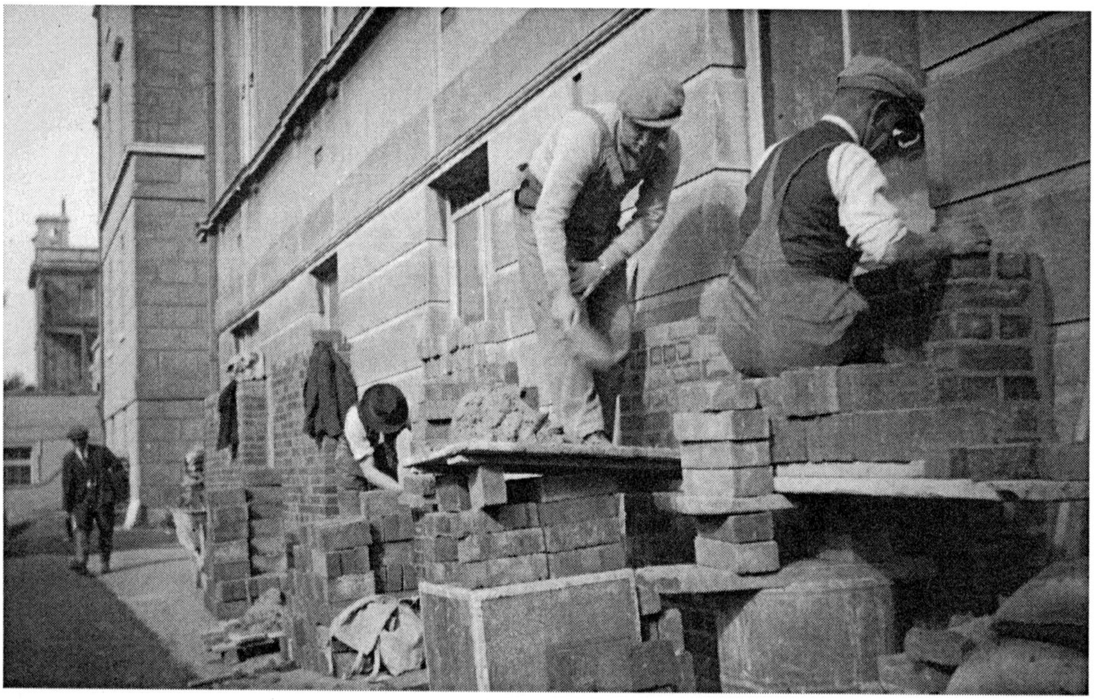

70. Workmen erecting blast walls outside the Barry Building that were another of the precautions taken against air raids. These also included blacking out the hospital's 1,496 windows.

and bedbound patients as near the ground floor as possible, and the County was no exception. Wherever possible, only ambulant patients were treated on the top floor wards. Nevertheless, the hospital had to devise a method of evacuating patients from the upper floors in the event of an emergency. In addition to using lifts, patients were also carried down the flights of stairs. To do this, the bedclothes were turned over the patient in bed, leaving the edges of the mattress free. A rope was tied over the patient's chest and pulled tight to the sides of the mattress, then tied below the patient's knees to form a cocoon in which four nurses could manoeuvre the patient down the stairs.

This evacuation drill was carried out during the blackout once a week using live 'patients'. It was so successful that nurses were able to clear a ward in ten minutes, and sometimes staff from other hospitals attended to witness the procedure.[4]

Civilian casualties were regularly brought into the hospital following the air raids on Brighton and Hove. Although the twin towns were never a target for large bombing raids such as those experienced by London, Portsmouth or Plymouth, for example, this part of the south coast suffered numerous so-called 'tip-and-run' raids. There were 56 air raids on Brighton borough between July 1940 and March 1944. 198 people were killed, 350 seriously injured and 433 slightly inured, a total of 988. In Hove, 24 civilians and six service personnel lost their lives, the total casualties being 190 civilians and seven service personnel.[5]

The hospital received its first civilian casualties following the first air raid on the 15th July 1945 when a single German bomber dropped nine bombs in the space of a little more than two minutes before flying back out to sea. (It later returned and dropped more bombs on Hove). Bristol Gardens and Whitehawk Road were among the streets near the County where the bombs landed, demolishing six houses and seriously damaging about 30 more. Two people died: one on his way to the hospital and the other died there the following day. Four others suffered serious injuries, but later recovered, three in the Sussex County and the other in the Sussex Eye Hospital.[6]

Possibly the worst raid by a single aircraft followed two months later on September 14th when adults and children were attending a Saturday afternoon matinee in the Odeon Cinema, just a few yards down the road from the hospital.[7] It was so close that the sister on Howard ward, who was resting in the nurses' home, looked out of the window and saw two bombs falling and thought they were going to hit the hospital. She later recalled the scene when she ran down to the hospital and saw the ambulances arriving:

> Most of the children were carried up by all and sundry: children with shattered limbs, guts hanging out, screaming; some were dead on arrival, there were bodies everywhere: on beds, on the floor, some cradled in the arms of passers by.[8]

The incident provided a severe test for the staff especially when parents and grandparents of the children began to arrive to add to the chaos. Three days later, a letter from Dr Donald Hall appeared in the *Sussex Daily News*. He praised the courage of the victims and recalled how the doctors and nurses had worked far into the night to deal with the casualties. He also enclosed £50 for the relief fund that had been set up for the victims.[9]

The hospital had to deal with many more air raid victims during the course of the war but the most unusual concerned a 20-year old naval rating, Henry Coates from HMS Vernon. He had been wounded during a hit-and-run raid by a lone Messerschmitt and admitted with what was recorded as a wounded leg.

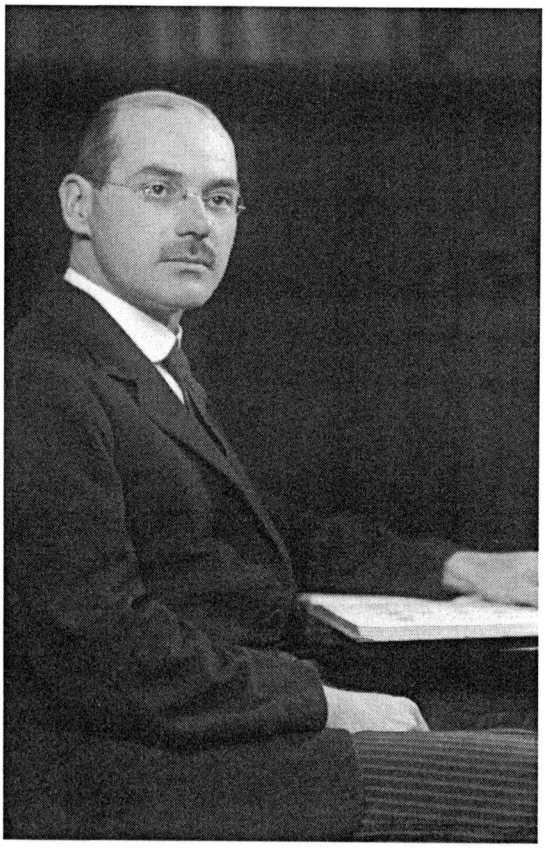

71. Surgeon Mr C.W. Beresford, who performed the dangerous 'miracle' operation on a sailor with an unexploded shell in his thigh.

Dr Donald Hall briefly related the ensuing 'thrilling and unexpected episode in the hospital's daily work with the "miracle" story that made the front pages of every newspaper in the country'. Speaking at a bazaar held in the Dome and Corn Exchange in aid of the hospital, Dr Hall said:

> Among the casualties from a south coast air raid admitted to one of our surgeons was a man with an injured thigh. X-rays disclosed that embedded in the tissues was an unexploded cannon shell.
>
> What was to be done? If the shell exploded, at best the man's thigh must be shattered and he must lose his limb – very likely his life. If it exploded during the operation for its extraction, there was a great risk to the surgeon and his assistant – almost the probability of their eyesight being injured and almost everyone in the operating theatre being wounded. The bomb disposal squad were consulted and they didn't know what to do. They had never heard of such a case.
>
> There was no hesitation on the part of the surgeon or his assistant, or the anaesthetist, or the nurses. And swiftly and successfully that surgeon of ours performed the most delicate and most dangerous operation of his career.[10]

A more colourful account headlined 'Surgeons Risk Death taking Live Shells from Patients' appeared in an Australian women's magazine. This identified the surgeon dealing with 'the delayed action time bomb' as C.W. Beresford and the four nurses present as 'Tall, slim theatre sister Page, blonde, buxom nurse Howard, petite brunette anaesthetist Anne Roulston and 18-year old probationer nurse Randall.' It quoted Sister Page as saying: 'It was just routine. There was noting heroic about it … it was a normal extraction of a bullet, of which we've had plenty of experience.' Another quote from chairman Dr Donald Hall emphasised: 'It is the duty of the hospital to take risks to save lives, and we're all in the front line here.' Then, under a crosshead 'Brave Charwoman', the story continued: 'Elderly grey-haired Miss Florence White (one of two sisters working at the hospital) [was] on duty when the patient was brought in, and even though she knew he was virtually a delayed action bomb, made him a cup of tea and held the cup while he drank it.[11]

There were not enough empty beds to accommodate the first five military casualties in the spring of 1940. They were naval personnel admitted from St Valery en Caux, some forty miles of Dunkirk, who had been blown up while attempting to rescue soldiers from the beach. They had been landed at Newhaven and transferred to Brighton by ambulance. Three civilian patients had to be discharged early, as there were only two available empty beds at the time. Soon after, the first major military challenge to the hospital was encountered as a result of the retreat from Dunkirk.

Four convoys of 105 seriously wounded solders were admitted. Mingled with the soldiers were a few French and Belgian civilians: one of these at the County, according to a local newspaper, was a Belgian peasant woman with gunshot wounds. There was an immediate appeal for magazines, periodicals, cigarettes, tins of sweets, handkerchiefs, games, writing pads, shaving mirrors and razor blades for the troops. The hospital's special needs included a wireless set for one of the wards, cash to buy newspapers for its 'numerous wounded patients', as well as fruit and cakes.[12]

At the monthly meeting of the management board the following week, the chairman, Dr Donald Hall, said that despite the short notice the wounded, who included many serious cases, were speedily admitted to the wards. Waiting list patients were not admitted for a short time and the children's ward, thanks to the co-operation of the Royal Alexandra Children's Hospital, was converted to receive adult cases.

According to Sister Howard (sisters were known by the names of their wards at that time):

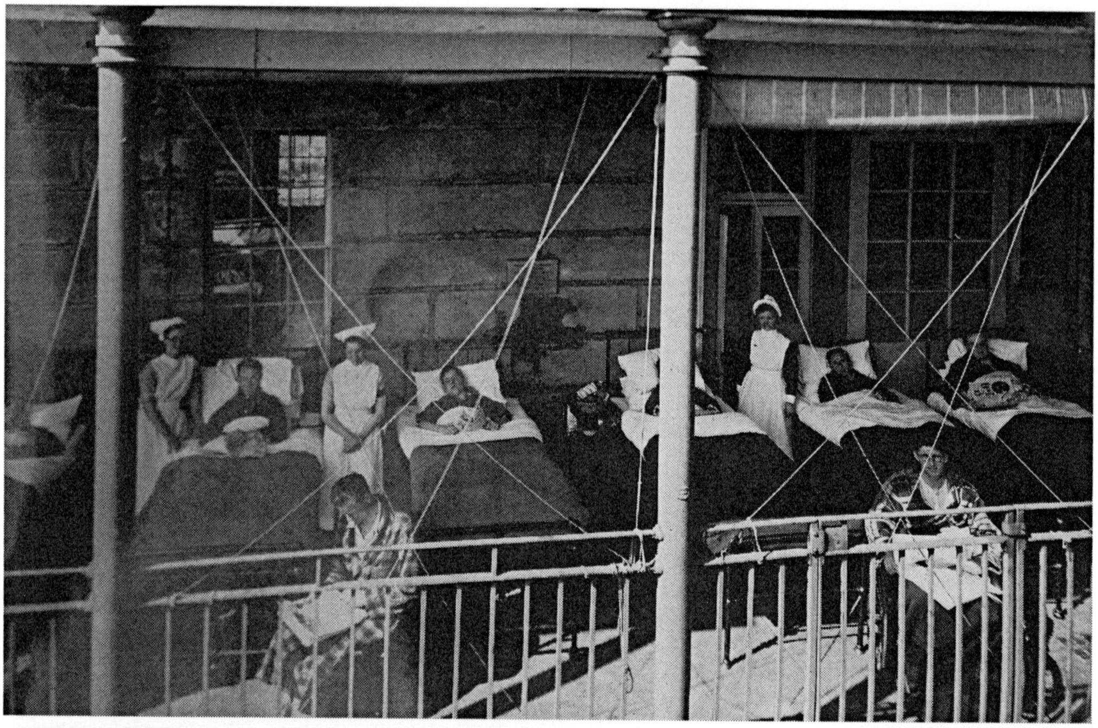

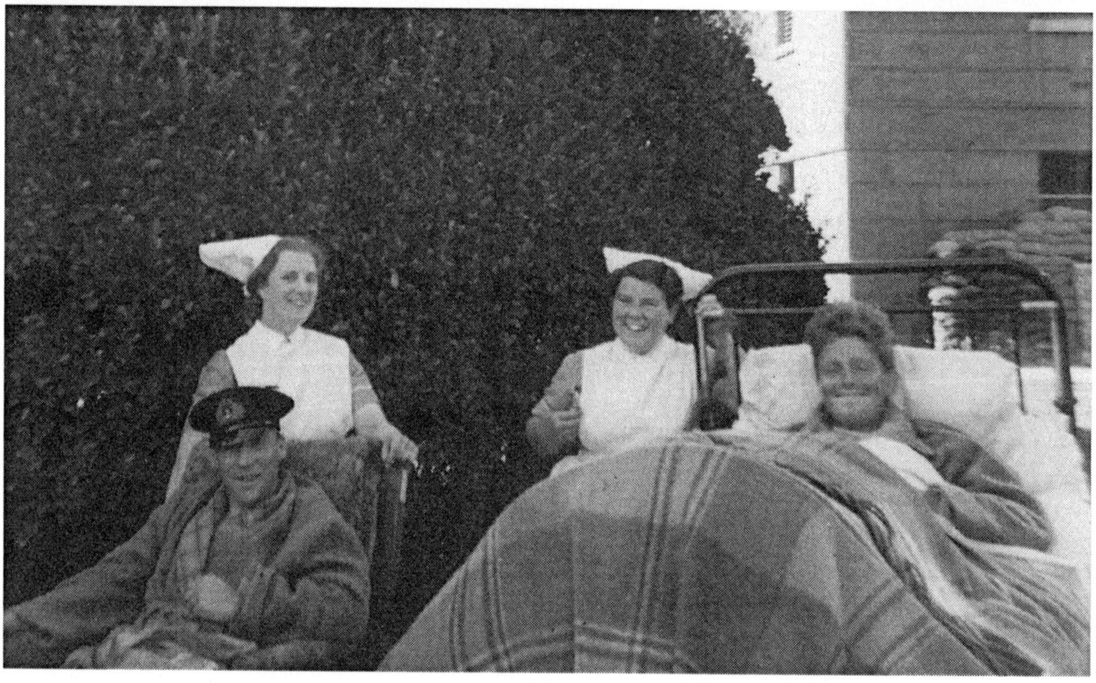

72. Weather permitting, wounded soldiers were moved out in their beds onto the balcony where the fresh air was believed to be especially beneficial for those with respiratory conditions and (below) a wounded soldier who has been wheeled out into the hospital grounds.

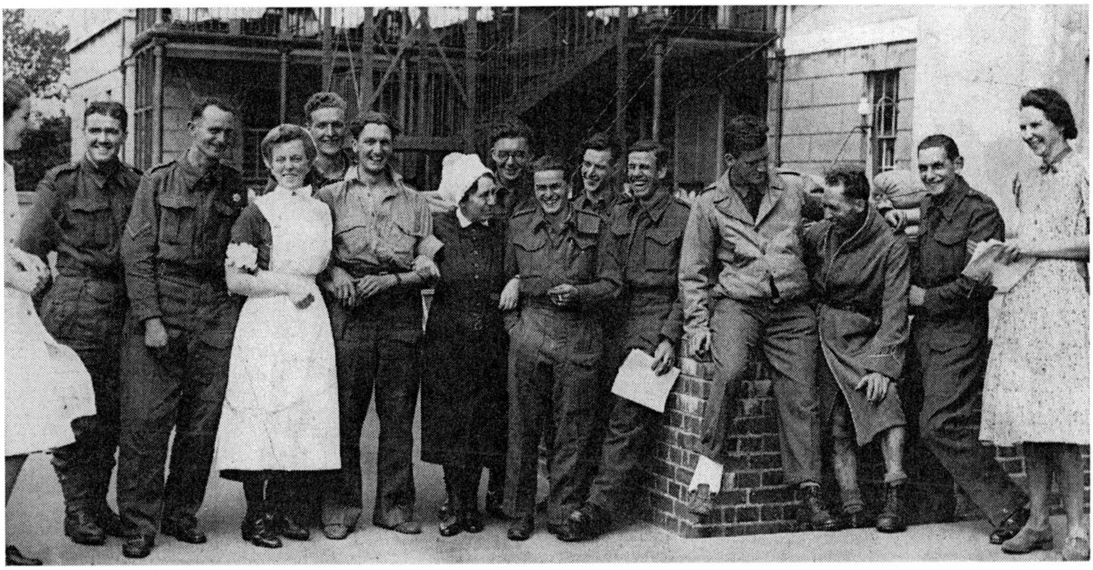

73. The matron, Miss Young, is in the centre of this group of soldiers from the Dieppe raid in 1942. On the right is one of the volunteers who provided invaluable help to the hospital during the war years.

> The men, all of them wounded, some very badly, had been waiting on the beaches of Dunkirk for two, three, four and even five days, waiting to be picked up and brought back to the south coast by the flotilla of small ships. The men, still in their uniforms, unable to move, had not seen a lavatory for days: I shall never forget the sight and smell that hit me for the first time I went over to the main wards ... The hospital was full to overflowing and the medical staff stretched beyond its limit ... As soon as the men were patched up and could be moved, they were transferred to military hospitals up and down the country.[13]

However, this was not the only occasion during which military patients were admitted in large numbers. In August 1942, the ill-fated raid on the Normandy town of Dieppe took place and the following day the survivors, many of them Canadians, were landed at Newhaven. Censorship meant that the full extent of the hospital's activities in connection with the EMS was not revealed until the end of the war. In the annual report for 1945, published early in 1946, it was revealed that 7,390 patients had been treated, including 352 air raid casualties. In addition, there were 57,995 attendances in the outpatient departments, including 3,222 by 435 air raid casualties.

One of the difficulties faced by the hospital during the war was the departure of a number of the honorary medical and surgical staff on military service. The first to go, in 1940, were physician, Dr C. Barrington Prowse, orthopaedic surgeon Mr R. Brooke, anaesthetist Dr J.E.C. Rouse, Dr G.H. Harper-Smith, medical officer to the early nervous disorders department, gynaecological and surgical registrar Mr Leslie Lauste and surgical registrar Mr G.A. Fraser.

Major Brooke was awarded the O.B.E. (Military Division) for gallant and distinguished service. Major Lauste was made a prisoner of war following the fall of France in 1940. He had declined the opportunity of being evacuated and returned from the coast to rejoin his unit to look after the wounded for which he was awarded the military M.B.E. Sadly Major Rouse was killed in action in 1941.

Assistant physician Dr H.G. McGregor was commissioned with the Royal Army Medical Corps (RAMC) in 1941 and was followed in 1942 by assistant physician Dr R. Kemball Price, dermatologist Dr J. H. Twiston Davies, Dr Windle, ophthalmologist Mr E.V. Oulton, surgical registrar and acting assistant surgeon Mr J.C.F. Lloyd Williamson, medical registrar Dr H.I.C. Balfour and temporary clinical assistant anaesthetist Dr F.R. Gusterton. Others who served during the war included medical registrar Dr John Beynon, clinical assistant anaesthetist Dr Rex Binning and Dr A.E. Drynan who was killed during active service as Colonel-in-charge of the 21st Eastern General Hospital.

The absence of these members of the honorary staff threw a considerable burden on those remaining. To some extent, this was alleviated by a number of temporary appointments and by medical officers from the RAMC and other services stationed locally. Dr Donald Hall, who had resigned as

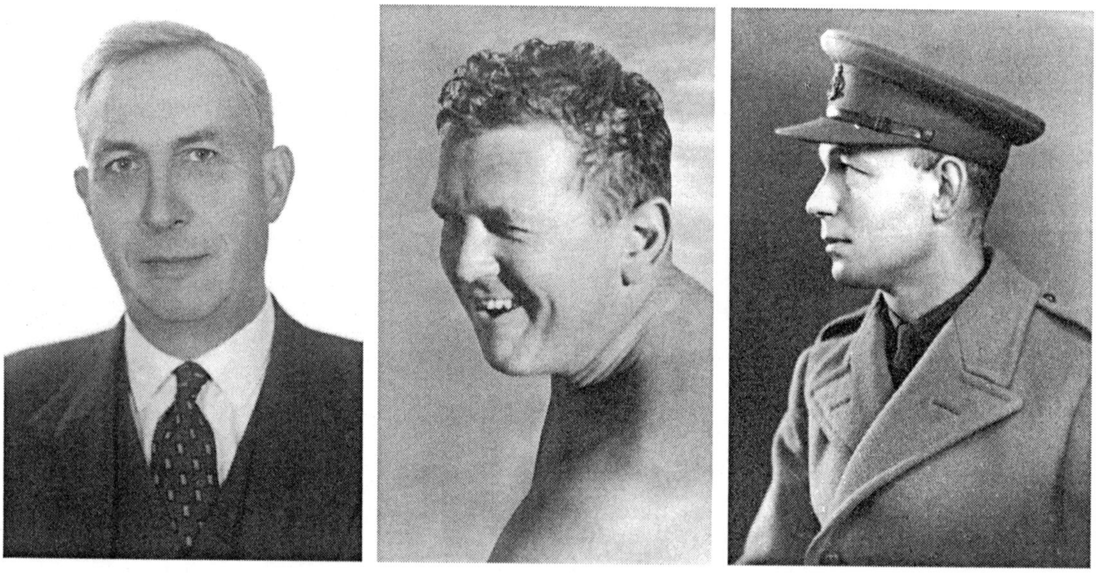

74. Two wartime medical medal winners; surgeons Mr Lauste and Mr Brooke and (right) physician Dr Rouse, who lost his life in action early in the war.

a clinician in order to concentrate on his role as chairman of the management board in 1938 resumed his professional duties as clinician in 1939. Like the rest of society, many women stepped in to fill the gaps left by the men away on war service: at the County Hospital they included medical registrar Dr Gladys Wauchope who took over Dr McGregor's outpatient work, dermatologist Dr Elizabeth Hunt, clinical assistant anaesthetist Dr Daphne Veale, gynaecological registrar Dr Constance Beynon and Miss Constance Mary Ottley.

In July 1946 a memorial tablet Roll of Honour for the five members of staff who gave their lives during the war was unveiled in the hospital chapel. It recorded the names of Miss V.M.S. Jones, QAIMNS, who was killed while working as principal matron in the Far East; Major J.E.C.Rouse, RAMC and Colonel A.E. Drynan, RAMC, and two members of the clerical staff, Sgt. Pilot J. Homewood, RAF, and Flight Lieutenant W. F. Barton. RAF.

Developments

It was not until the partial relaxation of certain wartime restrictions and air raid precautions in 1944 that the board was able to give serious consideration to the development of the hospital, which had been put on hold with the outbreak of hostilities. Even then, little progress could be made, any building work being subject to the issue of licences for the release of labour or materials. There was, however, one notable exception: during the war years the Latilla department continued to develop. By 1944, the original

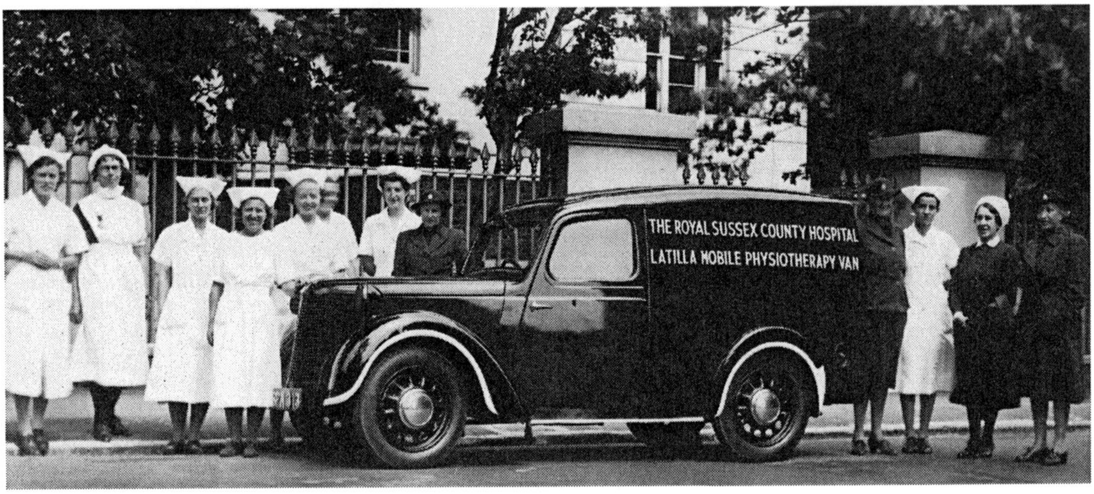

75. The Austin van that was used to provide physiotherapy treatment initially in four centres in Sussex, Newhaven, Hurstpierpoint, Woodmancote and Lancing. Steyning and Lewes were added later. It was provided with batteries for use when mains power was not available. The matron is pictured (right) with two of the Women's Voluntary Service members who acted as drivers.

massage department had continued its development from massage and electrical department, to physiotherapy department, department of physical medicine and finally to become the Latilla Rehabilitation Unit. Along the way the word 'massage' was dropped from the title of their professional body because it no longer played more than a relatively small part in current practice and the masseuses were now known as physiotherapists. When Mrs Latilla presented the hospital with an eight horse power Austin van in 1941 to take treatment to hospital patients in the country districts, it bore the legend: The Royal Sussex County Hospital Latilla Physiotherapy Van. It was equipped with apparatus for faradism, galvanism, ultra-violet and infra-red treatment, wax baths and sinusoidal current.

The following year an occupational therapy section was formally opened by the mayor in the upper floors of the Latilla building as part of the process of developing the unit into a rehabilitation centre. In 1943, urged to develop the unit still further by the Ministry of Health (although not accompanied by any funding) steps were taken to continue the expansion. Experts from the Ministry were closely involved in the planning of the development which one Ministry representative hoped would soon be running 'as further evidence of the progressiveness of the Royal Sussex County Hospital.'

The official opening by Lord Horder, president of the British Association of Physical Medicine, took place early the following year on 21st February. Lord Horder spoke of the rapid development of physical medicine that had taken place since the war while the chief medical advisor to the rehabilitation department of the Ministry congratulated the hospital, which, he said 'had been in the vanguard of the movement to establish similar departments throughout the country'.

To help in setting up these departments in Sussex and Hampshire and some other parts of the country, the Latilla department's sister, Miss K. Ward, was appointed by the Ministry to act in advisory capacity for six months while further recognition of the hospital's achievement was evidenced in one of a series of illustrated articles on the pioneering work in the field of rehabilitation in a leading hospital journal.[14]

In 1944, practical moves were taken to prepare for a reallocation of the hospital's 376 beds between medical and surgical cases and the re-establishment of the children's ward.

Approval was given to a plan to construct cubicles in surgical outpatients that would provide better facilities for the surgeons and gynaecologists and greater comfort for patients attending their clinics. Funds were provided by

Mrs G. Wisden and the approval of the Ministry of Health was obtained. However, progress was delayed while the approval of the Ministry of Works and Buildings was sought for the materials to be used. The board also sanctioned a reorganisation in the reception and treatment of outpatients aimed at reducing the time patients had to wait for their consultation with the surgeon or physician. This finally bore fruit in February 1945 when an appointments system was introduced and ended what a Hove general practitioner called 'the long, weary hours of waiting and [would] give great joy and relief to patients.' In some other hospitals in the area, he claimed, patients were waiting from three to six hours to be seen.[15]

Also in 1944, improvements were made affecting in-patients. A wartime regulation made in July 1943 restricted the number of friends and relatives visiting patients to a maximum of two on any *one visiting day.* This was relaxed reverting to the peacetime requirement of not more than two visitors *at the bedside.* More importantly, perhaps, was the attempt to secure improvements in the organisation of the patients' day. For a long time the pressure of the heavy medical, nursing and domestic workload had resulted in the day beginning 'at an early hour'. From June, this began a full two hours later. Advice was also sought from the Ministry of Health and the ministries of Food and Labour relating to catering for patients and staff.

Rising Costs

The financial situation continued to cause concern throughout the war years. Looking back in the 1939 annual report, the governors noted that it was the fourth successive year the hospital had depended on the receipt of legacies to cover running costs. Expenditure in 1939 reached a record high of £59,000 and by 1945 had almost doubled to just over £101,000.

The governors, concerned for the future, called for an increase in 'dependable income' in the 1939 report. Already, with the war just three months old, some reliance was being placed on payments from the Ministry of Health in connection with the EMS scheme. Presenting the report in March 1940, Dr Donald Hall said the hospital now came under the control of the Ministry of Health and added he found the Ministry 'a kind master and regular payer.'[16] Possibly this was not the wisest statement to make because later in the report for 1940 the governors declared that the belief in some quarters that the hospital was now 'subsidised by the state' was 'was misleading to those whose voluntary support is still so much needed.'

One of the more reliable sources of income, the annual fundraising fair, was an early casualty of the war. In 1938, the Sussex Market and Yuletide

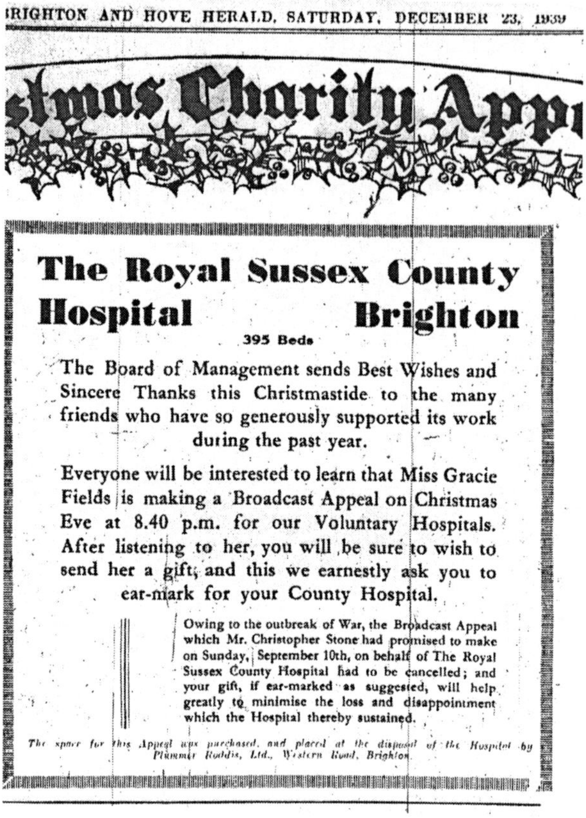
BRIGHTON AND HOVE HERALD, SATURDAY, DECEMBER 23, 1939

stmas Charity Appe

The Royal Sussex County Hospital Brighton

395 Beds

The Board of Management sends Best Wishes and Sincere Thanks this Christmastide to the many friends who have so generously supported its work during the past year.

Everyone will be interested to learn that Miss Gracie Fields is making a Broadcast Appeal on Christmas Eve at 8.40 p.m. for our Voluntary Hospitals. After listening to her, you will be sure to wish to send her a gift, and this we earnestly ask you to ear-mark for your County Hospital.

Owing to the outbreak of War, the Broadcast Appeal which Mr. Christopher Stone had promised to make on Sunday, September 10th, on behalf of The Royal Sussex County Hospital had to be cancelled; and your gift, if ear-marked as suggested, will help greatly to minimise the loss and disappointment which the Hospital thereby sustained.

The space for this Appeal was purchased, and placed at the disposal of the Hospital by Plummer Roddis, Ltd., Western Road, Brighton.

76. The cancelled 1939 Royal Sussex County Hospital Christmas broadcast appeal was an early wartime casualty so readers of the Brighton and Hove Herald were urged to support a general Christmas Eve Appeal for voluntary hospitals, ear-marking their gift for the County.

Fair held in the Dome and Corn Exchange raised over £1,523. In 1939, the event, now named a Christmas Market, was transferred to rooms in the Grand Hotel and raised only half that amount, about £800, and the following year the total fell to £770. However in 1941 there was a return to something like normal, a two-day Michaelmas Market in the Corn Exchange raising £1,179 and the following year's Hive of Industry and Horticultural Show realised £2,000. A steady improvement in results followed and reached a record total of £5,357 at the Great Expectations Market at the end of the war.

Subscriptions throughout the war years, which might be considered 'dependable income' were fairly constant in the region of £3,500 a year and reached £3,776 in 1945.

In 1943, voluntary income, on which along with legacies the financial health of the hospital depended, totalled £13,704, an increase of £2,569 over the previous year. The Golden Penny League remained a significant contributor, providing £2,516 of the total and the following year the annual report recorded that in the years to 1944 the total raised by the league had reached £17,751. Flag Days and, despite rationing, Pound Days continued to contribute to voluntary income. In addition, the Sussex Provident Scheme was contributing over £11,000 to hospital funds.

At the end of 1945, the final year of the war, the appeals department in Paston Place, 'led by the effective energies of the Hospital's Appeals Organiser, Miss Lilian Martin', was able to announce a record total of voluntary subscriptions of £23,547, an increase of £9,136 over the previous year. However, this included a donation of £3,000 by Mr D.J. James to enable a wing of Egremont ward to be converted for use as a children's ward, which was to be named 'Catherine James' in memory of his mother and formally opened in October 1946. A sum of £1,000 was donated by HMS Vernon for services to the ship's personnel during the war. (Vernon, the Royal Navy's torpedo, mining and electrical training establishment had requisitioned and moved to Roedean girls' school in May 1941, following the bombing of Portsmouth Harbour).

HMS Forward and HMS Aggressive were also associated with this gift. Smaller donations were received from HMS Lizard (£370), HMS King Alfred (£100) and South African forces in Brighton (£25). The total amount of voluntary collections for the year also included the annual box collections (£980), congregational collections (£272) and workmen's collections (£179).

Thanks in no small part to all the voluntary contributions received during the year, it ended with a deficit of only £2,440 but once again it was left to the receipts from bequests to balance the books and, in fact, actually show a surplus of £3,743.

Nursing

Like their medical colleagues, members of the nursing staff performed important roles during the war. Many nurses who had trained at the hospital served with the army, air force and naval nursing services or worked in areas of special danger in civil hospitals in Gibraltar, Malta and elsewhere in the colonies. In addition, a number of nurses temporarily left their posts at the hospital in the early years of the war to undertake active service.

Those nurses who remained worked under considerable pressure and were helped at first by members of the Civil Nursing Reserve and throughout by auxiliary nurses and volunteers. The hospital had been one of the first in the district to train auxiliary nurses, a hundred of

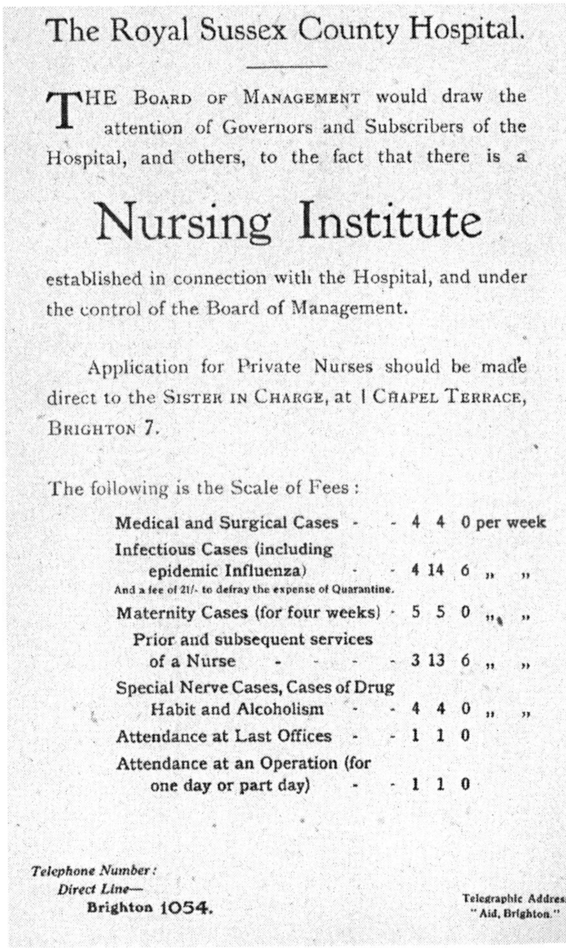
The Royal Sussex County Hospital.

THE BOARD OF MANAGEMENT would draw the attention of Governors and Subscribers of the Hospital, and others, to the fact that there is a

Nursing Institute

established in connection with the Hospital, and under the control of the Board of Management.

Application for Private Nurses should be made direct to the SISTER IN CHARGE, at 1 CHAPEL TERRACE, BRIGHTON 7.

The following is the Scale of Fees:

Medical and Surgical Cases	4 4 0 per week
Infectious Cases (including epidemic Influenza)	4 14 6 " "
And a fee of 21/- to defray the expense of Quarantine.	
Maternity Cases (for four weeks)	5 5 0 " "
Prior and subsequent services of a Nurse	3 13 6 " "
Special Nerve Cases, Cases of Drug Habit and Alcoholism	4 4 0 " "
Attendance at Last Offices	1 1 0
Attendance at an Operation (for one day or part day)	1 1 0

Telephone Number:
Direct Line—
Brighton 1054.

Telegraphic Address "Aid, Brighton."

77. This list of fees published in the annual report published in 1942 shows the range of work carried out by the Nursing Institute before its activities were suspended because of the wartime shortage of nurses the following year.

whom had completed their training and, when war broke out, there was an auxiliary nurse on duty in each ward both day and night.

In 1942, Miss Young retired as Matron after fifteen years at the hospital. She was later awarded the OBE for her services to the nursing profession and civil defence. Miss E.C. Eliott, matron of North Ormesby Hospital in Middlesborough, succeeded Miss Young. Soon after her arrival she submitted a scheme to establish a Preliminary Training School (PTS). This was opened in January 1943 in part of the Private Nursing Institute at 1 Chapel Terrace where there were now fewer nurses requiring the accommodation. The first group of twelve students commenced their eight week course in January; altogether, a total of sixty candidates entered the school during its first year. Miss Elliott resigned in March 1943 and was succeed by Miss I. Milne, Matron of Port of Spain Hospital in Trinidad, who was selected out of twenty-six candidates. Shortly after, in August, the activities of the Private Nursing Institute, which had found it impossible to retain sufficient nurses, were suspended. This meant the whole of 1 Chapel Terrace now became available for occupation by new students.

Nevertheless, a dire need for additional accommodation remained. Although the PTS met the needs of the County Hospital alone, the board hoped to receive proposals from other hospitals in the area to set up an 'economical' central school for preliminary training.

In addition, provision had to be made for a further substantial increase in the number of nurses in training in order to introduce a new 'block system' of training recommended by Lord Horder's Committee to the Ministry of Health. This was successfully accomplished shortly after the end of the war, an achievement that was to earn the hospital major coverage in the national nursing professional press.

12. *An End to Uncertainty, 1946 – 1947*

The future of the voluntary hospital system was a subject for debate for a number of years before the passing of the National Health Service Act in 1946. Even then, what the future held for the Royal Sussex County Hospital was far from certain. How would it fare in the new NHS? And what of suggestions that hospitals in Brighton should be concentrated on one site – how would it fare if, as suggested, that site should be on the edge of town at Falmer or Stanmer Park?

1946 and 1947 were the final two full years in which the County functioned as a voluntary hospital. Despite uncertainty over the future, however, it continued to develop, making up for time lost during the war and spurred on by the board's determination to hand over control to the new NHS management with the hospital as well equipped as possible.

During 1946, the surgical outpatient cubicles were constructed and put into use. Improvements to Grant Ward included the completion of altered accommodation for the reception and examination of ear, nose and throat outpatients while the beds in the ward were cubicled. The children's ward was completed and formally opened on the 7th October in the wing of Egremont and named Catherine Stewart. The Ministry of Health postponed a proposal to close in the balcony which would have increased the number of beds from 18 to 26 and provided more play space. Nevertheless, the new ward did include a number of cubicles as well as glazed screening for barrier nursing Also during the year, the wing of Defflis Ward was named Donald Hall in acknowledgment of the doctor's 43 year association with the hospital including eight successive years as chairman of the board of management. Much needed improvements also took place in the main kitchen and the laundry and at last a start was made on the exterior redecoration and repair of the buildings.

A number of other schemes which had been delayed pending Ministry of Health approval and the issue of necessary licences were completed in 1947 and included the reconditioning of York Block. Work began on modernising and enlarging the Stephen Ralli Pathological Department. While this work was in progress, the department also had to provide temporary accommodation for the nucleus of staff of another new department, the Public Health Laboratory being built in the grounds at the request of the Medical Research Council. A number of other schemes were started or planned during the year, which it was hoped would come to fruition in 1948. Plans for a completely new and more spacious diagnostic X-ray department awaited the removal of the existing building restrictions but steady progress was reported on the complete reorganisation of the radiotherapy department. This was expected to have an important role to play in the development of future cancer services of the region. The range of clinics in the outpatients department had been extended during 1946 and now included diabetic, endoscopy, varicose veins, chiropody and speech therapy. At the same time, a department of clinical photography was established under the aegis of the radiotherapy department.

All this work and planning went ahead hand in hand with the purchase of a large amount of medical and surgical apparatus and equipment intended to improve services and 'keep abreast of modern requirements' in accordance with board's policy regarding the hand over of the hospital.

Nursing

The hospital introduced the weekly block system of training on the 1st January 1946 on the recommendation of the matron, Miss Milne. It was designed to give the nurses six consecutive study days, 'long enough to settle down to some good work, and yet not keep them away from the wards for too long.' The decision to make the change showed that as in other fields, in nurse training the hospital was one of the leaders of institutions making innovative developments. As late as 1950, for example, the prestigious St. Bartholomews Hospital in London failed to introduce the system because it was found impossible to take nurses away from the wards for the necessary length of time.[1] Thanks to excellent recruitment results, this had not proved to be as problem at the County, which was in 1948 considered to be worthy of a well illustrated report over the two centre pages in one of the professional nursing journals.[2]

One of the immediate results of the introduction of the block system noted by the board was that it relieved the student nurses of strain and that this had contributed to a much lower incidence of sickness during the year. By the end of 1947, five schools were being held each year, usually of 14 or 18 students including students from Haywards Heath and Hove hospitals. This number was later increased to an average of 25 so that a new shift system for students consisting of an eight hour working day and a forty-eight hour week could be introduced. Plans were also made for the associated training of nurses with the Eliot Memorial Hospital at Haywards Heath which allowed four Brighton nurses to spend a period of three months there.

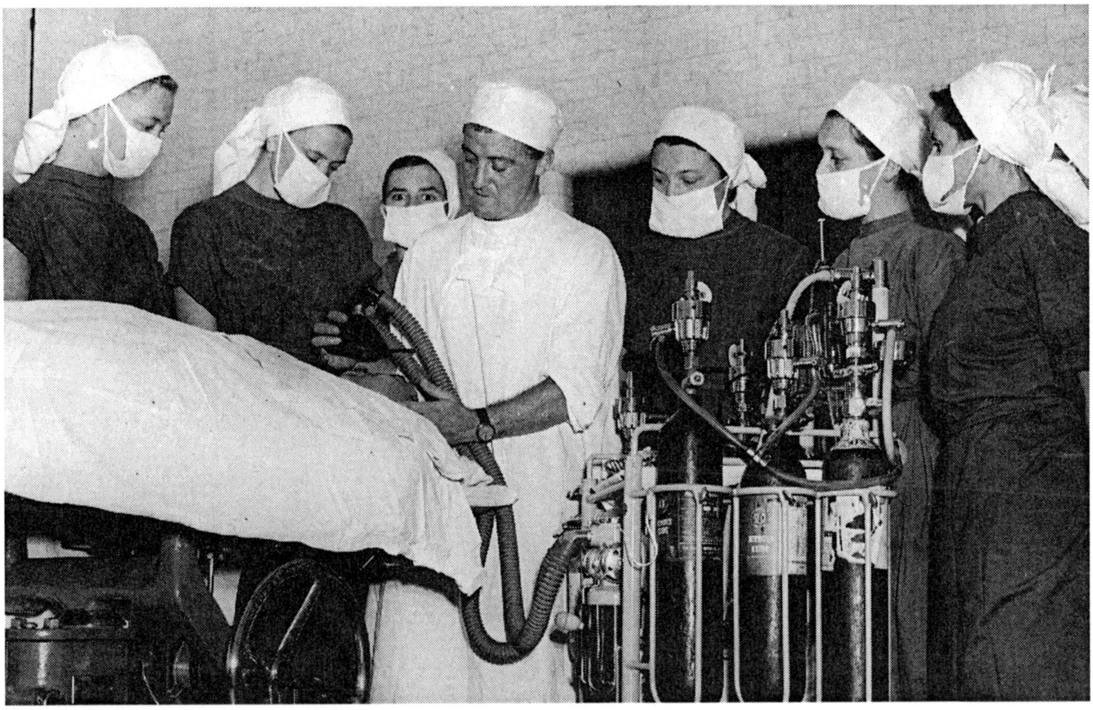

78. An anaesthetist gives a demonstration to nursing students in theatre.

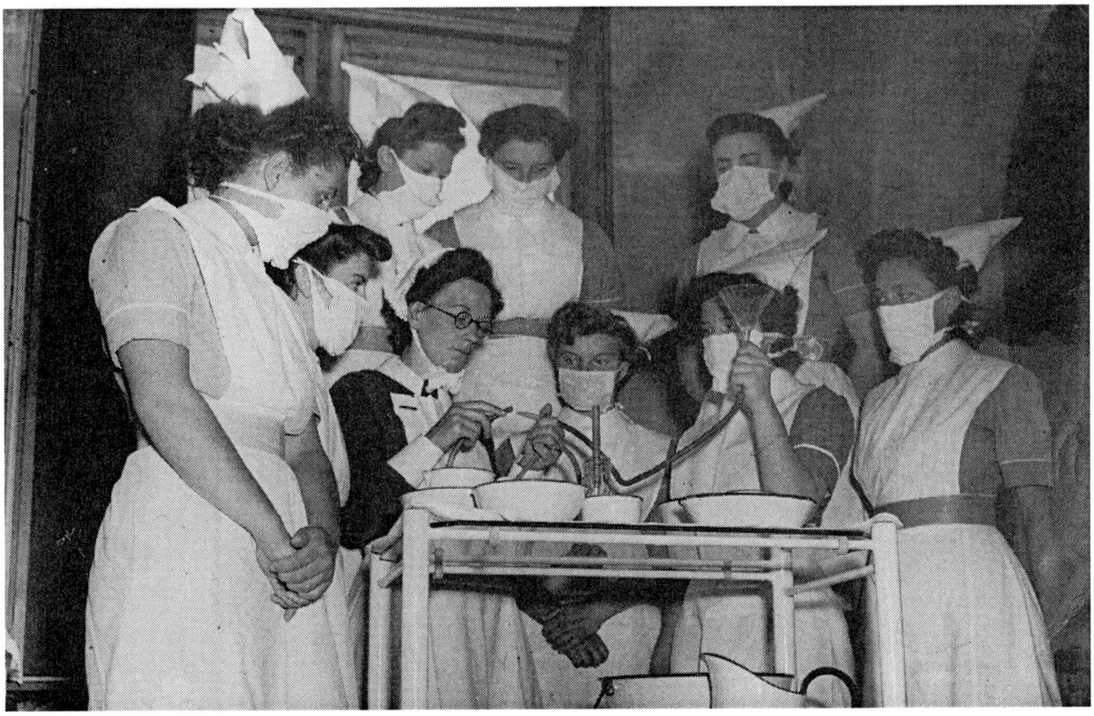

79. Sister Kirby gives practical tuition to a group of students.

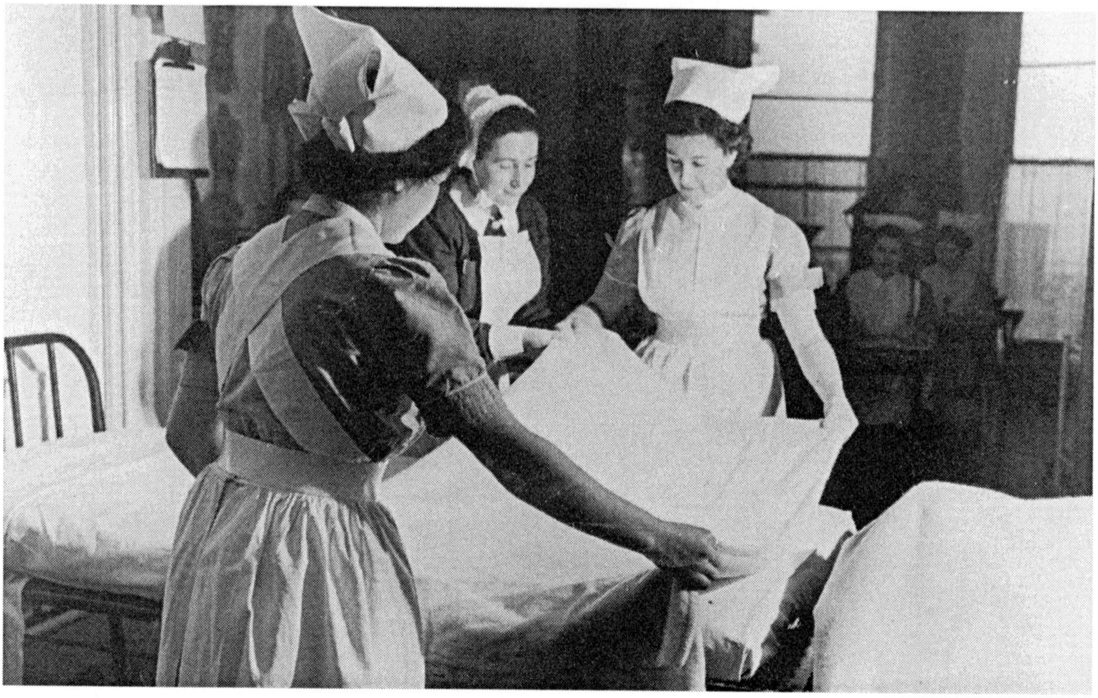

80. A demonstration of bed making.

The first nurses' reunion since the cessation of hostilities was held on the 4th July 1946 in the nurses' home. A Royal Sussex County Hospital Nurses' League was started. This was intended, said Miss Milne, to 'hold us together and keep alive the spirit and traditions of the "County".' It was also decided that the annual prize medals and badges presented to nurses completing their training would be struck to a new design in future. This would incorporate the Crown and Rose in addition to the other insignia that were officially used in the Arms of the Sussex County Hospital and General Sea Bathing Infirmary in the early years of its existence.

It had become obvious during the preceding years that with the increasing numbers of nurses, more personal accommodation was needed. Faced with the impracticability of securing permission to carry out any scheme involving an extension of the nurses' home, the board opened negotiations with the Ministry of Health in 1946 regarding the conversion of a property which they thought would be suitable as an annexe to the nurses' quarters. With financial assistance from the Ministry, 80/81 Marine Parade, formerly a small hotel, was eventually purchased and adapted into a Preliminary Training School. This provided accommodation for fifty students and included sitting and recreation rooms as well as lecture rooms and a personal laundry. The former training school then became a nurses' hostel.

Finance and the National Health Service

Not surprisingly, with the large number of repairs and renewals needed and increased salaries and wages resulting from national agreements for nurses, domestic staff, pharmacists, physiotherapists and others, as well as rising commodity prices, total maintenance expenditure in 1946 soared. It was 25 per cent higher than the preceding year, and totalled £131,950. The deficit was over £41,000 and once again was partly met by unrestricted legacies, although on this occasion these only amounted to some £8,500.

The financial situation worsened in 1947, not helped by further wage and salary increases, a general upward trend in prices and the continuing need to make up ground lost during the war years in the replacement, repair and renovation of equipment and buildings. Coupled with a diminution of voluntary income, the result was that ordinary expenditure exceeded income by nearly £100,000. Applications for grants to the Ministry of Health resulted in the receipt of £50,000 which left an overdraft of nearly £57,000 despite the receipt of legacies and selling off unrestricted investments.

Speaking to the Brighton and Hove Fabian Society in December, Mr K.I. Julian, who had succeeded Donald Hall as the board's chairman, referred to the financial deficit. It was becoming obvious, even before the war, that the voluntary system could not continue since people were prevented by taxation from contributing as generously as they did in the past, he said. At the same time, costs were rising because of 'very proper improvements for staffs and increases in their salaries'.[3]

The future organisation of the country's hospital services came under the spotlight during the Second World War just as it had during the First. On this occasion, however, it became firmly linked with proposals for social reform highlighted in the Beveridge Report of 1942 that aimed to attack the 'five giants of Want, Disease, Ignorance, Squalor and Idleness.' In the attack on disease in a reconstructed Britain, Beveridge assumed there would be a comprehensive National Health Service, including hospital treatment, freely available for the whole population and financed by insurance contributions. The effect this would have on the County was referred to by Ivor Julian in his talk to the Fabians: 'In the past there has been some class distinctions among people who used hospitals. People with incomes above a certain figure went to nursing homes. In future, hospitals will be used by a much wider section of the population.'

A survey of the national stock of hospitals in 1938 had shown that 'there was no hospital system ... instead there was a collection of individual hospitals, criss-crossed, separated, and enclosed by local government boundary barriers, legal and residential and occupational barriers, medical category and financial barriers.' In short, the hospitals were completely inadequate to the demands of war, and in June 1938 the creation of the regionally organised Emergency Medical Service effectively became the first step towards a National Health Service.[4]

So it was that the two strands came together in the National Health Act 1946: a national service organised on regional lines, financed by the state, free to all at the point of use.

What the supporters of the voluntary system had long feared, state control, had become a reality. However, some like Ivor Julian, took comfort from the possibility that the voluntary system would be continued in the control of hospitals through membership of the new hospital management committees. Referring to fears that voluntary hospitals would become 'institutionalised and lose the homely touch', he told his audience at the final fundraising fair in the Dome in October 1947: 'The hospital will be the same old firm, without the financial anxiety which has oppressed us for the last ten years.'[5]

Financial problems were also referred to at a farewell luncheon held at the Grand Hotel on the 4th July 1948 when Dr Donald Hall told his audience that the change had come about mainly because of the rising expenditure caused by what he called the prodigious improvements in the medical profession. 'We must recognise,' he said, 'although with sorrow, that the nationalisation of hospitals has become a stern necessity.'[6]

A new hospital?

A suggestion that there was a need to amalgamate the hospitals in Brighton first arose in the early part of the century, prompted by the competition for funds between the various charities. It was revived in the 1930s, prompted by the medical aspects of two Parliamentary Acts, the Local Government Act, 1929 and the Poor Law Act, 1930. The local medical profession found that none of the voluntary hospitals had sufficient beds for Brighton and Hove's population of 190,000 and that a least another 150 were needed: the time taken to clear patients off the waiting lists varied between hospitals from 10 days to three months. Among a number of proposals put forward was that the ultimate needs of the district would be met by just one 'general hospital' comprising all branches of medicine and surgery and that the existing special hospitals should be retained only temporarily or used for other purposes or even sold off.[7]

It seems unlikely that had the local British Medical Association (BMA) proposals been accepted the Royal Sussex would have been adversely affected, however this was not perhaps the case when proposals for amalgamation surfaced again in the wake of the National Health Service Act.

A preliminary report prepared by Dr Stanley Firth, medical superintendent of Brighton Municipal Hospital in Elm Grove, opened with references to the Act which permitted the Minister of Health, after consultation with the university concerned, to designate a hospital, or group of hospitals, as a teaching hospital; he also referred to the Gray/Topping Hospital Survey which called for the formation of a district hospital in Brighton, possibly around 'the nuclei provided by the Municipal and the Royal Sussex hospitals' with a single management committee.[8]

Whilst it could be argued that implementing Dr Firth's proposals would have left the County Hospital secure on its historic Eastern Road site, this need not necessarily have been the outcome – as subsequent events were to show.

In 1991 consultants argued strongly for a new hospital, which they believed, should be built on a greenfield site at Falmer. That this was a real possibility owed much to discussions some years earlier, at the outset of the NHS in 1948, when the local council was asked to reserve land on the Stammer Estate for the future development of a new hospital.

13. An N.H.S. Hospital: The Early Years

The introduction of the new National Health Service on the 5th July, 1948 did not result in the amalgamation of Brighton's hospitals. However, it did bring all the voluntary and public hospitals in the area under the control of a new body, the Brighton and Lewes Hospital Management Committee, which itself was answerable to the South East Metropolitan Hospital Board.

For administrative purposes, the thirteen hospitals and associated clinics in the Brighton and Lewes group were subdivided into a number of subgroups and as a result the County was linked with the nearby Sussex Eye Hospital and the Thomas Lye Convalescent Home. Although they shared an administrative officer (later named hospital secretary), the hospitals retained their individual matrons and separate house committees. There were also separate budgets for each unit. The County was allocated £281,630 for its first full financial year, 1949/1950, including anticipated income from private patients totalling £6,550. Howard One Ward was allocated 12 private patients in two single and five double rooms under Section 5 of the NHS Act. Howard Two included nine amenity beds under Section 4 with patients

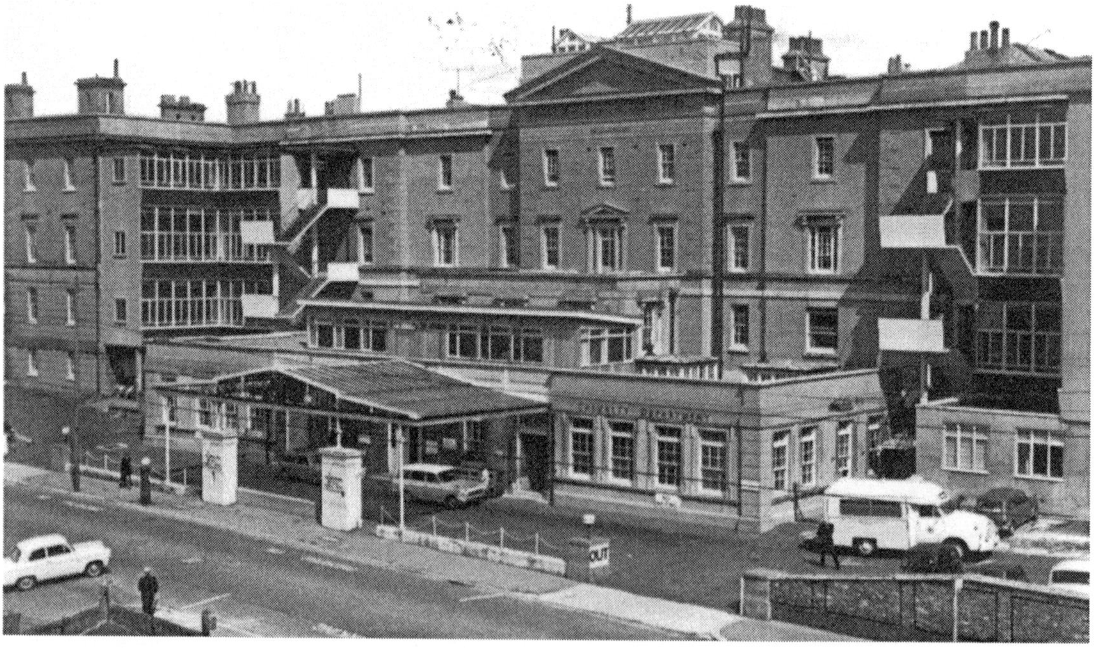

81. The hospital in the early 1950s before the ward balconies were enclosed.

paying for their accommodation but not for their medical care. The remaining four beds were used for general non-paying patients.

Another important change following the introduction of the health service was that the regional board now appointed the hospital's consultants. The board organised clinical services in various areas, one of which covered the Brighton and Lewes group and also included Mid Sussex. As a result, some consultant appointments were made jointly to both the County and Cuckfield hospitals.

The former voluntary hospital was well represented in the new organisation. Mr (later Sir) Ivor Julian became chairman of the regional board and another member of the Royal Sussex board, Mr J.C. Gaukroger, became chairman of the new group management committee while secretary/superintendent Mr F.G. Dawes was appointed as the new group secretary.

Attempts were made to harness voluntary effort to the new organisation, most notably by the formation of a league of hospital friends for the area. The league was formed in March 1949 and at an inaugural meeting held at the Grand Hotel in June. At the meeting plans were laid for a traditional fundraising event, a Fair held at the Corn Exchange on the 7th December. Twenty-seven stalls represented all the local hospitals at the event attended

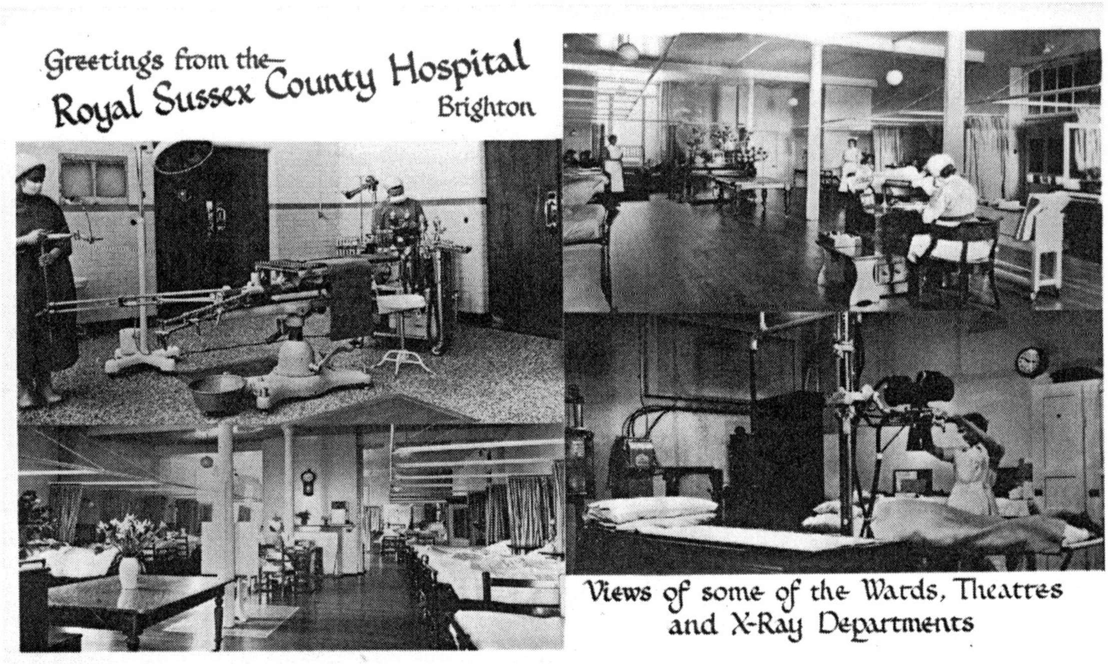

82. The hospital management committee revived the practice of allowing postcards of the wards to be produced. From the 1950s onwards they were sold from Red Cross trolleys priced 2d in aid of the League of Hospital Friends.

by 3,000 people that raised £1,561. The fair went from strength to strength and by 1954, still held in the Corn Exchange, a hospital ward 'complete with bed and patient' was erected to depict the work supported by the league.

In 1950, 'extras' provided for the benefit of patients and staff in the group included items such as bed jackets, caps for old men, card tables, confirmation veils, garden hammocks, harmoniums and wringers. Gifts specifically for the County Hospital in the early years included armchairs and Pillotones to enable patients to listen to the radio without disturbing others in the ward.

In 1956, bedpan washers were first installed in eight wards with the remainder of wards scheduled for the following year. Fifty hospital bedsteads were replaced by new beds with spring interior mattresses, an improvement on the hair mattresses previously supplied.

Endowment funds, largely made up from donations and legacies, played an important role in funding developments in the early years. Cubicle curtaining in the wards – Bristol, Overton and Egremont in 1951, and Peel, Stewart, Vallance and Jowers in 1952 were funded from endowments. £1,400 was approved for modernisation of the main outpatient department carried out in 1953 while £17,734, two thirds of the total cost, was approved for enclosing and reconstructing the ward balconies. These were officially opened on the 25th February 1956 by Professor C.W. Guillebaud, chairman of the Enquiry into the Cost of the NHS (the Guillebaud Report). Twelve additional beds became available to the hospital as a result of this scheme.

The prospect of major developments in Brighton during the first twenty years of the NHS largely depended on decisions regarding the building of a 'new' hospital, possibly by the redevelopment of the County site or alternatively a completely new building at Stanmer. In 1954, however, it was decided that 'owing to financial and other difficulties involved, detailed consideration be not given to a new Hospital at Stanmer, although its possible development could be borne in mind.'

In 1951, steps had been taken to purchase the School for Partially Sighted Boys (the Blind School) at 179 Eastern Road and while awaiting Ministry of Health approval for the purchase a sub-committee was set up to make suggestions for its future use. An early suggestion was that part of the building could be adapted as a radiotherapy department with a hostel, a gymnasium and a temporary linen room. Six months later, however, the regional board was told that there was insufficient space to form an up-to-date department and for hostel beds to be provided. It was also decided that it was unsuitable to house a linen room as it would be too far from the main building.

In 1964, the planning committee recommended that part of the site could be used to erect new buildings for a comprehensive orthopaedic, trauma and casualty unit with a minimum of 80 beds to serve the group as a whole. This was only possible because the Blind School, a four-storey, red-brick building in Venetia Gothic style had been 'needlessly demolished'[1] in 1952. According to Antony Dale[2] the demolition of the building was one of the principal architectural losses suffered by Brighton since the war. The 'diaper red and grey brickwork and ogee-headed windows and doorways gave it something of the make-believe air of the Royal Pavilion' so not surprisingly Brighton Corporation endeavoured to save the building by making a preservation order on it. However, in the case of Crown property this was not possible without the consent of the government department concerned. The Minister of Health declined to give this and the building, to the dismay of conservationists, became a casualty in the post-war expansion of the hospital.

The 1960s witnessed a number of changes at the hospital. In 1961, the so-called 'suicide steps' at the side of the main theatre were converted into rooms for the storage and preparation of radium, and also into a changing room for women doctors. By 1962, sterile supply departments were operating from rooms between Baily and Defflis wards supplying syringes, various kinds of dressings, swab packs and containers for instruments. During the year, an extensive enlargement and alterations were made to the X-ray department on the ground floor. In 1963, the hospital's endowment funds were used to upgrade Chapel Terrace, which was divided into five flatlets and five bed-sitting rooms for the sisters. During these two years, Baily, Jowers and Overton wards were also upgraded. The sluices were modernised and redesigned and to allow for the early ambulation of patients more washing facilities were made available. The existence of the central sterile department made it possible to remove the ward sterilisers leaving the wards steam free and much quieter. During 1964, Donald Hall and Catherine James wards were similarly upgraded. The sanitary annexes of Bristol, Chichester and Vallance wards followed in 1965 when four beds on Catherine James were used for intensive care pending the conversion of Egremont Ward as an intensive care unit. The pathology department, faced with ever increasing demands, was extended in 1964.

A development not directly connected with the redevelopment of the hospital but important in that it was to lead to the eventual establishment of a major

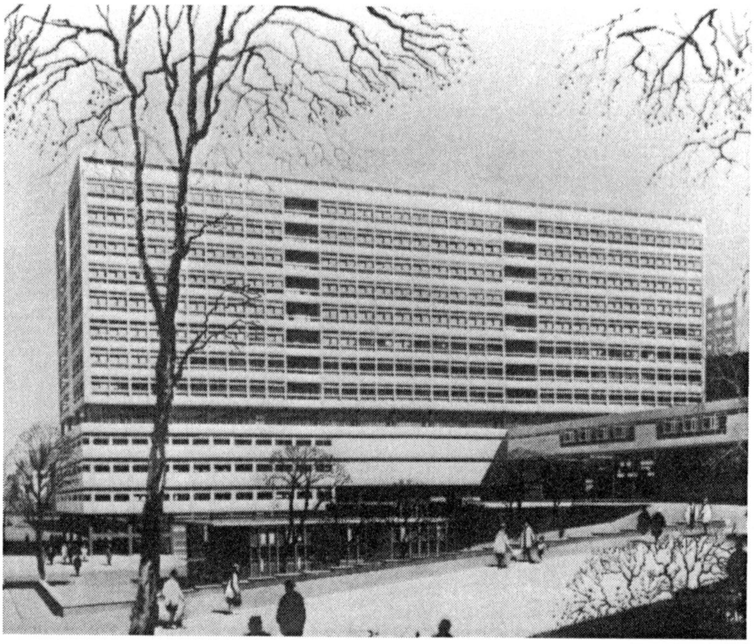

83. An artist's impression of the first part of the hospital's redevelopment as a district general hospital. This consisted of three linked blocks, but in the event only one of the blocks containing the new Accident Centre and the maternity unit was completed.

regional facility, was the regional board's decision to select Brighton as one of the first two provincial centres in the region for a chronic intermittent renal dialysis unit.

This opened in Donald Hall Ward early in 1967 and was viewed by the Minister of Health, Kenneth Robinson, during his three-day 'see-it-for-himself' tour of the South East. At a press conference held at the hospital on the 31st March he said 'substantial improvements are well under way all over the region'[3] One of these was the major development of the County as a district general hospital which, after some impassioned debate and delay got under way that year.

The main improvements suggested at the hospital formed part of a plan formulated by the regional board during the latter part of the 1950s for the redevelopment of the Brighton and Lewes group. Initially new casualty, trauma and orthopaedic departments were envisaged with the aim of eventually undertaking all casualty work at the County. A new outpatient department was also suggested. It was proposed that the children's beds at the County and Brighton General should be transferred to the Royal Alexandra Children's Hospital and the Sussex Maternity Hospital should be closed and transferred to Brighton General where all gynaecology, with the exception of the New Sussex Hospital, should be concentrated.

The hospital management committee responded in September 1960 recommending that the Royal Sussex and Brighton General should be developed, a third general hospital should be provided in Hove and that the order of the developments should be (1) Accident and Emergency and Orthopaedics, (2) a new maternity hospital within the 'area' of one general hospital and (3) the development of outpatient departments and supporting services.

Phase I of the redevelopment was announced in May 1963. It consisted of an Accident Centre with associated trauma and orthopaedic departments together that the promise that the following two stages were included in the Minister's 10 year programme which extended to 1972/73. Work was expected to start on site in the early summer of 1965 with the final result in 1973 being an almost entirely new hospital with the exception of the nurses' home and the comparatively new radiotherapy department.

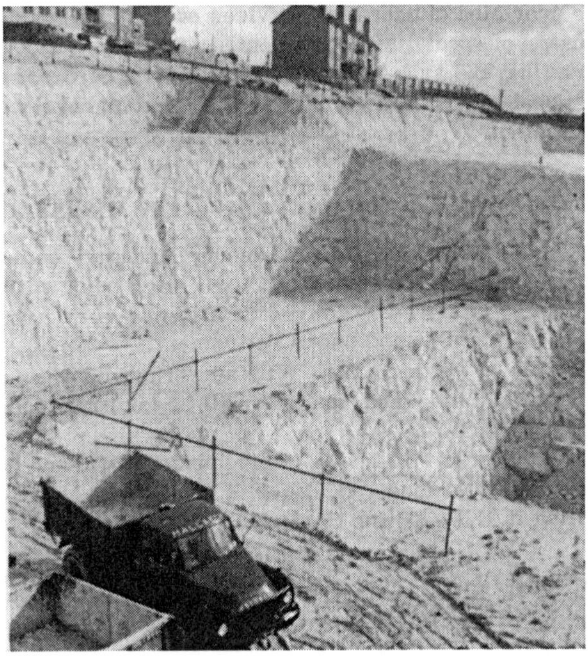

84. Early in the autumn of 1966, the bulldozers moved in to begin work on the new development and removed hundreds of lorryloads of chalk before construction of the new block could begin.

The first phase was to involve the preparatory work on the ground northeast of Latilla, previously leased to Brighton Corporation for allotments, followed by the construction of the Accident Centre with some 80 beds for trauma and orthopaedic cases. When the third phase was completed, the final hospital

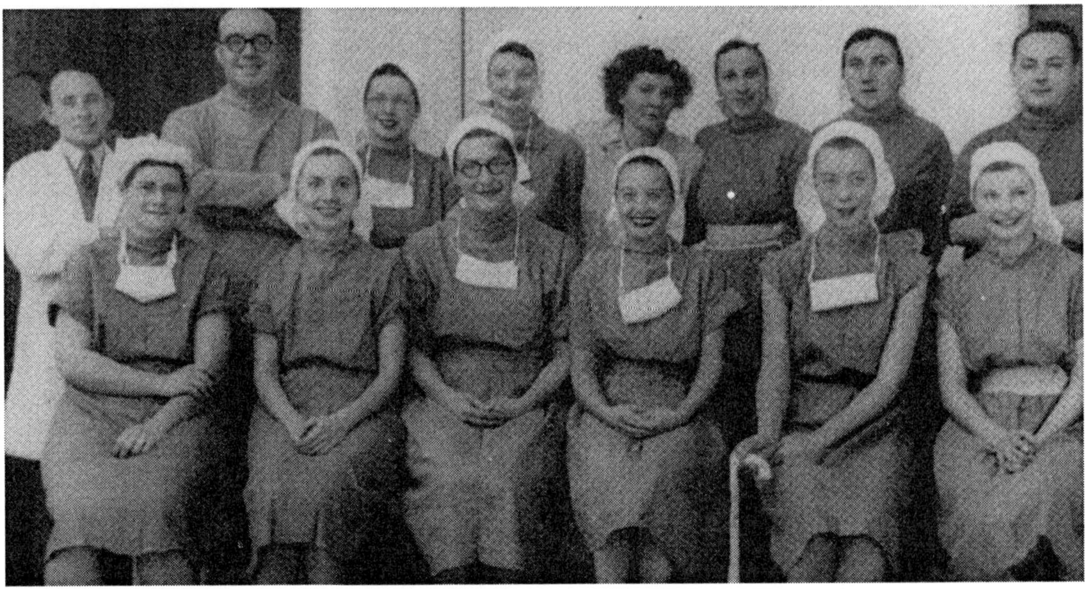

85.Theatre staff c.1949. Theatres were upgraded a few years later in one of the few schemes that were allowed to go-ahead despite a period of severe financial restrain nationally. Among those pictured are consultant surgeon Harold Park, Joan Humpherson, Sister Tyler, Dr Tom Copp, Dr Irene Stamford Cade, Pat Hope, Norah McCurrich, Geraldine Binning and Beryl Clarke.

building was expected to contain some 700 beds.

Preparations for the new building were well advanced when, in March 1965, the regional board announced that owing to the financial situation all its major schemes costing more than £100,000 were deferred, probably for two years. The delay did not disappoint everyone, however. For the consultant medical staff it provided an opportunity to press, not for the first time, for a building on a new site including a possible link with Sussex University. The consultants met members of the board and the management committee at Guys Hospital on the 14th April 1966 when the board promised to give further consideration to their proposals. However, at a second meeting held at the hospital their plan was rejected and despite the consultants who 'voiced strongly their disapproval of the board's decision' the Minister announced to the House of Commons on the 22nd April that work on the Accident Centre would proceed as planned with work being commenced in the autumn.

Accordingly, in early September, the bulldozers moved in and began removing the series of chalk cliffs where the allotments used to be. In the process, the hospital tennis court became a casualty, twenty feet of which were needed for the new development.

Financially, 1967 was a 'period of severe restraint' imposed on the country as a whole. Although Brighton was no exception, one or two developments did proceed during the year. As well as the opening of the renal unit, the hospital's twin operating theatres were closed for ten days for upgrading. One result which the staff particularly welcomed was the installation of two automatic autoclaves. These replaced 'the conglomeration of antiquated, hissing, noisy boiling hot water apparatus'[4] in the sterilising room.

Meanwhile, Glen Court, opposite the hospital, was purchased to provide increased accommodation for medical staff and the former domestic staff residence, 11 Walpole Terrace, was upgraded using endowment funds to provide accommodation for eleven staff nurses. This permitted a reorganisation of the main nurses' home to provide an additional doctor's bedroom as well as improved recreational and study facilities.

Changing times for nurses

A major challenge for the hospital during the 1950s and 60s arose from the shortage of nurses. This was a national problem and the County was no exception. Nurse staffing arrangements were under examination as early as 1953 and in December 1954 a working party reported that continuing falling intakes of student nurses at the hospital had resulted in difficulties in ensuring proper patient care and that extra burdens had been placed on trained staff. Consultations were arranged with staff and it was recommended that the students should be temporarily changed to a shift system similar to that worked by other groups. The students currently worked a three shift system with day staff coming on duty at 7.30 am, a late shift worked from 4 pm until midnight and night staff worked until 8 am.

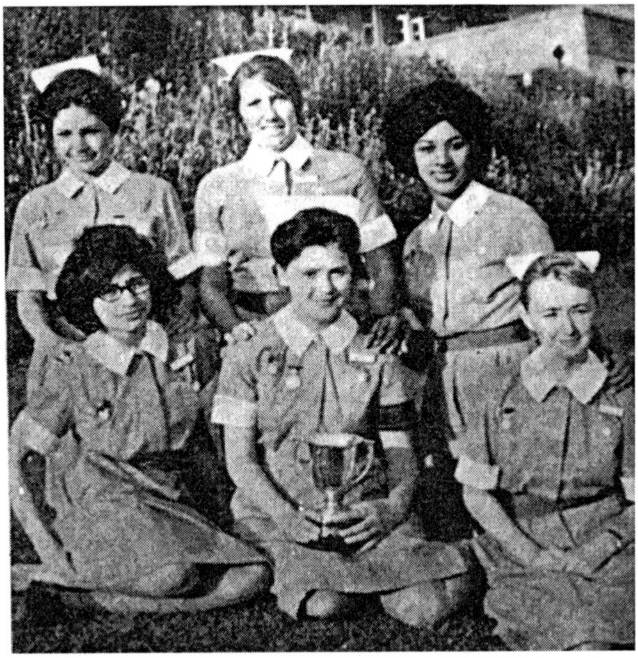

86. Severe nursing shortages nationally after the war led to recruitment campaigns for overseas nurses and the County was no exception, as this picture of their winning team at the Brighton and Sussex nurses' sports at Withdean in 1967 shows. Back row: Bobby Carr (India), Glynis Botting (England), Winsome Thompson (Jamaica); front: Habiba Kasam (Kenya), Jane Boakes (England) and Geraldine Moriarty (Ireland).

Some two years earlier an inspector from the General Nursing Council had drawn attention to a number of drawbacks this system posed for both staff and patients. Sixty per cent of the 135 student nurses attending the meetings voted for the change, which was to be kept under continuous review initially for a six-month period.

Meanwhile the management committee had been undertaking a campaign to increase recruitment to the group's various training schools which included a series of brains trusts and talks to Women's Institutes and Townswomen's Guilds across the county. By October 1955 the Preliminary Training School was able to report a record intake of 46, but the hospital's student nurse complement nevertheless remained below strength. Although split duty arrangements were working satisfactorily, Matron reported, the hospital was overtaxed because she had to supply 47 students to Hove General, the Sussex Eye and the Sussex Throat and Ear hospitals. At this time the nursing complement would have been 23½ ward and departmental sisters, 38 staff nurses, 166 student nurses and 16 ward orderlies.

The working party on nurse training continued its deliberations issuing periodic reports throughout the 1950s. In January 1960, Mr Dawes, the group secretary, wrote to the regional board stressing the need for immediate steps to be taken to fill nursing staff vacancies if the risk of closing beds were to be avoided. (Shortage of staff did in fact cause the temporary closure of

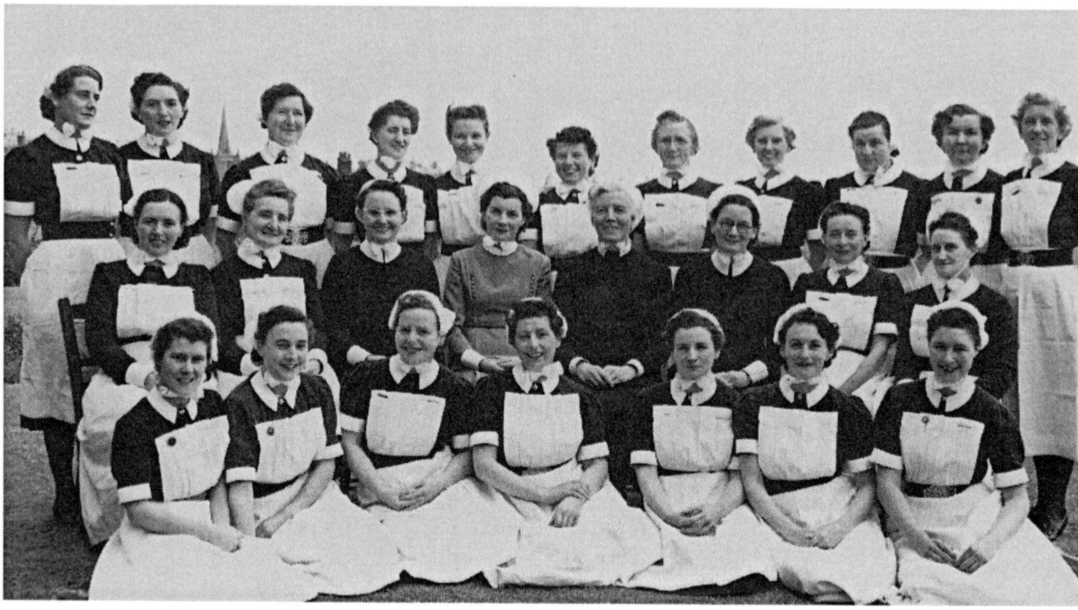

87 Ward and departmental sisters pictured with Matron in 1954.

the children's ward later in the year). At a time when advertising by hospitals was strictly regulated, the group secretary requested special permission to advertise locally and nationally using endowment funds. In a letter to the medical staff the following month, he said there was a total shortage of 50 nurses, 15 at Hove General and 35 at the Royal Sussex. Appeals would be made in the press and in advertisements, he said, for both part-time and temporary appointments.

At this time, there was a considerable amount of prejudice against employing married women and part-timers in the nursing profession generally, not least by full-time staff who regarded these colleagues as unreliable and resented the fact that they were able to pick and choose the times they were available to work. Despite changes brought about by the war, male nurses were unpopular, too. The County employed only one male nurse in 1950, Mr Allen, principally 'to do all the male preps for surgery plus one or two other jobs not seen as the thing that young gals should be doing.'[5] It was not until he retired in 1958 that three additional male nurses were employed on the male surgical wards, casualty and night duty. They replaced three female nurses and the nursing complement was increased to forty, made up of 36 females and four males.

Despite organising a mobile nursing exhibition during the summer in the Royal Pavilion grounds, Hove's Brunswick Lawns and on a site at Victoria Road in Portslade with shop window displays in gas and electricity board showrooms as well as distributing overprinted national posters to all churches and chapels in the area. According to the matrons the results of the campaign were 'generally disappointing'.

During 1961, in another attempt to stimulate further recruiting, students' friends were invited to talks by the tutors accompanied by an exhibition of 'coloured films and slides'. Consideration was also given to holding a 'Come Back to Nursing' course for married women and 34 former nurses attended the subsequent refresher course held during a week in November.

Despite the efforts to increase nurse recruitment, the matron, Miss Lynes, reported a critical shortage of staff in March 1964. A meeting was convened at which she joined the hospital management committee and nursing sub-committee chairman and four members of the consultant medical staff to discuss the situation. It was agreed to second four or five students to the children's hospital for paediatric training (this had been recommended by the General Nursing Council) and that there should be no change to the number seconded to Hove General. However, Miss Lynes was to be allowed to recruit by means of extensive local advertising an additional 30 unqualified staff in lieu of student nurses.

The new recruits, it was decided, should be given two or three days practical training before being allocated to the wards and further part-time instruction during the following two weeks. Additional sisters (eventually increased

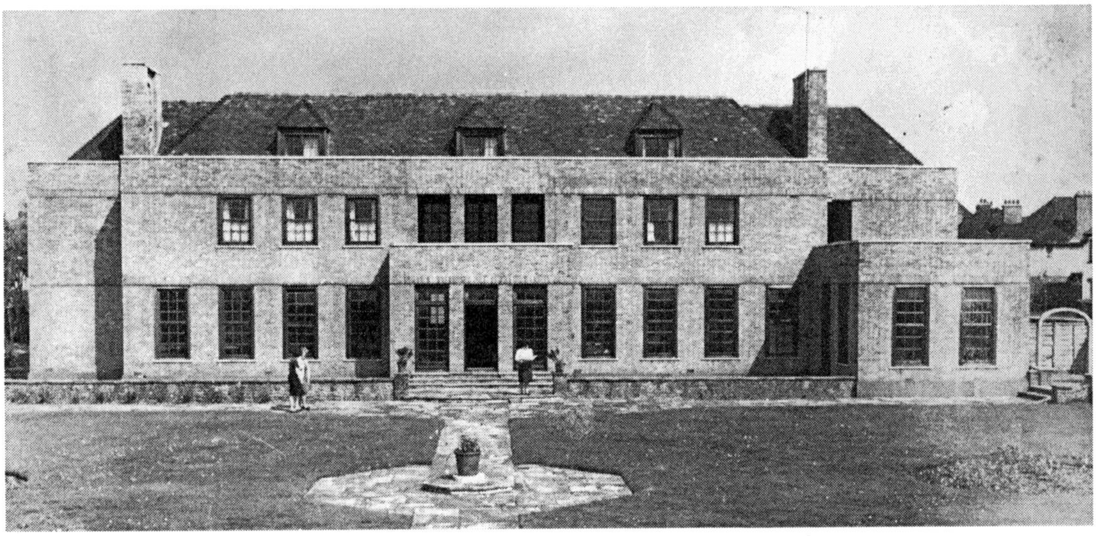

88. The new nursing school at 157 Kingsway opened in 1963. Previously the nurses' home for Hove General Hospital, the imposing grey building was set in extensive grounds with sweeping lawns and a sunken rose garden which, according to the principal tutor, Miss D.R. Kirby, gave 'a wonderful feeling of gracious living – and all this with the sea just across the road.'

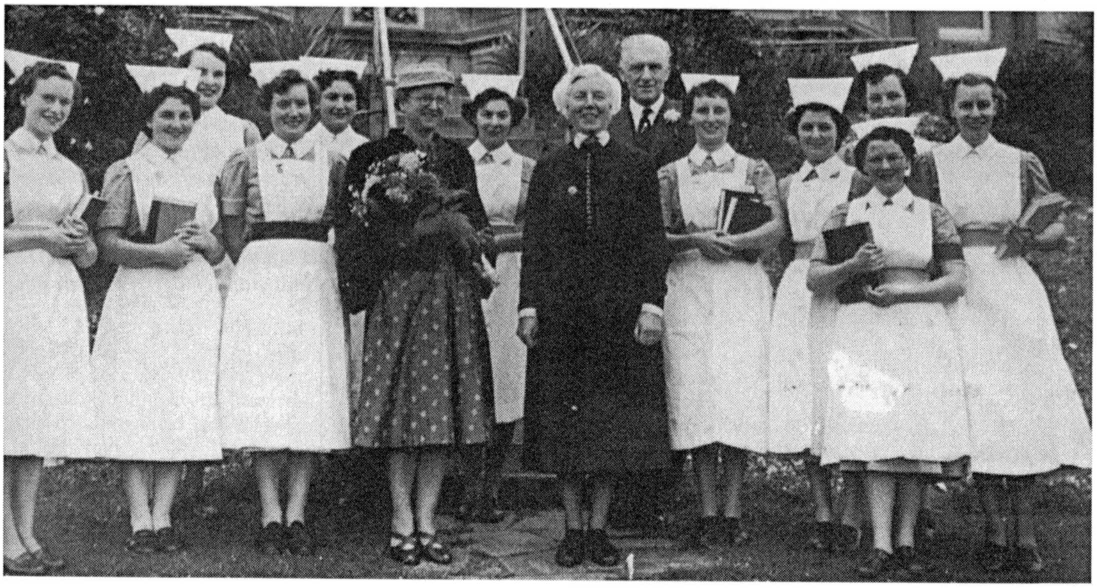

89. Prizewinning nurses at the hospital in 1954 with Matron and Mrs Donald Hall.

from three to seven) and unqualified staff were also to be employed on the wards at night in order to release student nurses for day duty. Finally, the matron was invited to submit proposals for the grouping of wards to enable a measure of progressive care to be introduced once sufficient unqualified staff had been recruited and trained. The hospital's long history as a successful nurse training school was undergoing a significant change at this time. Nationally there had been criticisms of shortcomings in some of the smaller nurse training schools and suggestions that these should be combined with the larger schools.

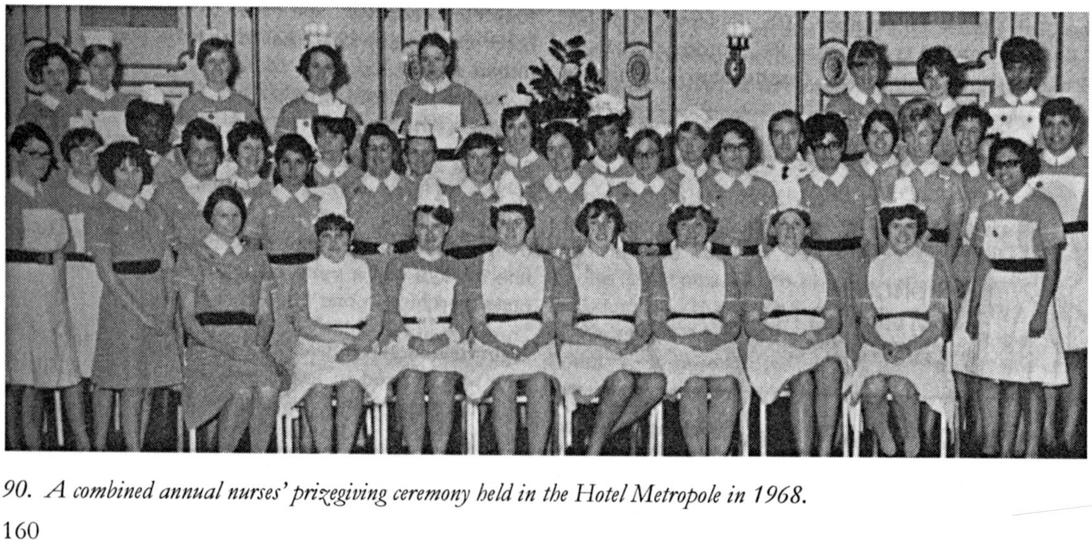

90. A combined annual nurses' prizegiving ceremony held in the Hotel Metropole in 1968.

A working party to consider setting up a group nurse training school in Brighton was established early in 1960 and a proposal to convert the Hove General Hospital's nurses' home at 157 Kingsway on the seafront for this purpose was submitted to the regional board. The aim was to provide formal classroom teaching for blocks of from four to six weeks for students from the County, Brighton General and the Royal Alexandra hospitals. The matrons of these hospitals would retain responsibility for recruitment of their student nurses who would continue their practical training work in their own hospital wards and departments. Eventually a plan for the ground floor to be converted and extended was approved and the first lectures were held in the new premises early in November 1963. As if to put the seal on this development, for the first time an annual combined nurses' prizegiving ceremony was held in the Royal Pavilion in October 1965.

During 1967 three new developments took place. Although the three year training programme for state registration continued at the County, a five year course was introduced consisting of three years studying for a degree at Sussex University followed by two years at the hospital. A four year integrated course was also introduced, with 2½ years spent with children and the remaining 1½ years on the adult wards. Finally, the hospital was also asked to establish an enrolled nurse training school, which opened in April in conjunction with the New Sussex Hospital.

By the end of 1968, the various measures to improve the hospital's nursing situation appeared to have been successful. Improvements to residential accommodation, the recruitment of nurses from overseas, the employment of more nursing auxiliaries and changed work patterns and improved recruitment of students were some of the factors that enabled the nursing sub-committee to report in December that the staffing situation had improved.

At the same time, with Phase I of the new development due for completion the following summer, the management committee looked ahead to the need to employ an additional 124 nurses, including 47 staff nurses, in the new Accident Centre. They also drew up proposals to establish a course in advanced nursing techniques, which, it was hoped, would attract nurses of the high calibre needed to work in the unit.

14: A New County Hospital or a New Site?

In 1968, the future seemed set for the development of an almost completely new Royal Sussex County Hospital on the Eastern Road site. The new building was already riding impressively alongside Bristol Gate and in 1969 Stage 1 of the first phase was completed and the new £1¼ million Accident and Emergency duly opened on the 15th September.

The new unit consisted of an accident floor, two major theatres and a plaster theatre, an intensive therapy unit and two wards. The theatres were on the same level as the accident department, but entirely separate, and for use only for emergency and orthopaedic surgery. A theatre sterile supply unit situated on the floor below served the complex. The intensive therapy unit (ITU), consisting of seventeen beds, was situated immediately above the major theatres. The two 28-bedded emergency wards were of the race-track design, unlike the Nightingale wards in the original building. They consisted of single and four-bedded rooms around the periphery with centrally placed service areas.

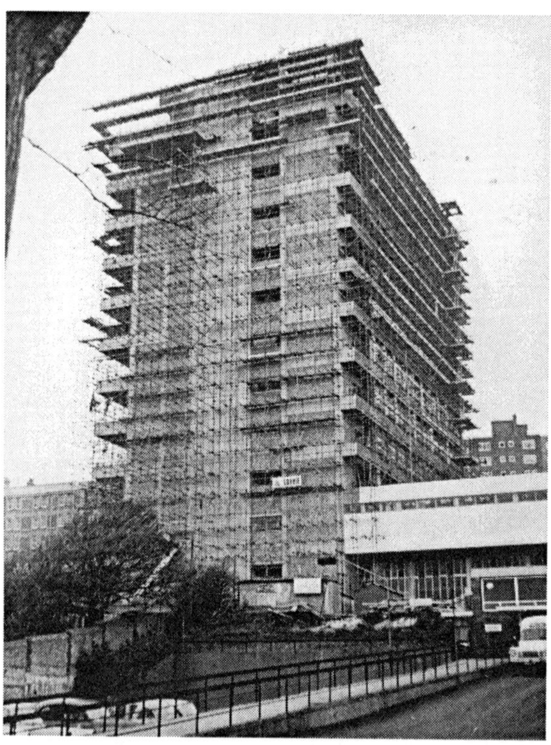

91. The new development in 1968 on course for completion the following year.

The casualty department transferred from the main building in September and ITU moved from Catherine James a few weeks later. Despite a delay caused by an outbreak of influenza, the traumatic and orthopaedic wards and the two theatres were soon fully operational. Emergency surgery cases were admitted to Emergency Ward One and transferred to the surgical wards in the main building after a few days. Emergency Ward Two was used for trauma cases and, supported by Peel Ward, for orthopaedic cases from the waiting list.

The new building was serviced mainly from the main building. A link corridor immediately north of the main theatre was used to transfer patients between the wards while the 100 yard stretch was also the route taken by an electric towing vehicle that contained the meals for patients

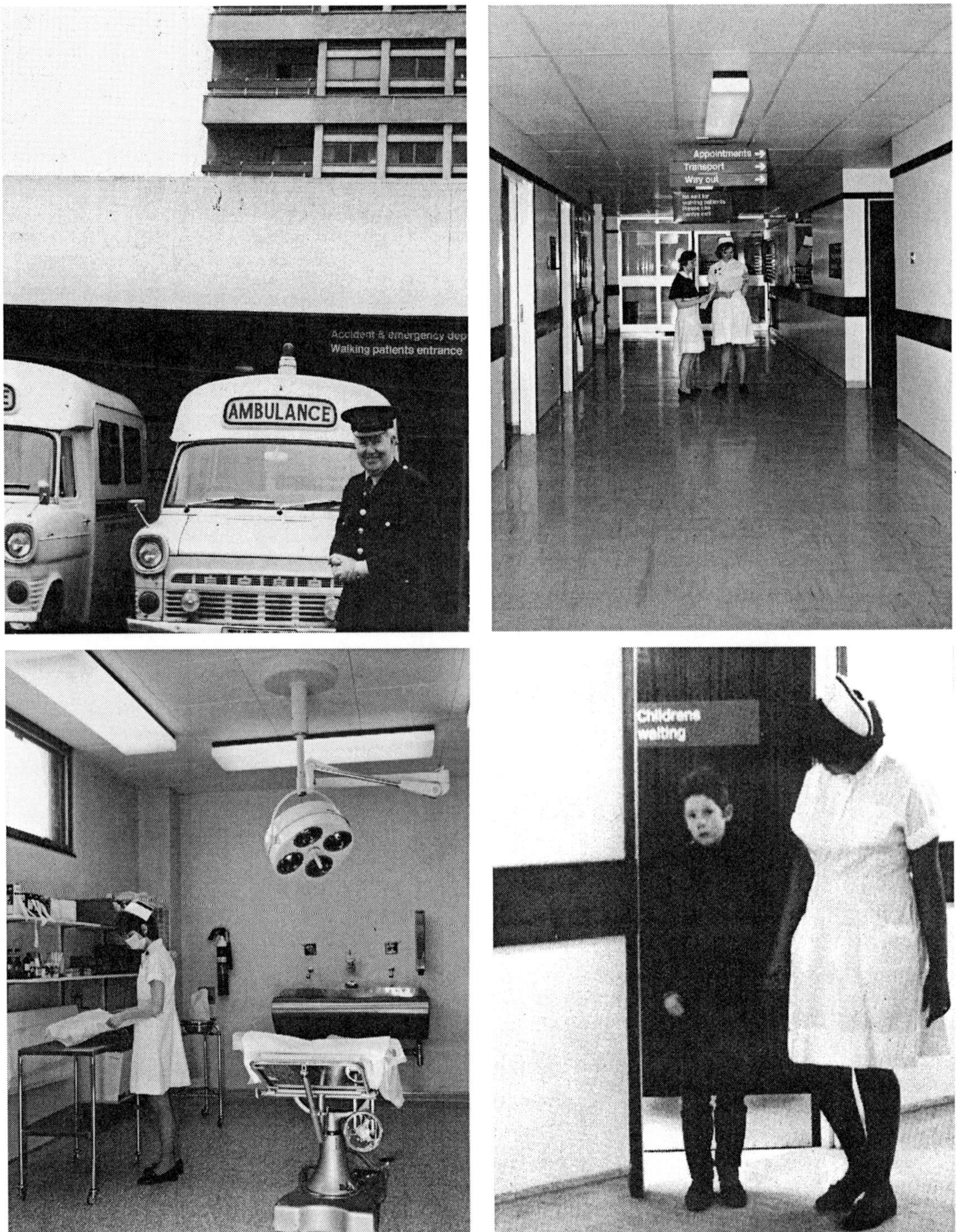

92. The new A&E department: Ambulances outside the new building; nurses in one of the corridors; (bottom) a minor operating theatre and a reassuring word for a young patient.

in the new block. These pre-selected plated meals were trayed up in the main kitchen using a specially installed 'Finessa' system. The system, used extensively in Europe, had been inspected in Switzerland by catering officer Ian Scott before it was decided to proceed with the purchase. The equipment, which was made entirely of stainless steel, used a special type of plate warmer and a specially designed colour card control to eliminate any chance of error in providing the hospital's wide range of special diets.

Stage 1a of the development, the top five floors, was completed the following year. The Sussex Maternity Hospital finally closed its doors on the 4th October and from that date the group's major maternity facilities were provided at the County. The new unit included an outpatient department, a 28-bedded ante-natal ward, a labour ward with an admission suite, eight single rooms and one four-bedded room. It also contained an abnormal delivery suite and a 24-bedded post-natal ward with three nurseries containing accommodation for 24 cots.

A special care baby unit contained three nurseries, each with places for seven cots or incubators. There was also a single cot isolation nursery and a self-contained suite with two single rooms and a lounge for mothers.

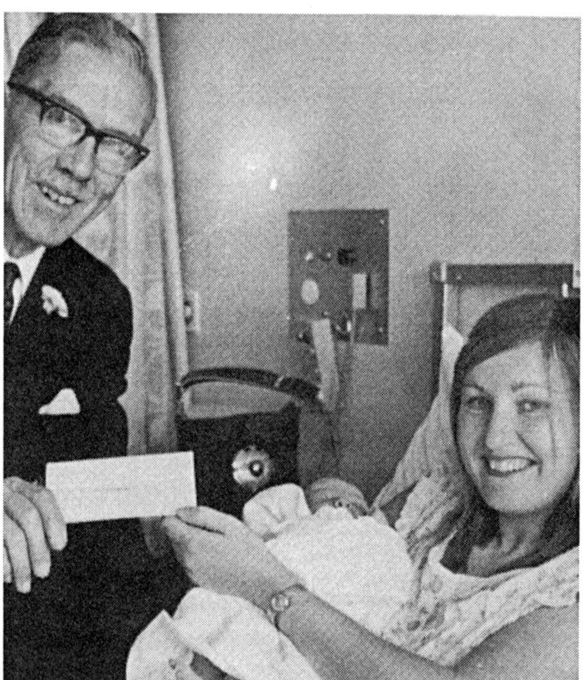

93. New arrival in a new unit. Chairman Clifford Gaukroger presents a premium bond to Mrs Mary Stubberfield, proud mother of the first baby, born in the new maternity unit, her daughter to be named Emma who weighed 8 lbs 3 ozs.

Finally, the unit housed a nursing administration and teaching unit for the Brighton group's midwifery division and a comprehensive teaching unit for pupil midwives.

Meanwhile, Phase II of the redevelopment was in the planning stage. This was to consist of a pathology laboratory and a second tower block with more operating theatres and an outpatient complex. But the dream was not to be realised. In the summer of 1971, the Brighton Corporation planning committee gave its approval for a new district general hospital to be built at Falmer on a probable site of 30 to 40 acres adjacent to the College of Education. The proposal marked a complete about turn in plans for hospital provision locally. It was believed the new hospital would replace Brighton General and Bevendean hospitals but Clifford Gaukroger, chairman of the group management committee, warned that 'wrapped around in the new hospital is the future of the County Hospital'[1] and the planned redevelopment of the hospital was put on hold pending the building of the proposed new hospital at Falmer.

In October 1972, plans for the new comprehensive hospital moved a step closer. The hospital management committee was told a feasibility study had confirmed that the Falmer site was suitable for the new development and that discussions concerning this were continuing between the regional board and the Department of Health. As further planning stages were being progressed 'with all speed', the regional board announced that no further major permanent building should take place until the Falmer project neared completion. The principal exception to this ruling was for three new operating theatres at the County, which were to form an extension to the existing theatre complex.

Knowing that the new hospital could not become operational for a number of years, the management committee undertook a review of the priority needs of the County and a fixed sum was set aside to carry out essential works in the interim. A project team was formed to draw up sketch plans of the proposed interim development with much of the work to consist of buildings in temporary fabric. Three phases were planned. Phase I consisted of new workshops, extensions to the group laboratory and main X-ray department, and the provision of a renal/metabolic unit. Phase 2 included a new main kitchen and staff restaurant, ante-natal and medical physics accommodation, on which proposals were well advanced. Phase 3 consisted of the three operating theatres and a central linen store. Work on the first phase costing nearly £300,000 got under way in September 1973 and was programmed for completion in December 1974.

The new workshop for engineering and allied staff, necessary because the increasing amount of complex equipment needed in a modern hospital, was built to the south of the tower block. Another prefabricated building was designed as a medical unit. This was to house the renal dialysis unit. Two additional X-ray rooms were provided as additions to the department in the main building.

Phase Two of the interim development looked in doubt in November 1974. A global oil crisis led to massive inflation and an economic crisis in the United Kingdom and as a result the government announced that all hospital capital schemes would be deferred. Fortunately, four high priority schemes were eventually given the go-ahead in the South East region. The exceptions included two schemes at the County, the extension of the pathology department and a new building for medical physics and an antenatal clinic.

To provide the extension to Pathology two floors were built over the animal house attached to the Public Health Laboratory, one for microbiology, the top floor for histology. The animal house was converted into a central wash-up for both laboratories. When these departments were fully functional, the aim was to use the Stephen Ralli Block with its extension almost entirely for biochemistry where there had been a considerable increase in demand. The second scheme involved the construction of a prefabricated building in the car parking area adjacent to the radiotherapy department. The ground floor was to be used by Medical Physics, mainly for work with patients that had been necessitated by advances in the fields of medical physics and nuclear medicine. The upper floor was to be designed as a maternity outpatient clinic. This would release Level 12 in the tower block for conversion to an additional ward.

The early 1970s witnessed a great number of other changes at the hospital. Some of these, but by no means all, reflected the number of medical advances at the time including heart and kidney transplants, computerised tomography (CT) and the development of whole body CT scanning. Moving Casualty to the new block freed space that was used as offices for the hospital secretary and his staff and for the haematology department. Wooden buildings on the roof were extended to accommodate a medical records office, a consultants' room, medical library and an enlarged junior medical staff lounge. Bristol and Overton wards were amalgamated to provide a system of 'progressive patient care' then in vogue.[2] Following the opening of the surgical wards in the tower block, male medical patients from Howard One were transferred to Egremont Ward and Howard One became a group staff sick bay. A wooden building was erected on the eastern side of Outpatients and became the Medical Photography and Illustration Department.

In September 1970, Catherine James was reopened as a urology ward, a new departure for the hospital marked by the appointment of two urologists. Early in 1971, two beds were opened in a new coronary care unit. In June, the smallest baby ever to pass through the maternity unit was discharged home thanks to a new technique. This involved pumping milk directly into a baby's stomach and was the first time the procedure had been used in Britain. Previously, the chances of survival would have been about one in twenty.

In 1974, the hospital enjoyed the best success rate in Europe for kidney transplant surgery and the same year it 'entered the space age' in the developing field of total hip replacement. This was regarded at the time as one

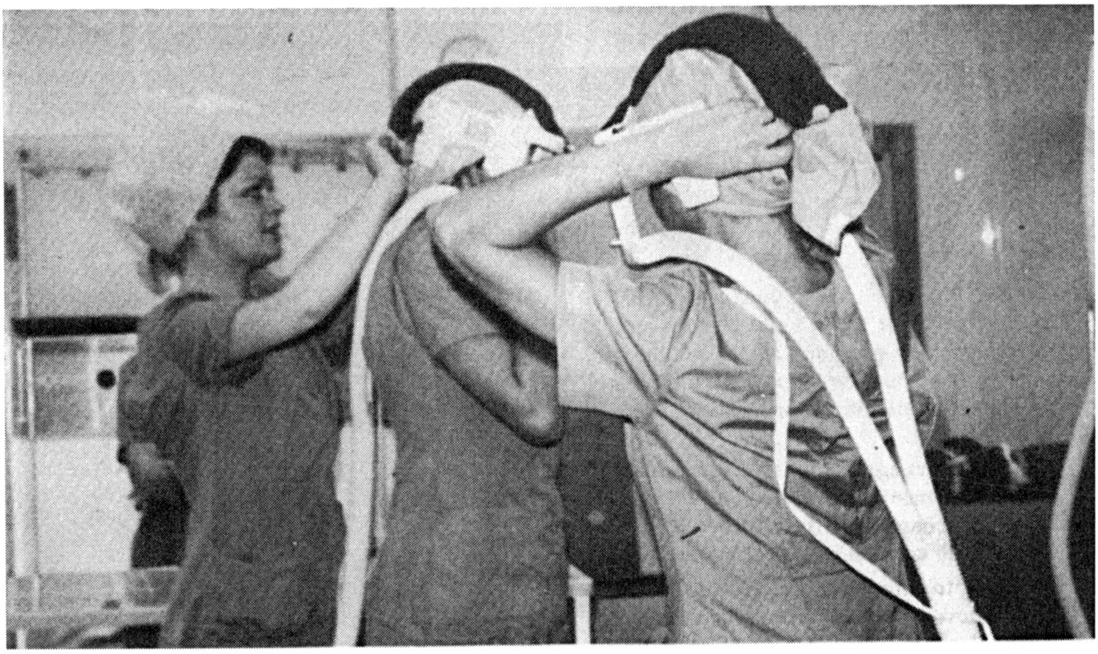

94. Space Age Surgery. Nurses preparing for a demonstration in the Charnley Howarth enclosure. During operations, staff communicated by means of a two-way radio.

of the most important developments of modern surgery. In November theatre staff demonstrated their Charnley Howarth enclosure that had been installed. This 'theatre within a theatre' made it possible to carry out the hip replacement surgery procedure while clean air was filtered through diffusers at ceiling level effectively locking out bacteria, an aseptic technique that was essential because of the amount of metal used for a prosthesis.

Probably the most important advance of the decade was the introduction of X-ray computerised tomography. Hailed as the most significant advance in radiology since the discovery of X-rays in 1895, the system provided television type pictures of thin, horizontal 'slices' right through the human frame, including the head. Research on EMI scanner systems had begun in 1967 and the first prototype brain scanner was installed in 1971. The first whole-body scanner was unveiled in November 1971 and just eight months later a new £285,000 X-ray unit incorporating a whole-body scanner, as advanced as any in the world, was officially opened at the hospital by Lord Mountbatten. The scanner was donated by Mr Charles Hunnisett, chairman of Hanningtons, the well-known Brighton department store. The unit, operating under the direction of senior consultant Dr Jan de Winter, was named after the donor as The Charles Hunnisett Department of Computerised Tomology.

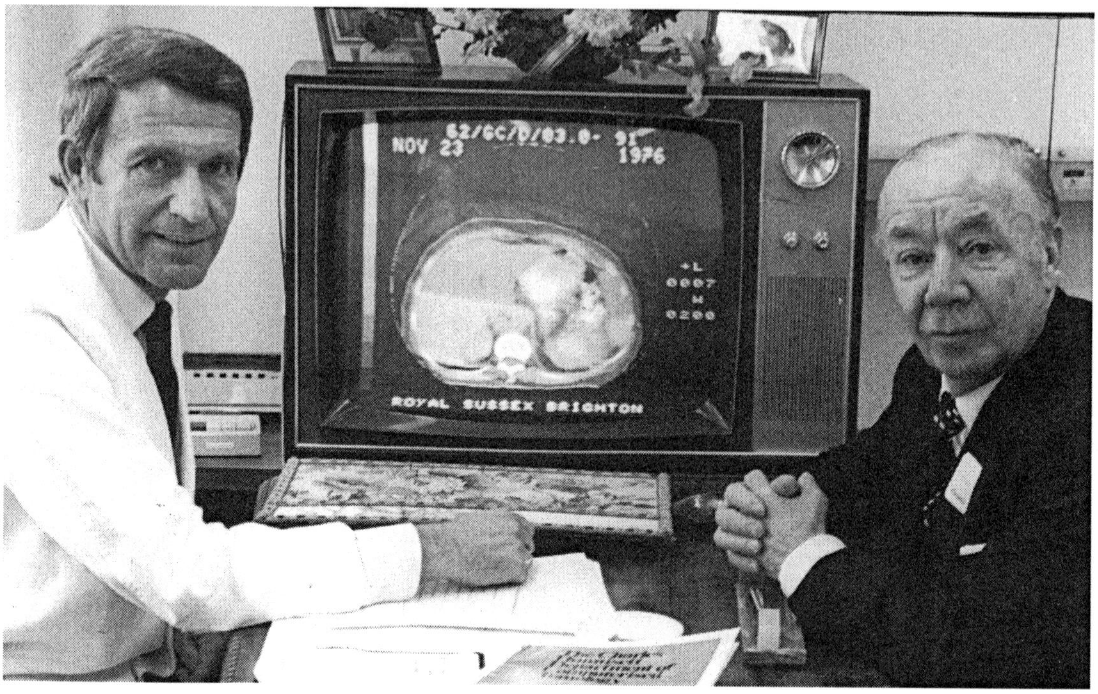

95. Consultant radiotherapist Dr Jan de Winter shows a read-out from the screen of the EMI scanner to its donor, Mr Charles Hunnisett.

During 1978, it became clear that the proposed Falmer development was a long way off and the Brighton district management team (DMT) undertook wide-ranging consultations with professional and staff interests on a three-part plan for the future accepted by the area health authority at the beginning of 1979. Believing that a new district general hospital at Falmer was still the best option for the future but that this could be some twenty years off, the team devised a mid-term, ten-year strategy which included the centralisation of acute services, and also detailed plans for 1979-1982.

Following the completion of the planned three new operating theatres at the County, the plan proposed transferring their out-dated surgical operating theatres from Hove General, the Sussex Throat and Ear and the New Sussex hospitals to the County. As there were insufficient surgical beds at the hospital, it was also proposed that more beds, both surgical and medical, should be provided which would permit the closure or change of use of Hove General, the Sussex Throat and Ear and the New Sussex. Subject to the availability of capital funds, the Phase Three of the Sussex County interim development – the provision of three new operating theatres and 38 extra beds – was seen as the principal planning activity for the next three years with completion of the work anticipated in the mid 1980s.

The district plan also included a number of smaller schemes. For the County Hospital, the most significant of these was the transfer of the GU Medicine Clinic from the hut at the back of Outpatients to Royal York Buildings. This scheme was included in minor capital works programme for the year approved by district health authority in May 1982.

Farewell to Matron

Nursing witnessed some significant changes at the hospital during the Seventies: uniform, for example, was a topic always likely to generate emotional responses, but it was the ending of the role of the matron had the greatest impact.

Admittedly the earliest matrons were not themselves nurses, but they had always been regarded as the public face of nursing. As the acknowledged figure of authority within the hospital, they were regarded with respect and admiration. All that changed with the implementation of the Salmon Report.

Early in 1963, a committee had been set up by the Minister of Health under the chairmanship of Brian Salmon to advise on the senior nursing structure in the hospital service, that is ward sisters and above. In its report published in 1966, the committee found that nursing occupied a secondary place in its partnership with medical and lay administration and recommended that a new pattern of nursing administration should be adopted. A feature of this, but by no means the only one, was that the position of matron should be discontinued. Salmon recommended an organisational structure with a nurse at every level in the hospital hierarchy, which reduced the historic power of matrons in large acute hospitals like the Royal Sussex County. In the new structure matrons were replaced with three tiers of nurse managers, and at the top of the tree a chief nurse who represented nurses at the highest level but without the intimate involvement matrons had previously enjoyed. Brighton's chief nursing officer was appointed in 1971.

Nurse management in Brighton was divided into four divisions, controlled by principal nursing officers who took up their posts in 1972. The 361-bedded County was placed in one of two general divisions and was itself divided into four units, medical and outpatients; surgical; accident and emergency; and nights, each one controlled by a nursing officer. The nursing officers in turn were responsible to a senior nursing officer who effectively replaced the matron but was herself answerable to the principal nursing officer. There was another complicating factor because theatres in the hospital, for example, now came under control of their own senior nursing officer

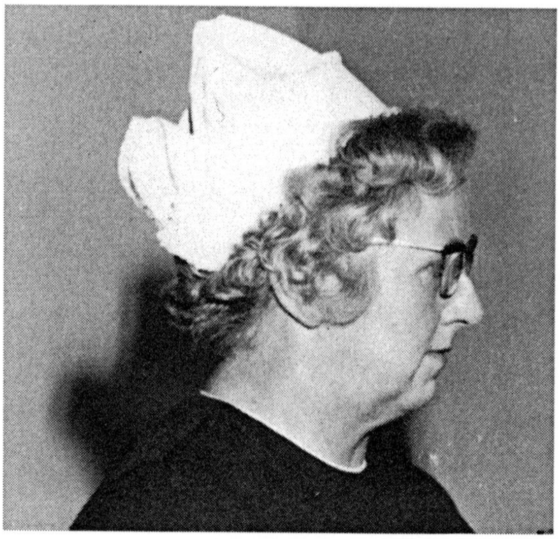

96. Barbara Lynes, the last Matron of the County Hospital.

who was responsible for all theatres in the group. Following the introduction of the new structure, Matron, Miss Barbara Lynes, was appointed senior nursing officer for the hospital's acute area. She continued in her new role until her retirement at the end of November 1976 after seventeen years at the hospital. Helen Brennan was appointed to replace her as senior nursing officer, taking up her new post in January 1977.

The new nurse managers brought with them a range of new uniforms but uniforms for nurses generally at the hospital had already been in the process of change, something not welcomed by everyone.

Towards the end of 1969 there were unconfirmed reports in the press about recommendations made by a working party set up three years before to enquire into nursing staff uniforms for a new standard dress for female nurses in French blue lawn and short sleeved with a hemline just above the knee. Function and rank were to be identified not by the colour of

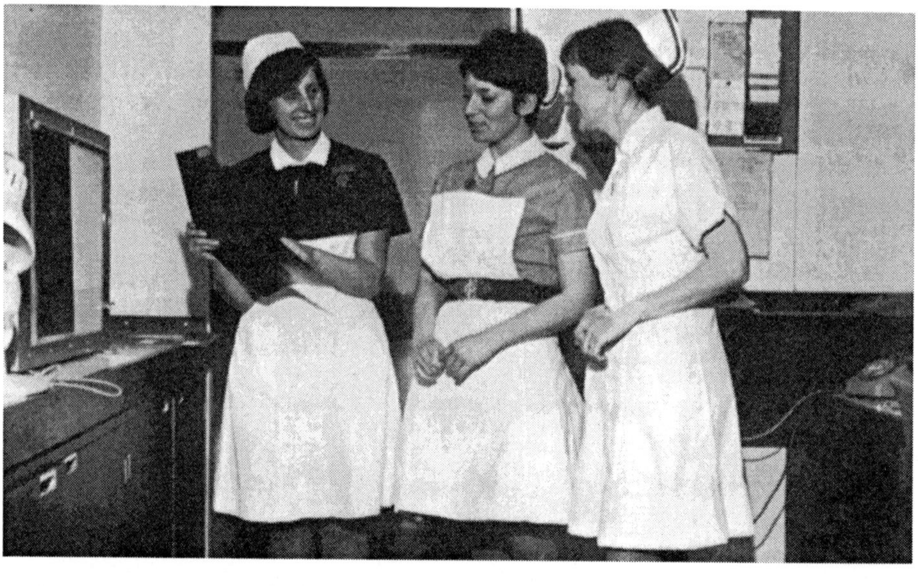

97. The Nursing Mirror illustrated the change in nurses' uniforms with Sister A. Sawyer and staff nurse L. Attree in the new basic white dress and staff nurse J. Dade wearing a traditional uniform. Tippets were worn to denote the grade of sister while a blue band round the cap indicated the staff nurse grade.

the dress but by a plastic badge. Questions were asked in Parliament and the national press vigorously pursued the matter. Brighton's *Evening Argus* columnist, Collie Knox, commented that the recommendation found 'no welcoming niche in my heart ... indeed it disgusts me'. He was by no means alone and probably typical of many who would 'miss the rustle of starch and the little white cap that would disappear'. So far as Brighton senior nurses were concerned, a straw poll found no one in favour of the change.[3] Their views were confirmed the following June when their misgivings were conveyed to the regional hospital board as the official view of the hospital management committee. Nevertheless, change was in the air. When the new accident and emergency unit opened its doors in September 1969, all nursing staff there regardless of grade wore a new white terylene mixture dress that formed part of an experiment by the regional board and which was expected eventually to be adopted throughout the hospital.

Opening the doors

On the 1st April 1969, five hospitals in Brighton, including the County, took a step into the unknown. The date was the beginning of an experimental three-month period when visiting, previously restricted to Wednesday and Sunday afternoons, was to be permitted for varying periods every day. At the County daily visiting was to be allowed between 2.30 and 4 pm, except on Mondays and Fridays, and between 6.30 and 8 pm in the evenings although visitors would be requested to stay for no longer than thirty minutes.

As with many significant changes in hospital routine, it received a mixed reaction from patients, staff and visitors. One Brighton consultant said it was 'not in the interests of anyone' if members of the public and consultants were on the ward at the same time. Another likened the milling hordes of visitors under the traditional system to visitors at the zoo![4]

As early as 1962, more liberal visiting arrangements had been recommended in a Ministry of Health circular which stated that it should be regarded as an important contribution to the patient's recovery. However, until relatively recently few hospitals had given effect to the recommendation. At the end of the three-month experimental period, patients were surveyed to obtain their reactions to the change, which were to be an important factor in deciding whether it should be continued. In the event, the management committee agreed that the new arrangements should become permanent and extended to four more local hospitals, with the continued proviso that visitors should continue to be requested not to stay longer than thirty minutes during any one visiting period..

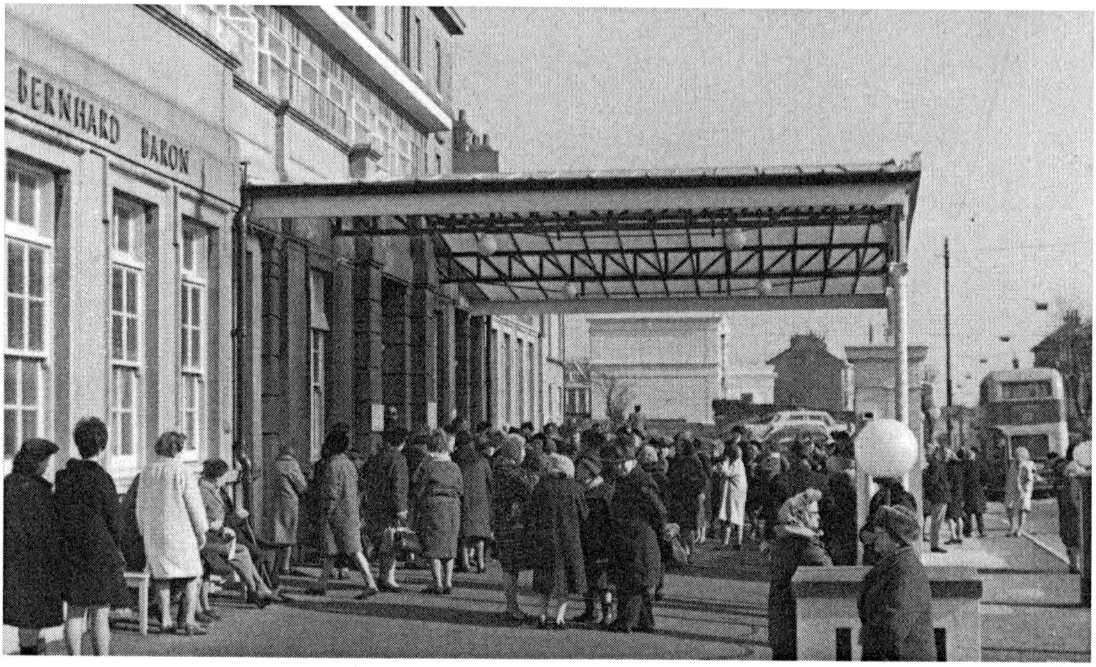

98. Visiting day. Ten minutes before the doors open yet another bus load of visitors is seen swelling the crowd blocking the main entrance to the hospital on a fine winter's day a few weeks before the experimental change in visiting arrangements. The Wednesday before it had rained heavily; the week before that it snowed!

The doors were opened to more visitors in June 1978 when an event was launched by the mayor to celebrate the hospital's 150th anniversary. One of the first of the many other events held was a jumble sale in the outpatient department that raised £150 for the League of Friends. A sponsored walk was expected to raise a further £500. Special football and cricket matches also took place, as well as a musical concert, a buffet and dance at Hove Town Hall, a coffee morning in the board room and a church service attended by the local mayors and the Member of Parliament.

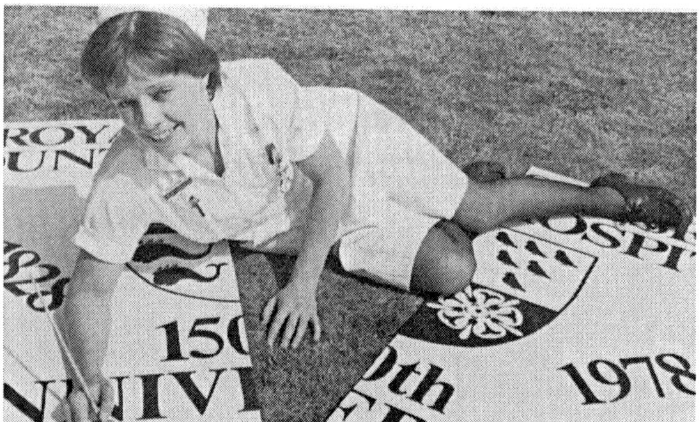

99. Student nurse Sue Jellis used her experience in graphic design to create a placard advertising the hospital's 150th anniversary celebrations.

The 1978 events, however, in no way compared with the first open day held in April 1982 when an estimated 5,000 people flocked to the hospital and toured the wards and departments. Visitors were asked

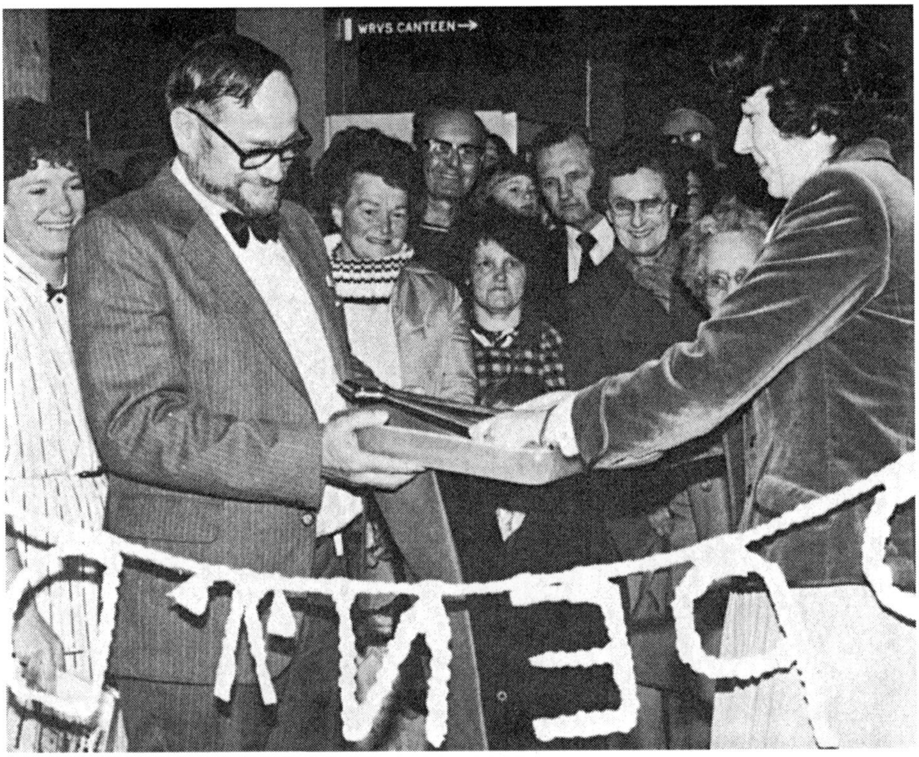

100. Health authority chairman Mrs Julia Cumberlege performs the opening ceremony at the 1982 open day with Pathology's Dr Doug Flowers, chairman of the organising committee.

to select from six tours that showed all aspects of the hospital's medical care as well as its support services. It was planned to clear the site by five o'clock but some of the tours were so popular that it was not until six thirty in the evening that the final visitor left.

Although not primarily intended as a fund-raising event many visitors made donations. One elderly visitor, perhaps recalling earlier Pound Days, donated tea, sugar and two tins of soup. The only record of disappointment by a visitor was of a man who thought he was being taken to a seaside bar called 'The Tiller' but found himself visiting Latilla.

15. The Debate Ends and a Decision is Made

The future of the Royal Sussex County Hospital hung in the balance for another ten years. That change was needed, there was no doubt.

The County Hospital, like so many former voluntary hospitals established in the nineteenth century, was no longer suited to modern medicine Their city centre sites may have been accessible (for public transport, at least) but were on the whole too small or difficult to be developed. The fabric of their aging buildings was poor, their wards ill suited to meet twentieth century needs. One alternative, and one with much to commend it, was to start from scratch and build a completely new district general hospital. How would this affect the existing general hospitals? One possibility was that it would lead to their eventual closure. Nearby Eastbourne provided a good example of this. There, the Princess Alice Hospital, opened in 1883, was replaced by a new district general hospital. The Princess Alice wards were reconstructed and in 1978 it entered the final stage of its existence caring for elderly long stay patients. Eventually it was closed and the site was sold.

Building a new hospital at Falmer, deferred by the economic crisis of the 1970s, was still seen by many as the ideal solution but might equally well have led to the eventual closure of the Royal Sussex County for which there was a strong sentimental attachment. Not surprisingly, despite the consultants' continuing campaign for a new hospital on a greenfield site, there were those who wished to retain the County as the town's major hospital if at all possible. One such attempt was evident in 1984, when a health authority member, Mr Derek Hunnisett, whose family were renowned for their financial support, commissioned at his own expense a feasibility study to fully develop the Eastern Road hospital.

However, neither of these views found favour with the combined regional and district team currently reviewing the options for the future shape of hospital services in the Brighton district, which no longer included a one site district hospital in its options. The cost of building a large hospital at Falmer was deemed 'prohibitively high'; as for developing the County 'the problems caused by its restricted size, together with the enormous disruption such a huge development would involve, effectively ruled out the notion'. In spite of this, Brighton Health Authority agreed that the Hunnisett proposal should be evaluated. If this was eventually adopted, the hospital's tower block abandoned in 1969 would be completed and the County could then have 1,342 beds together with a 1,300 place car park.

An eventful year

1984 was an eventful year for the hospital. The Hunnisett family matched the contribution made by the late Charles Hunnisett by providing £350,000 towards the £450,000 cost of a replacement of the EMI scanner purchased in 1976 with what was described as 'the most advanced body scanner in Europe'. It was officially opened in September by Lord Romsey, grandson of the late Lord Mountbatten, who had opened the original scanner.

A more modest but nevertheless welcome development was the facelift in the main outpatient department. This was funded by the League of Hospital Friends and the Women's Royal Voluntary Service. The WRVS also financed a facelift for the hospital's main entrance.

However, the event that drew attention to the hospital locally and nationally was the way the staff coped with the aftermath of the IRA bombing of the Grand Hotel on the 12th October.

This was clearly directed at the Prime Minister, Margaret Thatcher and members of her cabinet who were attending the annual Conservative Party conference in the town. Although Mrs Thatcher and her husband narrowly escaped injury, the explosion caused four deaths and serious injury to 34 others. What followed was 'a baptism of fire' for the accident and emergency department's first consultant in charge, Carlos Perez Avila, who had only

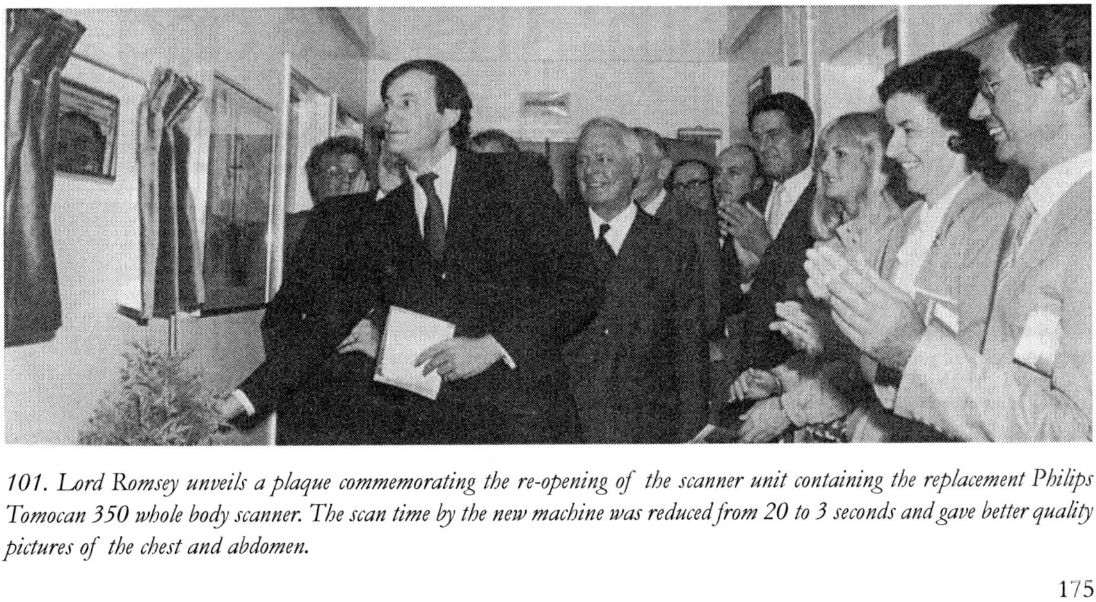

101. Lord Romsey unveils a plaque commemorating the re-opening of the scanner unit containing the replacement Philips Tomocan 350 whole body scanner. The scan time by the new machine was reduced from 20 to 3 seconds and gave better quality pictures of the chest and abdomen.

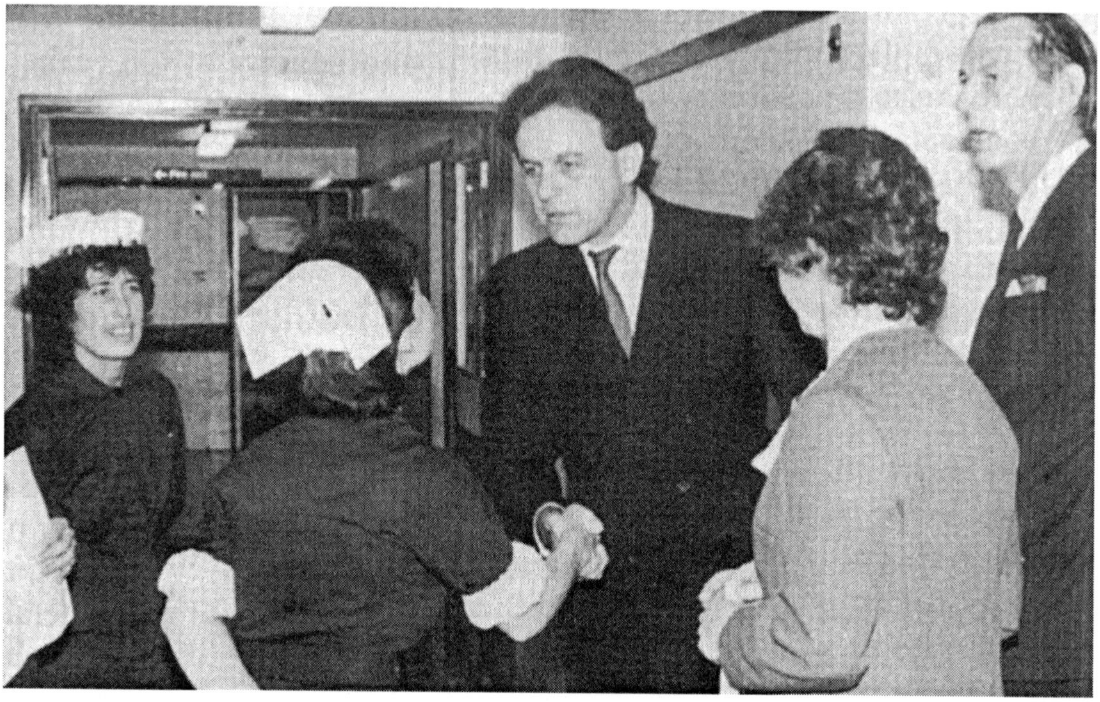

102. Junior health minister John Patten thanks staff working in A&E the morning the bomb went off in the Grand Hotel.

been in post for a few weeks. The decision to make such an appointment had been a contentious one, the health authority chairman acknowledged later, 'but events on Friday proved it to be the right one'. In the few weeks following his arrival, the new consultant had already reviewed the hospital's major accident procedure and reorganised the A&E department.

The ambulance service arrived at the Grand Hotel within four minutes of the alert being given and conveyed the injured, who included the Trade and Industry secretary Norman Tebbitt and his wife Margaret and the government chief whip, John Wakeham, to the hospital. The way the County handled the crisis brought praise, tributes and thanks from all quarters.

The chairman, Mrs Cumberlege, praised the skill of the doctors and nurses: 'Every single person who witnessed the events, every patient, every visitor from the Prime Minister downwards has remarked not only on the efficiency, but on the humanity and compassion which permeated the County Hospital.'

She also referred to the great many 'unsung heroes' who unstintingly gave themselves – 'administrators, technicians, radiographers, those who slogged away for long hours on the switchboard, catering staff, porters and cleaners

… they carried on cheerfully. They, like others, were put to the test and did not fail.'

A letter from Mrs Thatcher was later framed and hung in the department:

> The explosion at the Grand Hotel, Brighton, last Friday morning, inevitably put enormous strain on the emergency services and I am writing to tell you how marvellously my colleagues and I thought that those concerned with caring for the injured responded.
> I have had reports from every side of their speed, efficiency and humanity. And I had the opportunity of meeting some of those concerned when I visited the Royal Sussex County Hospital.
> We owe an incalculable debt of gratitude to all the men and women who dealt so professionally with the crisis.

In her autobiography, Mrs Thatcher recalled how she went to the hospital the following morning to visit the injured, among whom was the unconscious John Wakeham whose legs had been 'terribly crushed'.

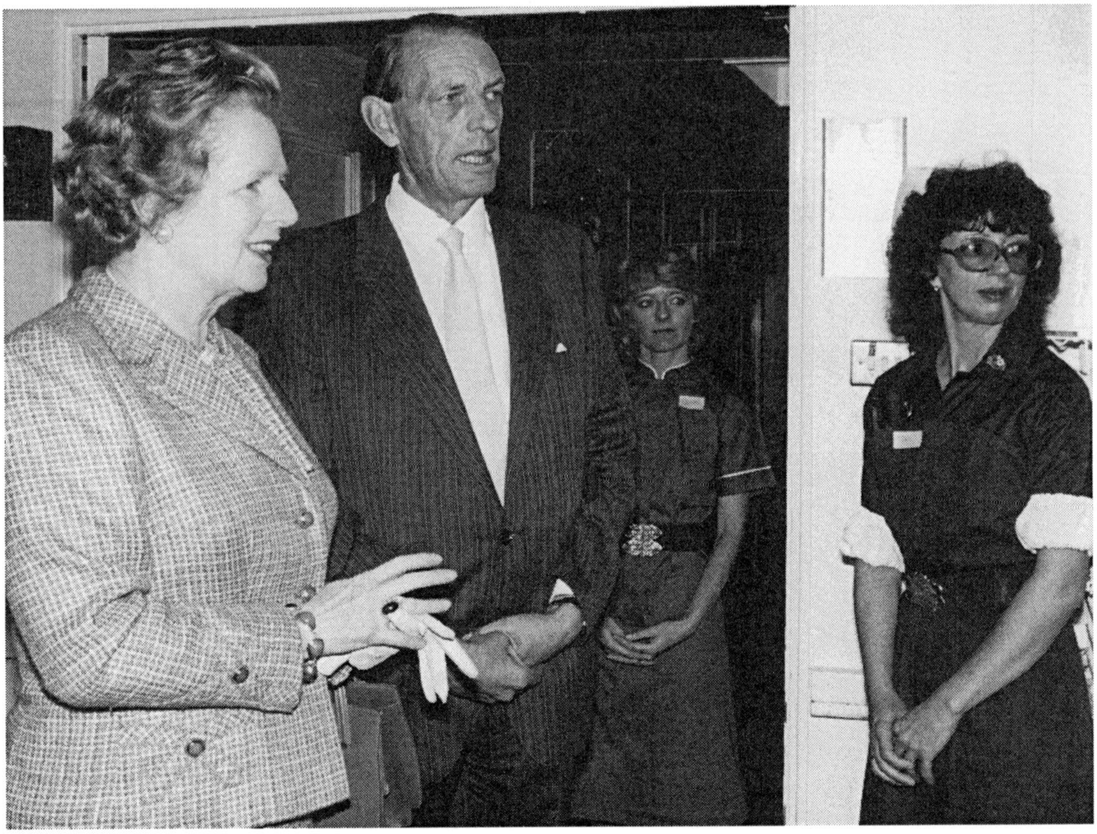

103. Prime Minister Margaret Thatcher tours the Renal Department extension with consultant physician Sir Anthony Trafford.

> By chance we all knew the consultant in charge: Tony Trafford, who had been a Conservative M.P. I spent hours on the telephone trying to get the best advice possible from experts in dealing with crush injuries. In the end it turned out there was a doctor in the hospital from El Salvador who had the expertise required. Between them they managed to save John's legs.[1]

There was an unexpected sequel to the events of the 18th October the following year when the Queen's Birthday Honours List was announced. Dr Tony Trafford received a knighthood. The 'doctor from El Salvador', A&E consultant Mr Perez Avila received an honorary O.B.E. Registrar Dr David Bellamy and director of nursing services Eileen Brennan were both were awarded M.B.Es. Also in the list was Mrs Cumberlege, who was made a C.B.E. for her services to political and public life.

Options for the future

In July 1986, the regional health authority issued a consultation paper outlining seven main options[2] for developing health services in the Brighton district.

Option 1 was based on providing acute services at the County (536 beds) and Brighton General and a new 151-bedded hospital at Hove on a 20 acre site at Holmes Avenue purchased earlier in 1981. Option 2 was similar but without a new hospital at Hove. Option 3 consisted of the County, Brighton General and Bevendean. Option 4 was the only one to include a new hospital at Falmer intended to work in conjunction with the County. However, this was rejected early in the process because of problems of accessibility and of obtaining planning permission. Option 5 linked the County with a smaller Brighton General and 296 bed hospital at Hove while Option 6 contained variations on the proposed bed numbers at Holmes Avenue and Brighton General. Option 7 was similar but excluded Hove and included Bevendean.

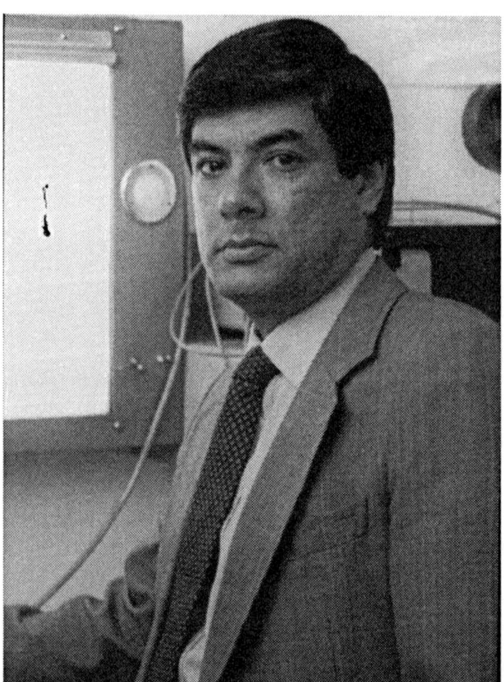

104. Carlos Perez Avila: awarded an honorary OBE.

Debate on these options continued throughout the 1980s, much of it focusing on the proposals for Hove that were strongly supported by residents and other interested parties, including the town's MP, Tim Sainsbury. However, it was not until 1991, nearly five years later,

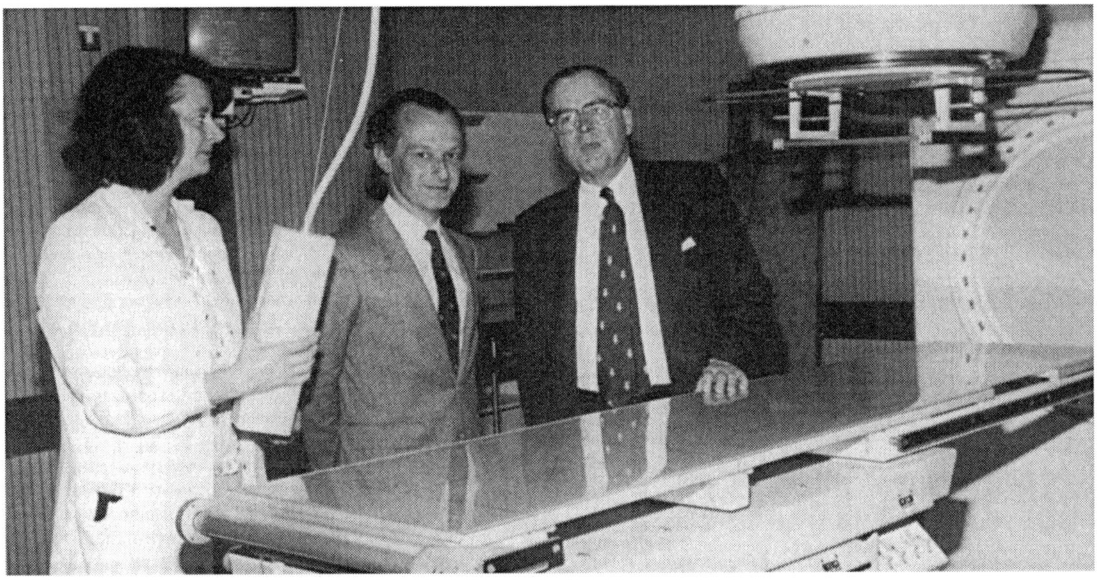

105. MP Sir Andrew Bowden (right) with consultant Dr George Deutsch at the opening of the new £1 million linear accelerator suite. The six million volt computer controlled accelerator represented the latest in cancer treatment technology at the time.

that a decision to recommend one of the options to the regional authority was finally taken.

In the meantime a number of smaller developments took place at the hospital. In 1986, for example, the renal unit was extended and the Sussex Throat and Ear department opened following the closure of the hospital in Church Hill.

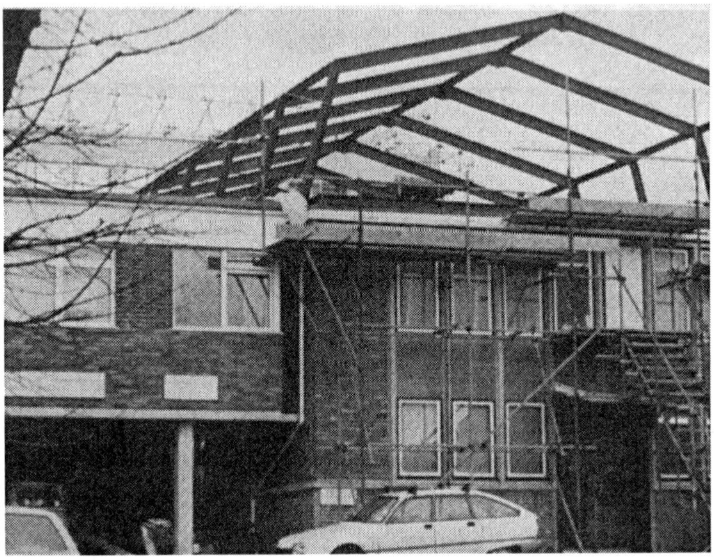

106. Work gets under way on building an extension to the Radiotherapy Department.

The radiotherapy department witnessed considerable expansion during 1987. At the beginning of the year, work began on a £250,000 extension funded by the Sussex Cancer Treatment Fund, another voluntary body that was adding its support to the hospital and which had spent over £1.5 million on cancer treatment facilities and equipment over a period of three year. Later in the year a new £1 million linear accelerator suite was opened in the department which was then treating 2,000 patients a year, 500 more than five years earlier.

During 1987 there was considerable press publicity about conditions on York Ward, described by one clinical nurse manager as 'a crumbling environment'. York Ward that had traditionally catered for diabetic patients had also catered for patients with the HIV/AIDS virus during the preceding two years and it was acknowledged that the staff had worked in challenging conditions in the ward that was scheduled for demolition. Fortunately conditions improved considerably the following year when staff and patients moved to an upgraded Grant Ward where the diabetic unit was named after former consultant, Dr Joanna Sheldon.

Time to celebrate

The 5th July 1988 was a very special day in most Brighton hospitals and the County was no exception. Plans to mark the fortieth anniversary of the NHS had been prepared earlier in the year. One suggestion was to offer staff a Forties style meal at the 1948 price of 2s 1d, just eleven pence in 1988 currency. This would be based of a 1948 meal when typical items included Spam or luncheon meat fritters, boiled beef and dumplings or toad in the hole with stuffed apples, prunes or spotted dick with custard to follow. Demand was so great at the County, that forty members of staff were selected by ballot to sample the anniversary menu. Another suggestion

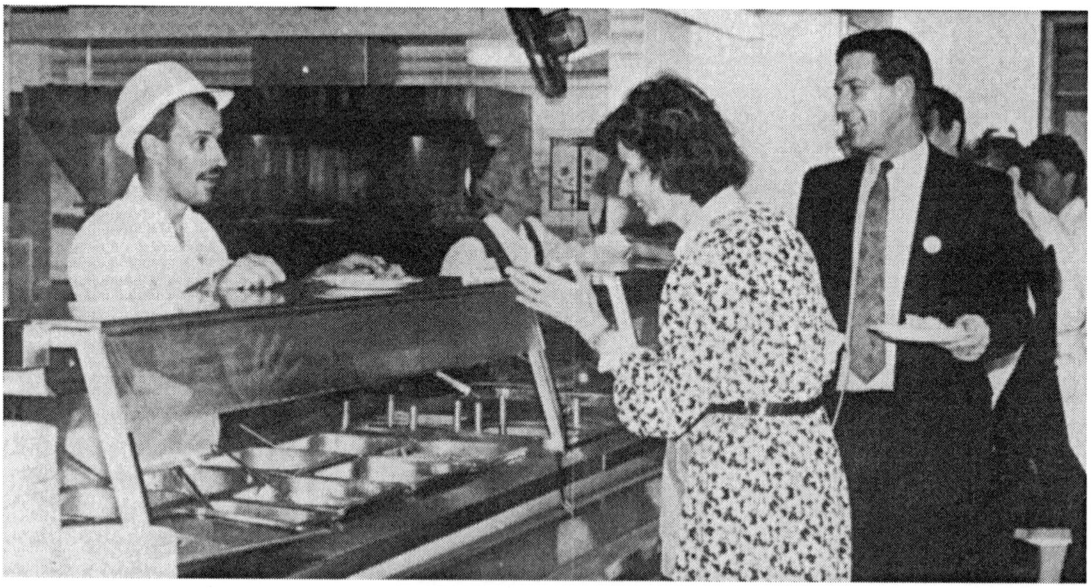

107. The chairman, Mrs Julia Cumberlege, and district administrator David Bowden in the staff canteen selecting their celebratory '1948' meal.

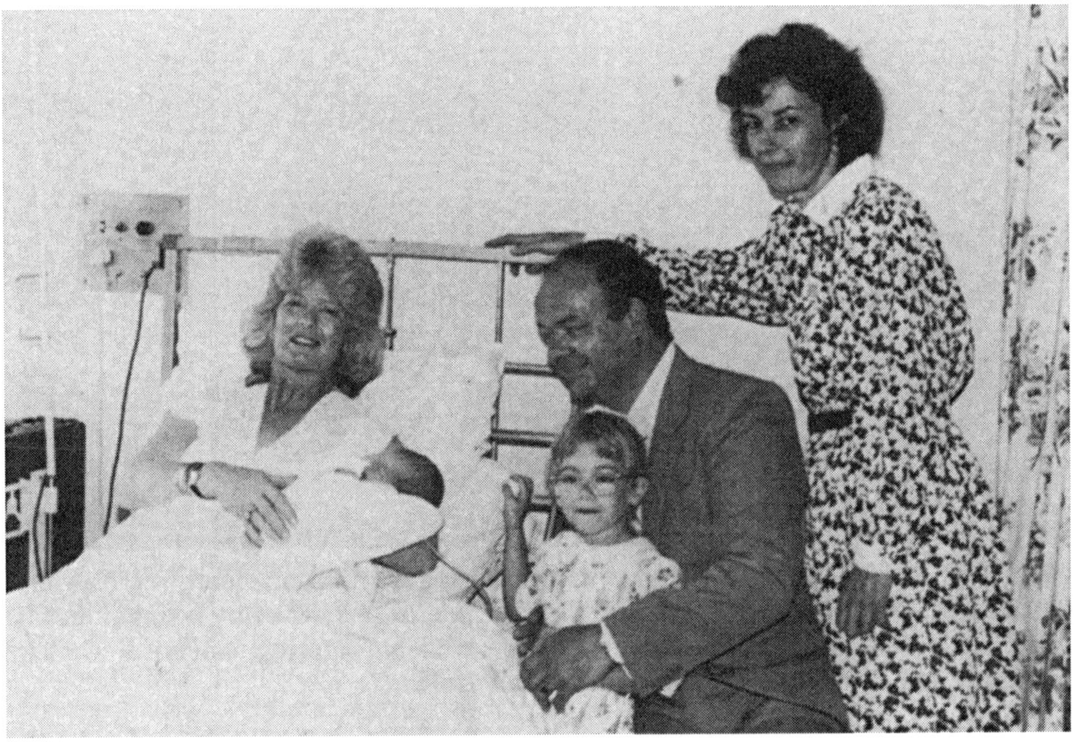

108. Anniversary babies: John Sudbury, Brighton hospitals' first NHS baby meets Mrs Anne Forde with her daughter, the first baby born in the hospital earlier in the day of the fortieth anniversary.

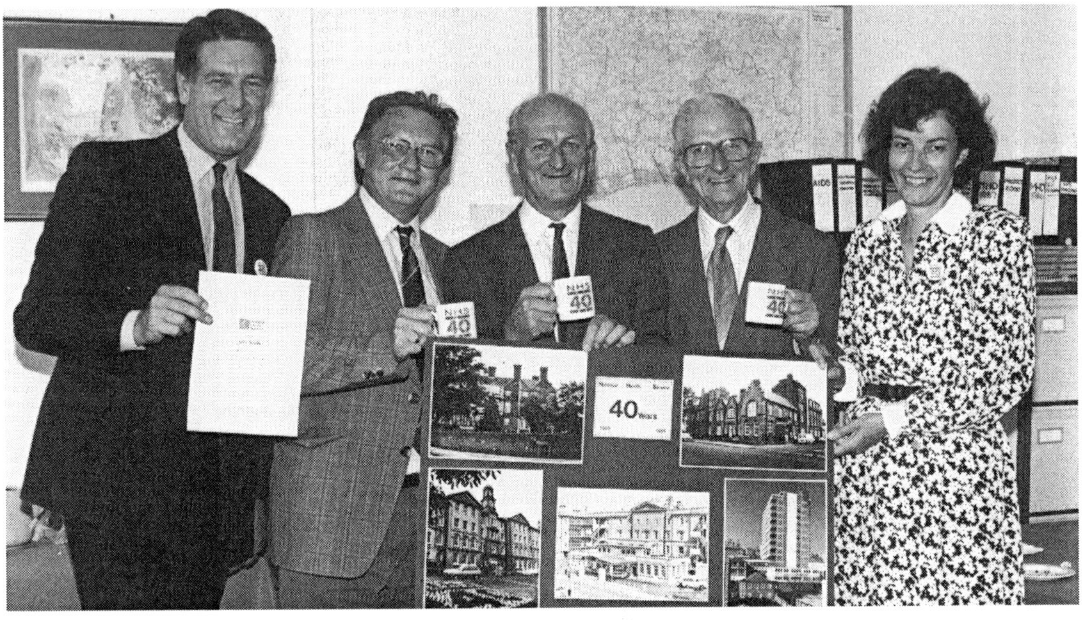

109. Three hospital staff who had worked in the NHS since the Appointed Day in 1948 with their awards: John Kimber, Mick Collins and Ken Tapson, with the district administrator and the health authority chairman.

that hit an unexpected snag was to hold a gathering of people born on the day at local NHS hospitals, at that time Brighton General and the Sussex Maternity. It transpired that only two babies were born in Brighton on the day, and only one of them in hospital. The League of Hospital Friends also announced plans to mark the occasion by donating a £2,000 birthday bed to the maternity unit, the second presented to the hospital within a few months.

The day itself was marked appropriately by a visit to the Maternity Department from Mr John Sudbury, who had been born at Brighton General on the appointed day, 5th July 1948, together with his family. During his visit he met Mrs Anne Ford of Hove and her daughter, the first baby born in the unit earlier in the day. All babies born in the hospital on the day had a TSB deposit account opened in their name, the TSB donating a £250 deposit to each. As well as the promised League of Friends gift, TSB Trustcard also donated a pair of rocking chairs to the unit as a birthday present.

Three members of staff attended a reception to mark their employment since the appointed day. They were the unit personnel manager, Mick Collins, John Kimber, chief medical laboratory scientific officer (MLSO) and senior MLSO Ken Tapson. Administrative assistant Angus McLeod was unable to be present but like the others he received a certificate to mark his achievement as well as a photographic collage and a souvenir mug. Mick Collins and John Kimber also attended a reception given by the Department of Health in London on the eve of the anniversary.

On the following morning, the chairman made the presentations to all the babies born in Maternity during July the 5th. In the afternoon there were talks on the accident department and on changing diets over the forty years as well as demonstrations of imaging (the new term that embraced X-rays and more modern developments in the field) and hip and of knee replacement surgery as well of tours of a number of different departments.

One of the best

1990 started promisingly for the hospital with the news that it had been named as one of fifteen hospitals highly commended for the quality of care provided in the 1989 *Sunday Times* Best of Health competition which 212 hospitals from every English region as well as Scotland, Wales and Northern Ireland had entered. A project to improve customer satisfaction in Accident and Emergency earned the certificate of commendation, which was hung in the entrance to the hospital. According to the judges: 'Among the examples of success reported were 90 per cent of patients under twelve being seen by a doctor within one hour and ninety per cent of all other patients being seen within two hours.'

However, the news was not so good three months later when the slump in the property market caused a number of planned developments to be put back including the construction of a proposed renal and pathology block and a new ward block. Locally, the health authority had been looking forward to receiving the proceeds of the sale of Pouchlands Hospital at Chailey and the School of Nursing on Hove seafront. Improvements to the outpatient department and pharmacy were also deferred for a year as a result of the slump.

Fortunately the situation did not delay the £2.5 million scheme to provide additional lifts in the 14 storey tower block and work started in October. On completion, the scheme was expected to alleviate some of the problems caused by the failure to complete the other two tower blocks in 1969, which would have included several more lifts. Refurbishment of the block was planned to follow the completion of installing the new lifts at a further cost of £4 million.

On October 31st there was a small ceremony to name another of the hospital's departments, named like some of the wards earlier in the hospital's history, in honour of a doctor. In the presence of his widow Geraldine, a former nurse at the County, and her son Peter, the Department of Anaesthesia was named after former consultant anaesthetist Dr Rex Binning. A general practitioner and anaesthetist before the start of the NHS, Rex Binning opted to become a specialist anaesthetist after his return from war service. He became well know nationally and internationally within his specialty and locally was very largely responsible for putting the department on a sound footing in the 1950s and 1960s.

1990 was also the first of two good years for Endoscopy. The Women's Voluntary Service continued their support of the hospital by donating £90,000 from their hospital canteen profits to mark the Queen Mother's 90th birthday. The gift was made help purchase new equipment, which was on view in October 1991 when the department moved to new accommodation in the accident and emergency department, using funds from a bequest to pay for the transfer

The time to decide

Future development of the hospital largely rested in the hands of the members of Brighton Health Authority on Wednesday the 24th July 1991. On that day they had to decide on their recommendation to the regional health authority for future hospital development in the area. By then the options for change had been reduced to a shortlist of three: a revised Option 5 for a major acute hospital at the County site of 989 beds supported by a community rehabilitation hospital at Hove; a revised Option 8, the County with four supporting community units at Newhaven, Holmes Avenue, North Brighton and Lewes; and finally, a revised Option 14: a 1,179 bedded hospital on the greenfield site at Falmer plus supporting units.

That Option 14 was included, despite the original decision of the regional authority not to include the Falmer proposal, undoubtedly owed much to Brighton's medical consultants. On the 19th December 1990 they had written to health secretary William Waldegrave inviting him to visit Brighton and see for himself how he district's three adult hospitals, largely built in the previous century, were falling apart because of a £23 million maintenance backlog, while money set aside for new building had 'largely disappeared.' They asked Mr Waldegrave for help with the short-term financial problem and to consider their plea for a greenfield site hospital development which

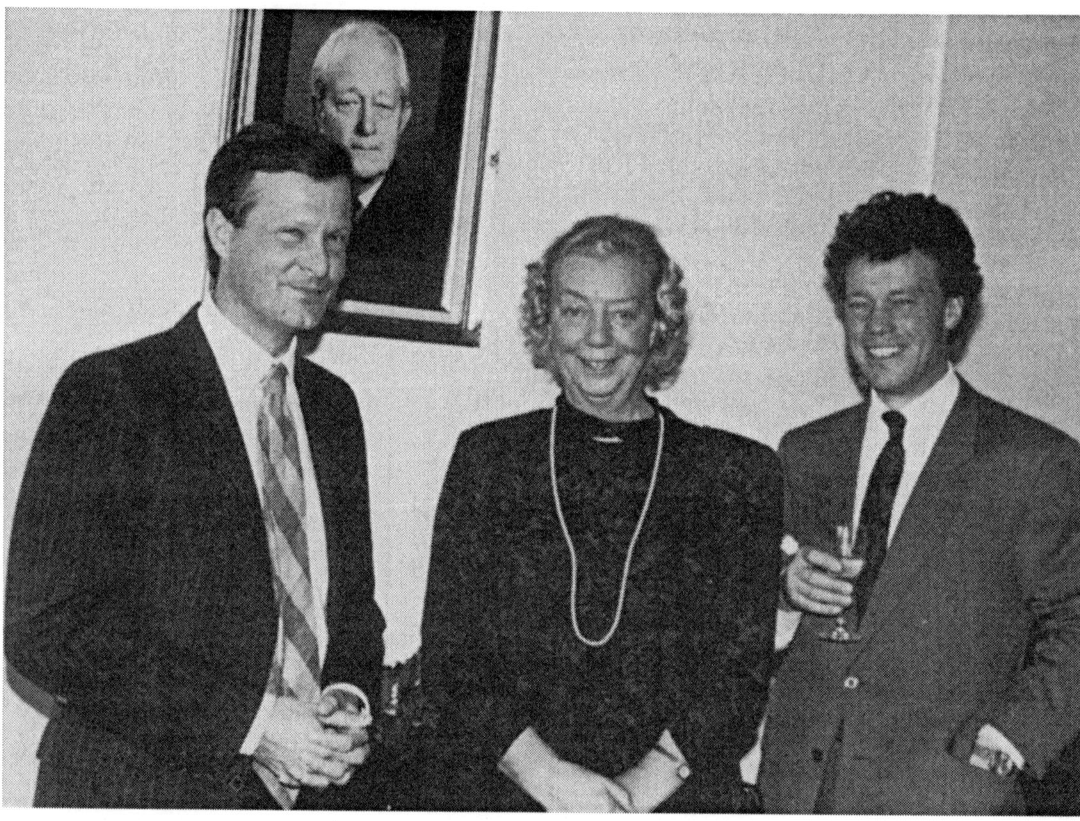

110. Consultant anaesthetist Dr Mike Twohig with Mrs Geraldine Binning and her son Peter stand before the portrait of her husband, Dr Rex Binning, that hangs in the department that now bears his name.

was 'unanimously supported by the consultant medical body'. In February the district health authority (DHA) learned that the Minister of Health had requested a complete re-assessment of the strategy for developing the major hospital services and the result, in the form of a 160 page report containing 14 options ranging from doing the minimum to building a 1,181 hospital on a greenfield site, was presented to the meeting. The consultants again pressed their case for building on a greenfield site. This was considered by the DHA but the members were reluctant to give it unqualified backing.

The debate continued throughout the following months, much of it in the media; one suggestion made in a letter to *The Health Service Journal* was to transfer one of the London teaching hospitals, of which there was a surplus, to the site adjacent to the Sussex University campus.

The debate on July 24th lasted three and a half hours. Once again consultants attending the meeting pressed their case for the greenfield site. But it was against the background of an earlier statement by the regional authority and the Department of Health that there was unlikely to be sufficient capital to develop a major new hospital providing all the district's acute services, estimated to cost over £200 million. The alternative, however, developing the County with a 260-bedded hospital at Hove, would be more in line with the likely availability of capital. Although several members believed the case for Falmer 'was exceptionally strong', they appeared to agree with view of the finance officer. His 'gut reaction was for bricks and mortar on a greenfield site', but he believed that by going for that 'we could well end up with nothing.'

When the vote was taken eight members voted for the Sussex County/ Holmes Avenue option. One member voted for the County with four supporting community units. None voted for the greenfield site.

And so the way was prepared for the development of the County. This, subject to regional approval, was expected to be the subject of an information campaign and public consultation exercise in due course.

16. First Steps towards a New County, 1992 – 1996

In the Summer of 1992, detailed plans for a £57 million redevelopment of acute hospital services began to take shape. Approval for the redevelopment was given by the regional health authority in July, although discussions on the final amount of capital that would be made available were still taking place.

At this stage the intention was to concentrate acute services at the Royal Sussex County in top quality purpose built accommodation. Work was expected to start on site the following year with completion by 1999. The plan envisaged closing outdated facilities at Hove General and Brighton General hospitals so that by the turn of the century the Royal Sussex would be offering new wards with some 300 beds, improved pathology facilities, better catering and more car parking. In addition, there were to be extra theatres and day case facilities, expanded clinical support services and a new postgraduate centre. And, what was perhaps the most exciting prospect for the future, a plan to submit proposals for a new cardiothoracic suite able to carry out a thousand open heart procedures a year.

The programme for the main developments with their anticipated completion dates was in two phases. Phase 1: pathology department (1995), clinical inpatient block, approximately 130 beds (1996), extended catering facilities, postgraduate medical centre and multi-storey car park, all for completion 1996; Phase 2: 236 bed ward block with theatres, day case unit and endoscopy suite, clinical support block for diagnostic and other support services and a second multi-storey car park, all for completion in 1999.

However, as events over the next five years were to prove, there were still many obstacles to be overcome before a start could be made in bringing these ambitious plans to fruition.

Only a few months were to pass before changes were made to the plans to meet the concerns of local residents and the council's planning officers. More than five hundred people attended an exhibition run by hospital staff in the hospital car park as part of the normal planning process. Possible increases in traffic and the proposed new car parks were particular causes of concern and the car parks seemed likely to be reduced in size as a result. Other likely changes included modifications to the clinical block proposed to the north of the existing tower block while the relation of some buildings to the boundary of the site were being re-examined. Despite this, the principal problem to progressing the scheme remained a financial one: although the regional authority pledged continued support and had funds available, the government had announced a review of its spending plans.

Fortunately this was resolved a few months later when the health secretary, Virginia Bottomley, announced that the Treasury had approved the expenditure of £35½ million on the first phase. This left only one remaining hurdle, final planning consent from the local authority. Shortly before Christmas, details of the scheme were submitted for planning approval and the hospital trust's chief executive announced that the next year, 1995, would see a start made on site. This, he said, would include 'the new 198 bed clinical block (which includes a new cardiothoracic centre), a complete refurbishment of A&E and Orthopaedics on Level 5, improved catering facilities, a new pathology department and, at long last, improved car parking facilities.'

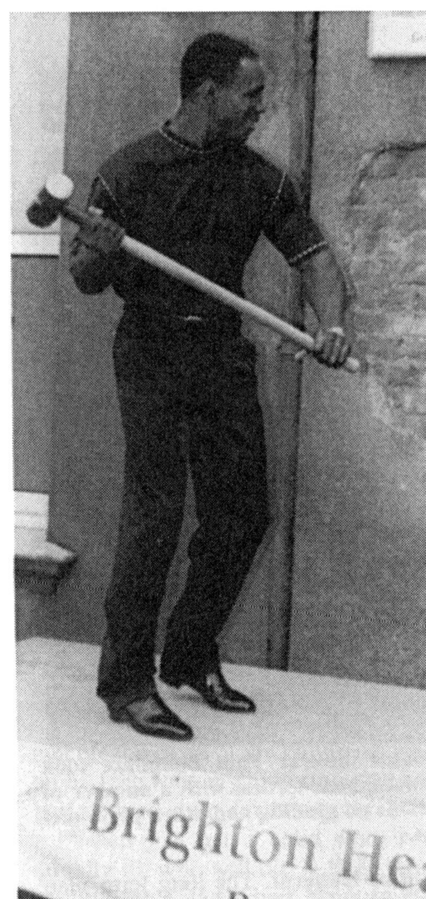

111. Former world champion boxer Chris Eubank uses a sledgehammer to knock out the first bricks in the demolition of the nurses' home.

In fact, work had begun before Christmas on what was effectively the start of the redevelopment with the construction of a new computer department behind the Barry Building.

By February this was up to roof level, but progress on the redevelopment proper was slower than expected. It was not until the autumn that the first visible signs of a start to the scheme were seen with the demolition of the nurses' home that was needed to make way for the car park. Watched by an invited audience, which included a number of nurses, Hove's former world champion boxer, Chris Eubank, swung a sledgehammer to knock out the first bricks from the building. The ceremony was followed by a reception in which the trust's chairman, Dame Audrey Emerton, wielded a knife to knock out the windows of an iced cake modelled in the shape of the nurses' home that stood for nearly 100 years.

With the demolition completed, work began in earnest excavating 35,000 cubic metres of chalk and installing piling round the north perimeter of the site needed as a retaining wall and as a basis for the foundations of the new car park and clinical block.

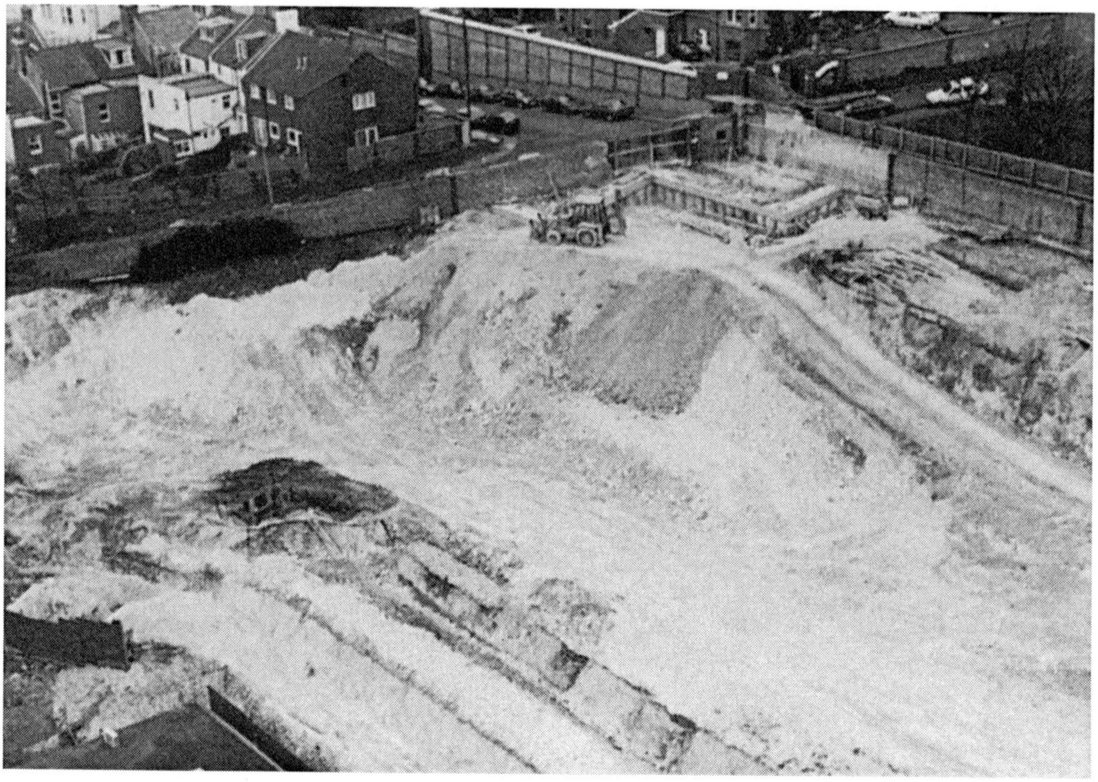

112. The long-awaited development gets under way early in 1995 when some five hundred lorry movements daily were needed to remove the vast quatities of chalk excavated in readiness for the construction of the car park and the new clinical blocks.

Five Years of Progress

Although a great deal of attention was focused on the major redevelopment, many other developments were taking place at the hospital during the five years up to 1996.

In April 1992, a staff nursery opened at Rosaz House, partly funded by a staff lottery. Previously hospital staff had relied on an 18 place nursery at Brighton General Hospital. The County Hospital nursery added a further 33 places for staff working in the health district. Unlike the Brighton General Hilltop Nursery, it was also able to accept babies from three months old and upwards.

Rosaz House, situated in Bristol Gate opposite to the tower block, was formerly the Brighton and Hove Girls' Orphanage established in the early nineteenth century. It was later used as an educational holiday home for London children before conversion to its new use. The nursery was situated on the ground floor while the first floor of the house was adapted to provide a staff training centre.

April also marked the completion of the first phase of the redevelopment of the X-ray department with the opening of a new screening room. This was followed by the completion of two more phases, new ultrasound and vascular intervention suites.

Meanwhile, the main outpatient department was being upgraded. In 1973 it still resembled:

> a huge barn with a very high ceiling [where] in the waiting room all the chairs were arranged in regimental rows. Patients were resigned to waiting and sat patiently staring into space, waiting their turn to see the doctor.[1]

The first major change to take place utilised the huge amount of space in the ceiling where a second floor was erected. Although originally intended as offices, extra consulting rooms were provided making it possible to transfer gastroenterology clinics there from Brighton General Hospital.

December 1992 saw the start of work building a completely new department at the hospital. Appropriately, for a former voluntary hospital, this provided yet another example of the way the voluntary tradition had been carried on, and had by no means been extinguished by the introduction of the National Health Service back in 1948.

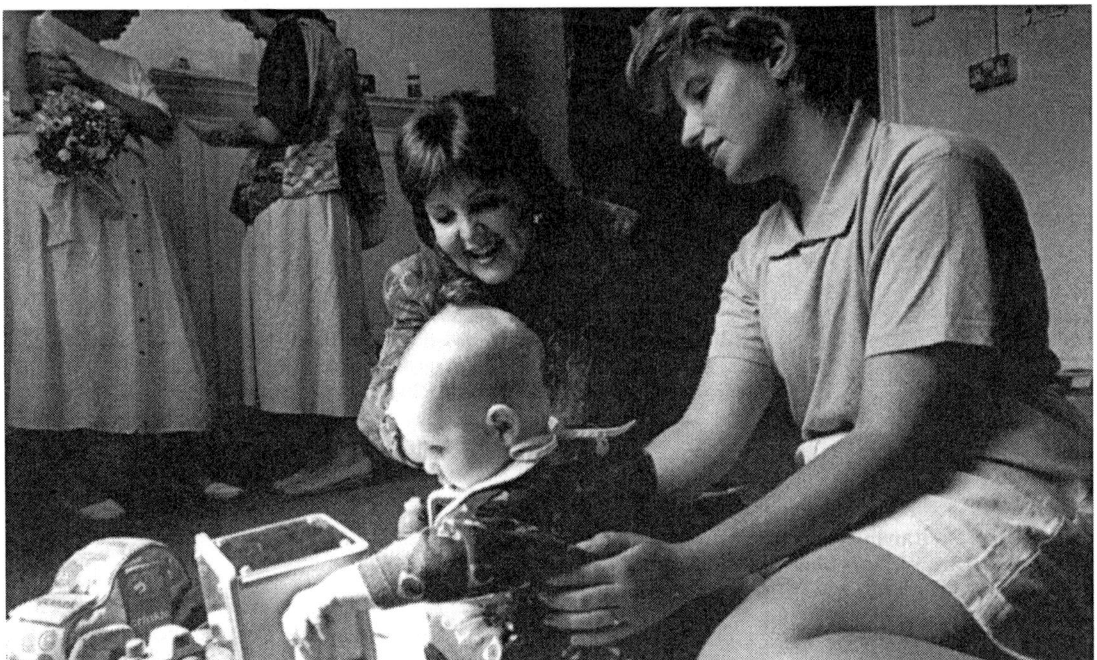

113. Actress Pauline Collins (centre) plays with one of the children after officially opening the Rosaz House nursery and staff training centre.

Some eighteen months earlier, two consultant surgeons, Brian Hogbin and Bob Gumpert, launched an appeal to raise £195,000 to provide a purpose built breast care unit in the grounds of the hospital. At the time, breast care work was carried out on different sites in Brighton and some of the facilities were very poor. The new purpose built unit was to be sited adjacent to the existing breast assessment unit. The appeal got off to a good start with a well-attended ball at the Hotel Metropole and when the sum of £170,000 had been raised it was decided to begin building work on site. However, with a further £30,000 needed to furnish and equip the unit, a final push for funds was launched with a visit by actress Barbara Windsor (who was appearing as the Fairy Godmother in pantomime at the Theatre Royal!). Her visit to the breast assessment unit and the rubble-strewn site of the new breast care unit resulted, as intended, in gaining television and press publicity for the appeal. Within four months, the unit was completed and opened and named the Nigel Porter Breast Care Unit after consultant surgeon Nigel Porter who worked in Brighton from 1963 to 1985.

The transformation of what had become known as the Sussex Oncology Centre was completed early in 1995 and the £½ million new-look department was officially opened by the Duchess of Gloucester. As well as the landscaped new entrance in Bristol Gate, the unit featured a tranquil oriental-style garden with flowing water, a wooden bridge, rocks and flowerbeds. Access to the garden was from the waiting lounge, which contained driftwood sculptures, while murals with a sea theme lined the walls leading to the linear accelerator room.

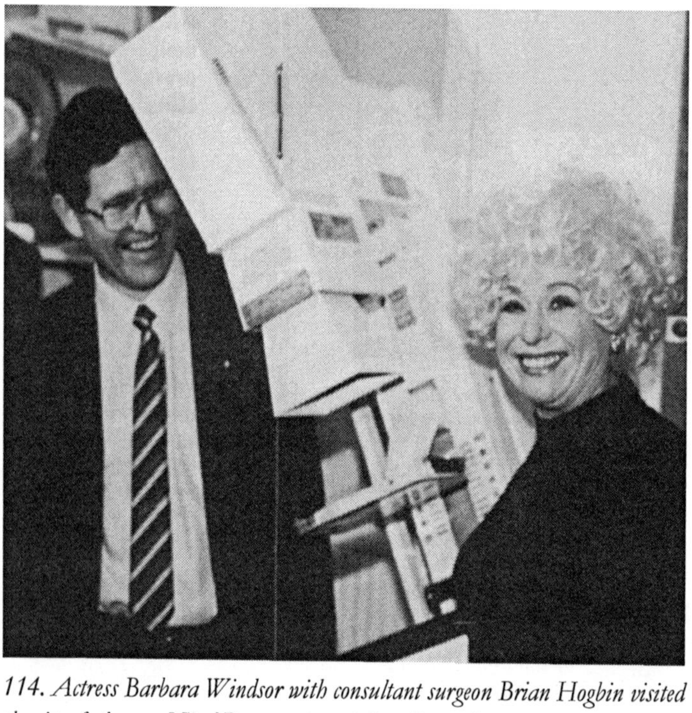

114. Actress Barbara Windsor with consultant surgeon Brian Hogbin visited the site of the new Nigel Porter unit and the adjacent breast assessment unit to publicise the need for more funds to equip the new unit.

There were more celebrations in the X-ray department in 1994 when it became the first in Sussex to be provided with a new MRI Scanner. The magnetic resonance imager marked a major step forward being safer than X-rays but able to produce considerably more information. Using a

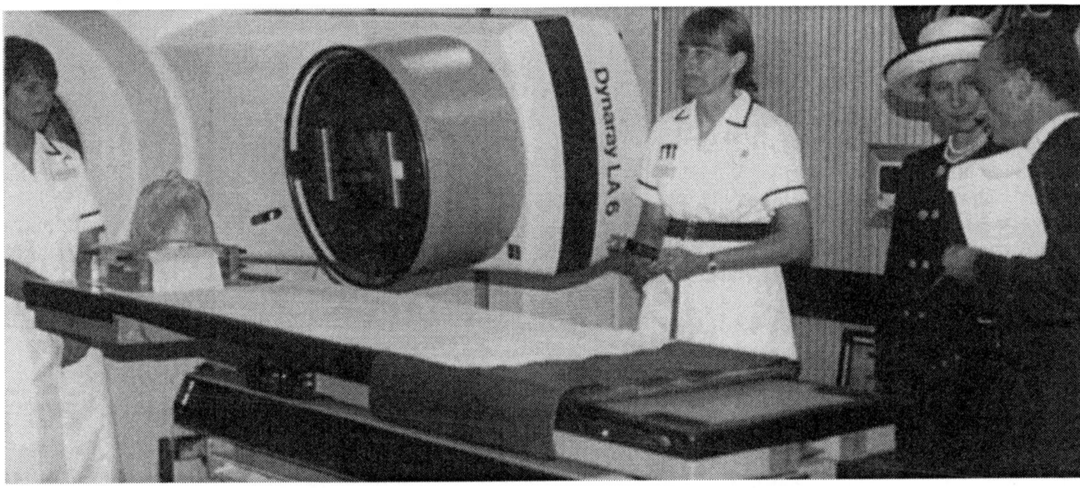

115. Radiographers Lorraine Young and Angela Hammond demonstrated the unit's linear accelerator during the visit by the Duchess of Gloucester to the transformed Sussex Oncology Centre.

giant magnet used to create a magnetic field, the machine was capable of producing very detailed pictures of body tissue. A technical problem on the morning of the day in May when it was meant to go into service delayed the scan for the first patient until the afternoon. Fortunately there were no more problems with the £1 million machine, which was officially opened by health secretary Virginia Bottomley on the 22nd June. She described it as 'a fine example of how innovative technology brings real benefits to patients' adding that 'this and other developments which are in the pipeline … will ensure that your hospital continues to go from strength to strength.'[2]

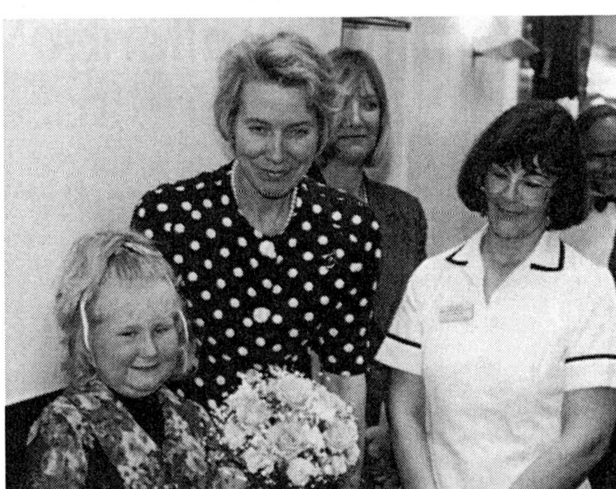

116. Nine year old Katie Symes was chosen to present a posy to health secretary Virginia Bottomley who opened the new MRI unit. Katie, the youngest person to be scanned with the new equipment, would previously have had to travel to London for her check-up.

One of these developments was unveiled a few weeks later in August when actor Adam Faith launched the new trauma room in A&E. He posed for pictures on one of the Traumex trolleys to demonstrate the extraordinary manoeuvrability of the £¼ million system, one of only two installed in the world outside the USA at the time.

During her visit, Mrs Bottomley also praised the pioneering work in the hospital in developing patient focused care as part of its drive to improve the

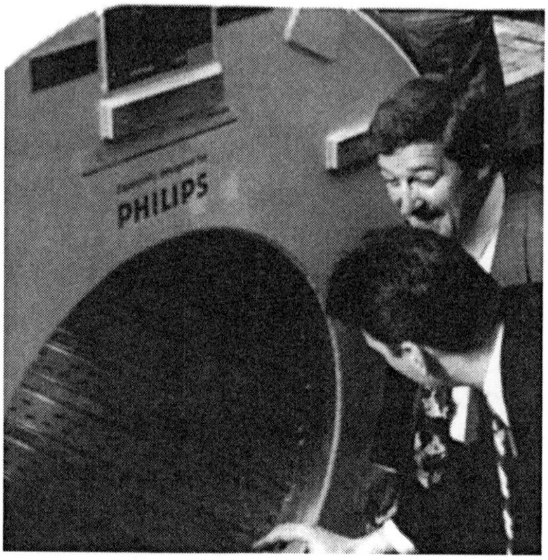

117. Consultant anaesthetist Dr Tim Doyle (top) inspects the giant magnet on its arrival at the hospital. More than six feet high and weighing 2,800 kilogrammes, the magnet was hoisted into position using a special crane.

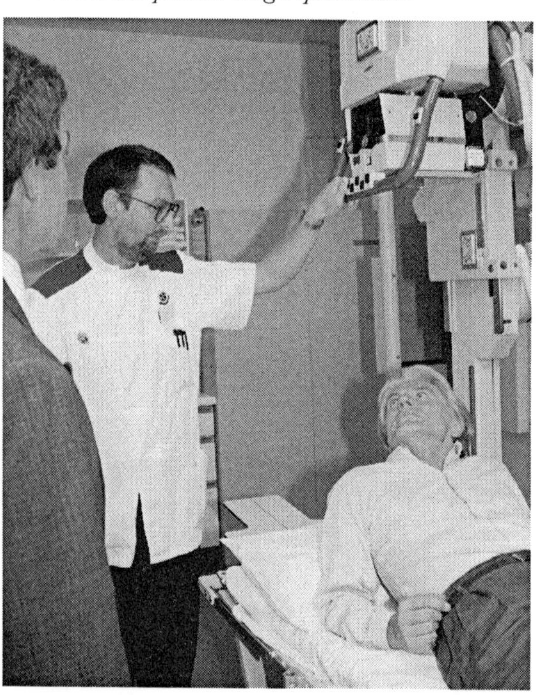

118. Actor Adam Faith climbed on one of the new Traumex trolleys in A&E to demonstrate its manoeuvrability – something that was not available when he suffered a serious road accident in 1973.

quality of care offered. Work on this new approach had begun the year before when Brighton was awarded a £250,000 grant by the Department of Health. This enabled the hospital to join about half a dozen others investigating and implementing the new system that was also being developed in the USA and Australia.

Patient focused care was based on the fundamental assumption that everything a hospital does, and its physical layout, is best centred around the needs of the patient. Surveys had shown that doctors and nurses spent several hours a day walking round hospital corridors on activities not devoted to patient care while patients had to travel around hospitals for procedures such as X-rays and blood tests. Moreover, according to the survey, on average 45 individual members of staff came into contact with a single patient during a five day hospital stay. These were just some of the problems patient focused care was intended to tackle.

In October 1993, the board of the newly formed Brighton Health Care NHS Trust gave the go-ahead for a pilot care centre for gastroenterology. This specialty was chosen because of the range of patients catered for – medical and surgical, elective and emergency, inpatients, outpatients and day cases. The board was told that there was a revolutionary move away from invasive surgery as a result of the development of new technology. In the field of diagnosis, endoscopy for example was replacing the barium swallow.

A principal aim of the change was to draw all of the work together in one department, making it possible to offer a holistic approach by a familiar group of staff. Events were to prove, however, that praiseworthy though this aim was, bringing this work together in one place was not easily going to be achieved until more progress was made in the major redevelopment of the hospital.

Nurses and nursing

Changes in care were already in evidence, however, largely through the initiatives of staff, especially nurses. In 1992, for example, aromatherapy was introduced into the high tech world of intensive care. A qualified aromatherapist offered her services to the unit which members of staff who had attended reflexology courses were more than happy to accept. It was claimed that improvements to even unconscious patients were visible on the monitors as a result of receiving massage with essential oils. A staff nurse from London who arrived to take the six month intensive ITU course, undertook a research project into the treatment. She assessed three different groups of patients thirty minutes after their treatment that demonstrated its effectiveness compared with the alternatives which were massage without essential oils or a curtained off rest period.

Staff in the Trevor Mann Special Care Baby Unit trod a similar path when they encouraged mothers and their partners to overcome their anxieties by taking an active part in the care of their very sick or premature baby

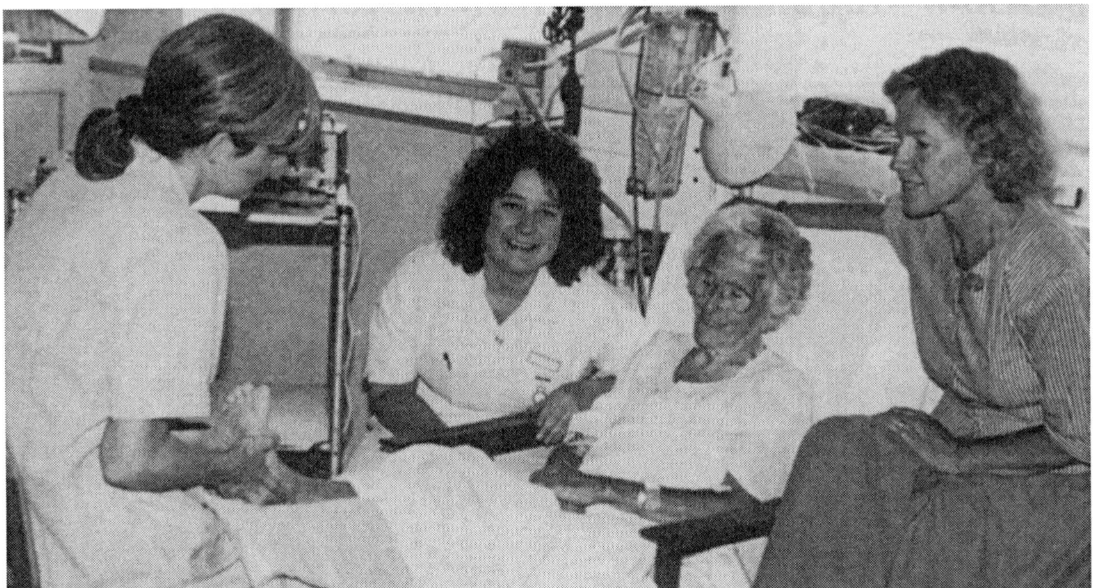

119. A patient receives a foot massage in the coronary care unit where staff nurse Dawn Hewitt (centre) carried out research on the effectiveness of aromatherapy for patients in intensive care.

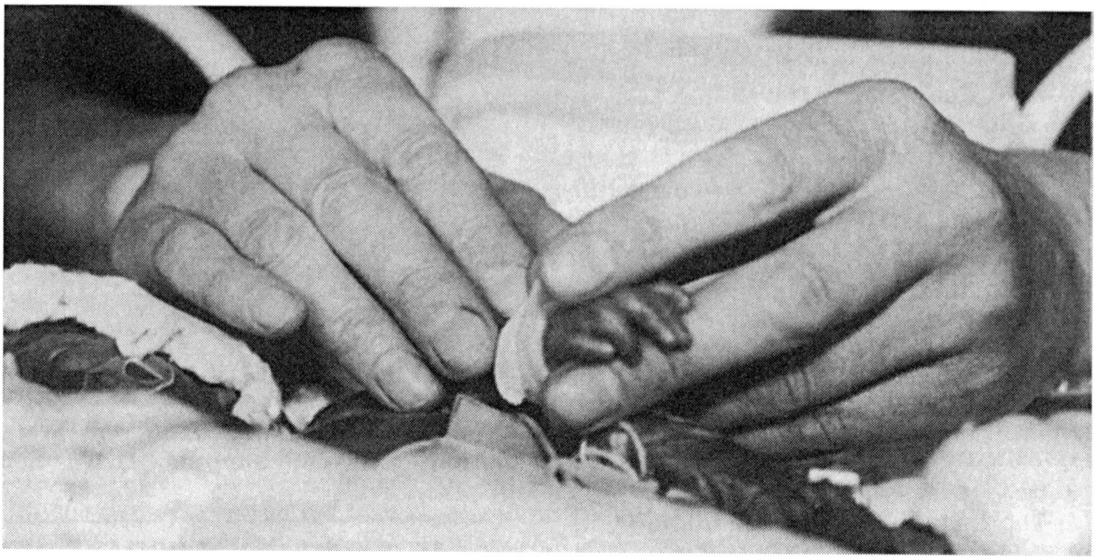

120. A Trevor Mann Baby Unit staff nurse strokes the fingers of a seven days old 24 week premature baby to describe the benefits of positive touch for babies in the unit that was featured in a television programme.

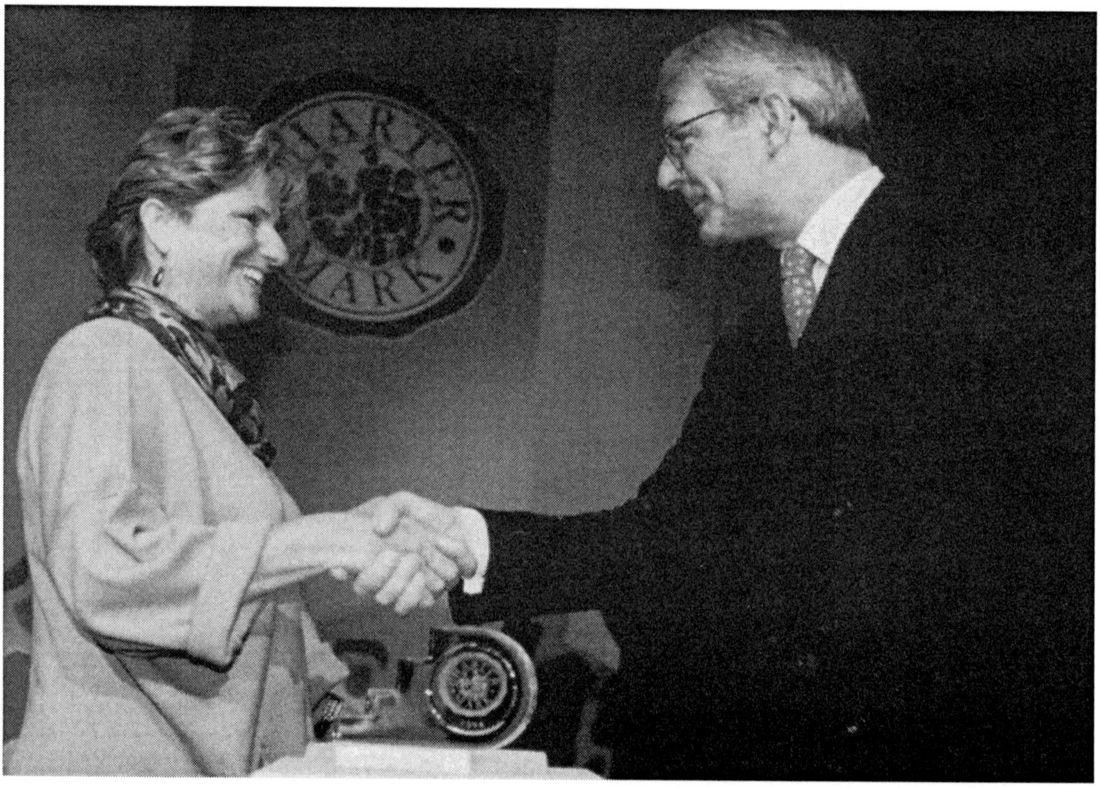

121. Head nurse Jane Stach receives the Charter Mark award for the Sussex Oncology Centre from the prime minister, John Major, at the ceremony in London's Festival Hall.

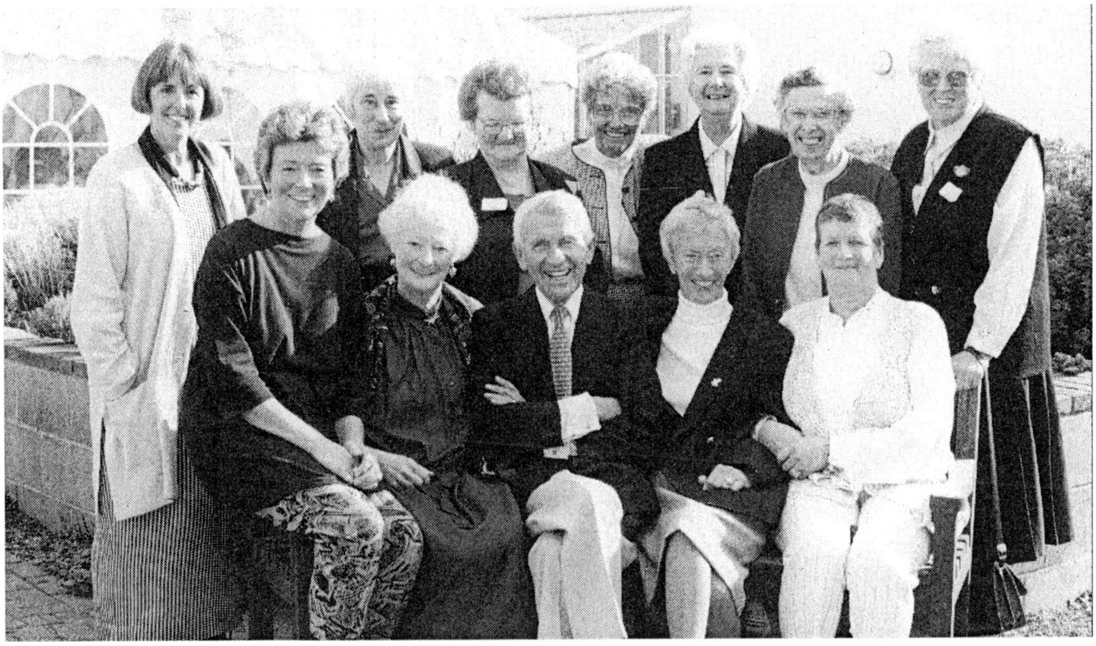

122. Nurses with retired consultant Dr Jan de Winter who celebrated their league's 50th anniversary.

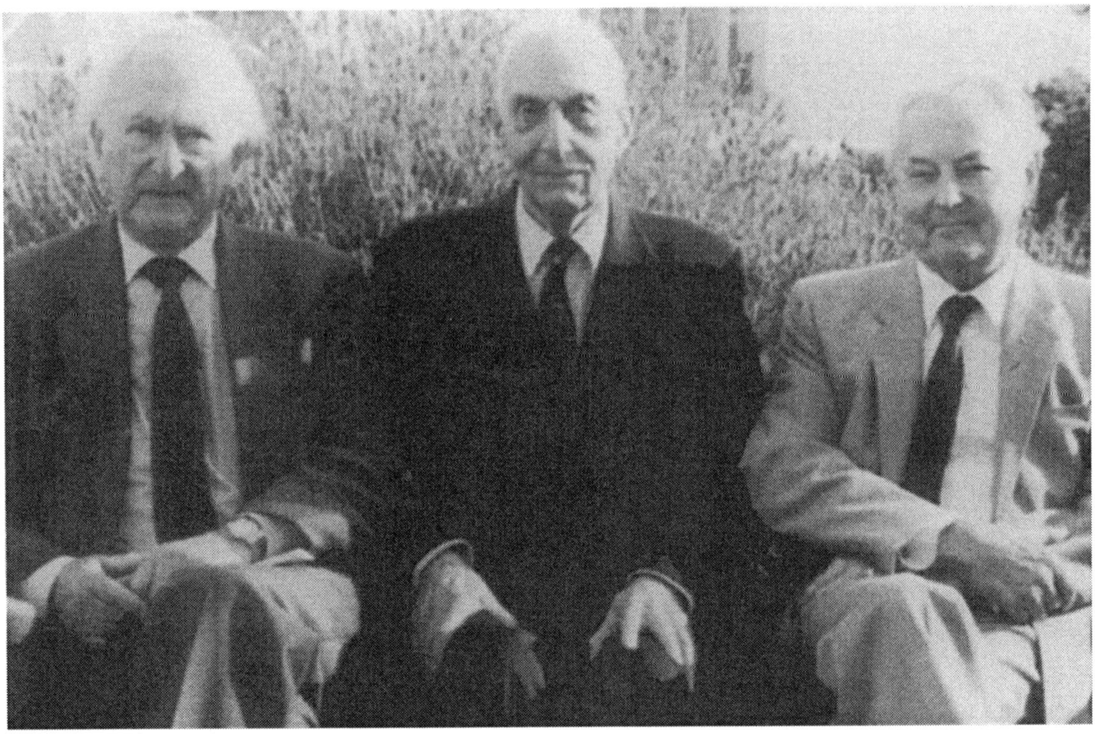

123. Former consultants Nick Lawrence, Leslie Lauste and Dr Tom Copp. who joined in the nurses' anniversary celebrations.

through the use of touch in the form of massage and stroking. Their work was featured in a special televison programme in June 1995.

Alternative therapies were also introduced by staff in other hospital departments including Howard 1 for their cancer patients and in the Nigel Porter Breast Care Unit while books on complementary therapies were included in the wide range of information available to cancer patients at the hospital. It was because of the excellent standard of advice, support and treatment, including a 24-hour helpline for patients, a resource pack and range of leaflets, that the hospital's Sussex Oncology Centre won the first-ever Charter Mark awarded to an oncology centre in the country. This was presented in October 1994 by the prime minister at a ceremony in London.

The closure of the hospital's nursing school and subsequent changes that led to introduction of nursing diploma and degree courses at the University of Brighton had its effect on the hospital's nurses' league. In October 1996, more than a hundred former nurses from as far afield as the USA and Ireland visited the hospital to celebrate the league's 50th anniversary. It was about this time that membership of the league, previously restricted to nurses who has trained at the hospital's school or had held a post as ward sister or higher for more than three years, was changed to encourage membership of all trained staff who had worked at the hospital.

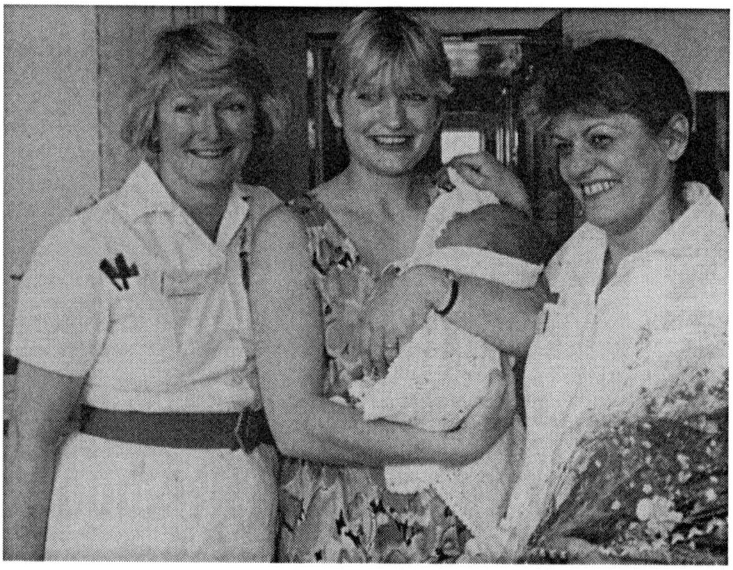

124. To celebrate the birth of the new Brighton Health Care NHS Trust, Level 11 was renamed George Miles Ward after tthe first baby born in the hospital on the day. Baby George is held by his mother Ros, who is accompanied by midwives Pauline Tarrant and Jo Hill.

Enlarging the hospital

Change was a continuing feature during this five year period, none less than the organisational change that took place on the 1st April 1993 when Brighton's acute hospital services came under the control of the newly formed trust. This was marked at the hospital in several ways.

There was a ribbon cutting ceremony in the main entrance, Level 11 in the tower block was renamed the George Miles Ward after the first baby born in

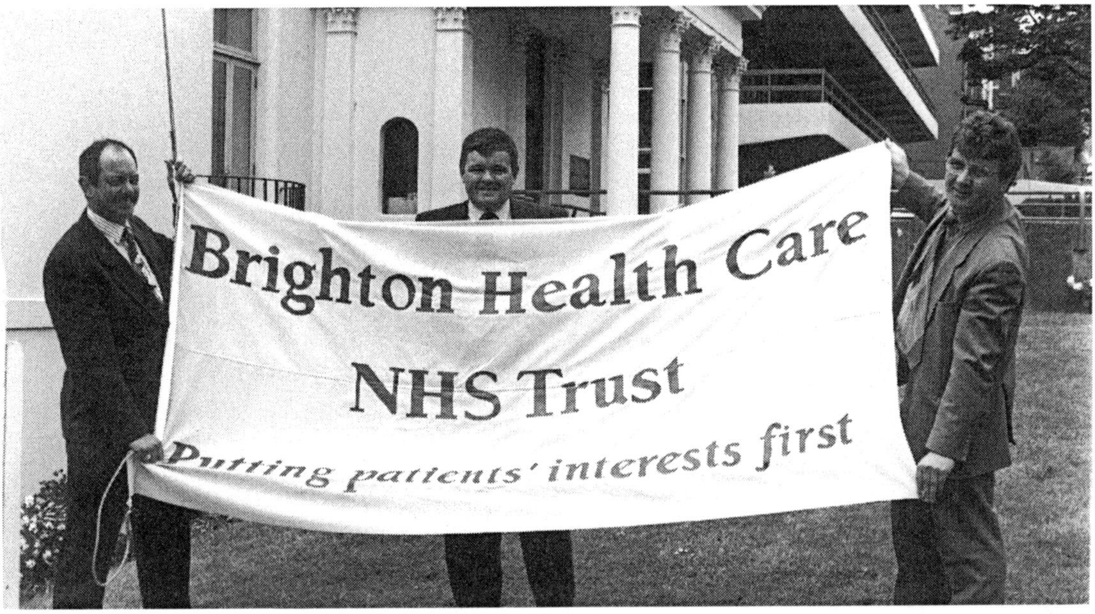

125. Glenn Hewlett, Lee Soden and Bartley Quinn raising the flag to mark the renaming of Pearson House to Sussex House.

the maternity unit that day, and there were exhibitions of old photographs and hospital artefacts.

There was a special menu for patients and staff and patients and visitors were offered a non-alcoholic cocktail, the Trust Tonic, to toast the new venture. Outside, the Union Jack fluttered from twin flagpoles over the hospital; inside, a major programme of upgrading began with the opening of refurbished facilities on Level 5 of the tower block.

April 1st also marked the return of the GU Medicine department to the hospital. When the department was transferred to Royal York Buildings towards the end of 1984, it had been renamed the Claude Nicol Centre. Now, instead of a hut at the rear of Outpatients, the centre was incorporated at the west end of the department. The Lawson Unit for HIV/AIDS patients (named after Dr Lawson, medical officer of the original GU clinic in 1918) was then established adjacent to Claude Nicol and opened on April 1st two years later in 1995.

There was a major boost for the hospital early in 1995 when the trust purchased a listed building, Pearson House, the St Dunstan's property more or less on the hospital doorstep in Abbey Road. Because the trust was not allowed to retain the existing name, a staff competition for a new one was held (with a £50 prize or dinner for two at the Grand Hotel) and on the

5th June the building was vacated, handed over to the trust and renamed Sussex House.

The purchase of the building eased the pressure on space at the hospital and also occurred at a very convenient time with the prospect of work due to start on the major redevelopment when it was expected to alleviate some of the inevitable short term problems. Early plans for the property included a seventy-one place staff nursery, a board room, staff social club and dining facilities on the ground floor. The lower ground floor was to be used for urology, the first floor for thirty units of staff accommodation and for the department of medical photography and illustration, while the second floor was to contain a sixteen roomed patient hotel and additional staff residences.

The Patient Hotel, the first of its kind in Sussex, was officially opened on the 17th November when the first patient to arrive was greeted with flowers and a bottle of wine. The hotel was expected to free hospital beds for patients requiring investigations such as X-rays and scans prior to surgery or for an overnight stay prior to early morning surgery. It was also hoped to benefit patients who needed to travel long distances for outpatient treat-

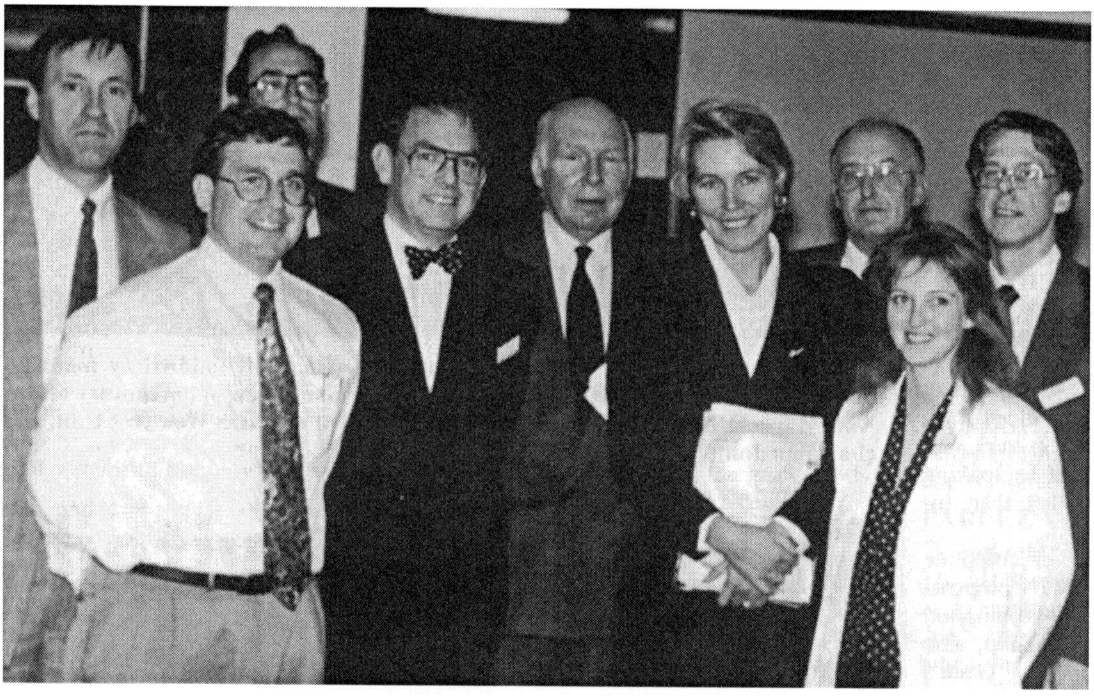

126. Medical staff who urged the health secretary Virginia Bottomley to consider their case for a new medical school in Brighton. Consultants from left: Matthew Fletcher, Dr Charles Turton, Dr Nick Bishop, Dr Patrick Hall Smith, Colin Strachan and Professor Richard Vincent with (front) junior medical staff representatives Dr Simon Biggart and Dr Alison Taylor.

ments such as radiotherapy as well as for others waiting for discharge who perhaps needed equipment or services to be set up at home.

Thanks to the efforts of staff who worked throughout the weekend, the staff nursery was also transferred to Sussex House during the month without any interruption to the service previously provided at Rosaz House.

Towards a university hospital?

The five years from 1992 to 1996 also witnessed events that were eventually to have a significant impact at the hospital.

These began in October 1992 when consultants and other medical staff took advantage of a visit by health secretary Virginia Bottomley. Taking time away from the annual Conservative Party conference that was being held in Brighton, she rounded off a tour of Brighton General Hospital at the Sussex Postgraduate Medical Centre. There, over a cup of tea, she met a number of consultants and representatives of the junior medical staff and discussed a number of issues including redevelopment in the district, junior doctors' hours and the possibility of establishing a medical school locally.

This was only the beginning of what was to prove a long running saga. The two local universities joined the trust in putting forward proposals for a new-style medical school that they believed would meet the needs of the 21st century. The redevelopment of the County Hospital was another factor used in support of the bid since the hospital would provide the principal base for the students' clinical experience in acute medicine.

Although the proposal was unsuccessful and the prospects for the establishment of an undergraduate medical school locally appeared to have faded, all was not lost. A few years later it became known that bids were being sought to establish a new medical school outside London. There were four known contenders for the new school – Plymouth, Wirral, Keele and Hull – and determined to join them, the local universities joined forces with the two Brighton trusts with the intention of submitting a costed proposal in April 1996.

There was no real prospect of any further developments until after the forthcoming general election, which was anticipated in 1997 – and that was also the year when it was confidently expected that first fruits of the hospital's major redevelopment programme would be seen.

17. Towards the New Millennium, 1997 – 2000

The years leading up to the new millennium witnessed an intensity of activity probably never seen before in the history of the hospital that culminated in the Royal opening of the Millennium Wing on Friday the 17th November 2000.

1997 began with what promised to be a two year period of disruption for staff in the A&E department. The year opened with one of the busiest weekends of the winter when icy conditions led to a veritable flood of casualties with broken limbs. There followed an even more testing time when on the 20th January the redevelopment of the department began which was scheduled to least for 135 weeks.

Temporary buildings were erected in the car park to accommodate decanted staff and facilities and a temporary canopy was erected over the ambulance and walking wounded entrances. On completion in 1999, the new facilities in an enlarged department would include a trauma X-ray room, a CT suite, a new fracture clinic and treatment areas.

In the meantime, a service for an anticipated 165 patients a day had to be provided in much reduced accommodation and a public appeal was made for prospective patients to visit their GPs rather than visit the hospital. GPs

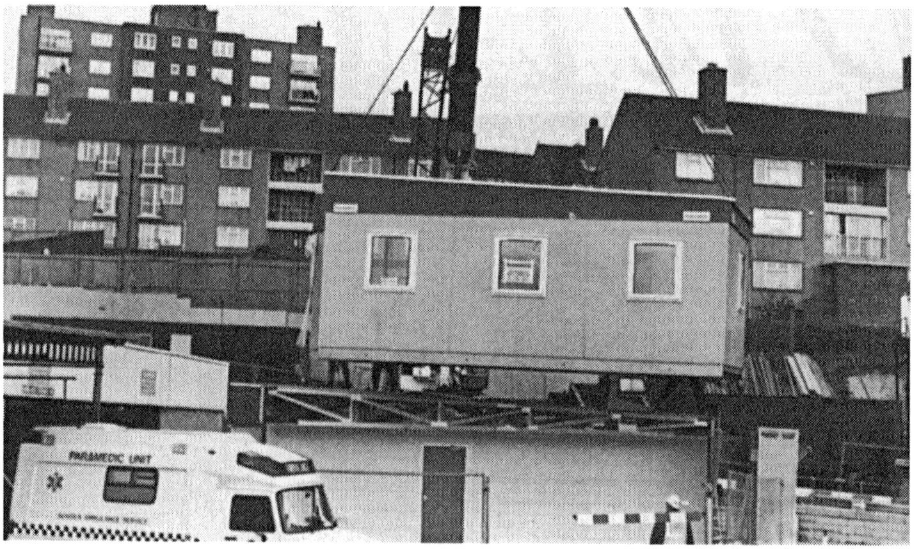

127. A Portacabin is lifted by crane into the A&E car park in preparation for the redevelopment of the department.

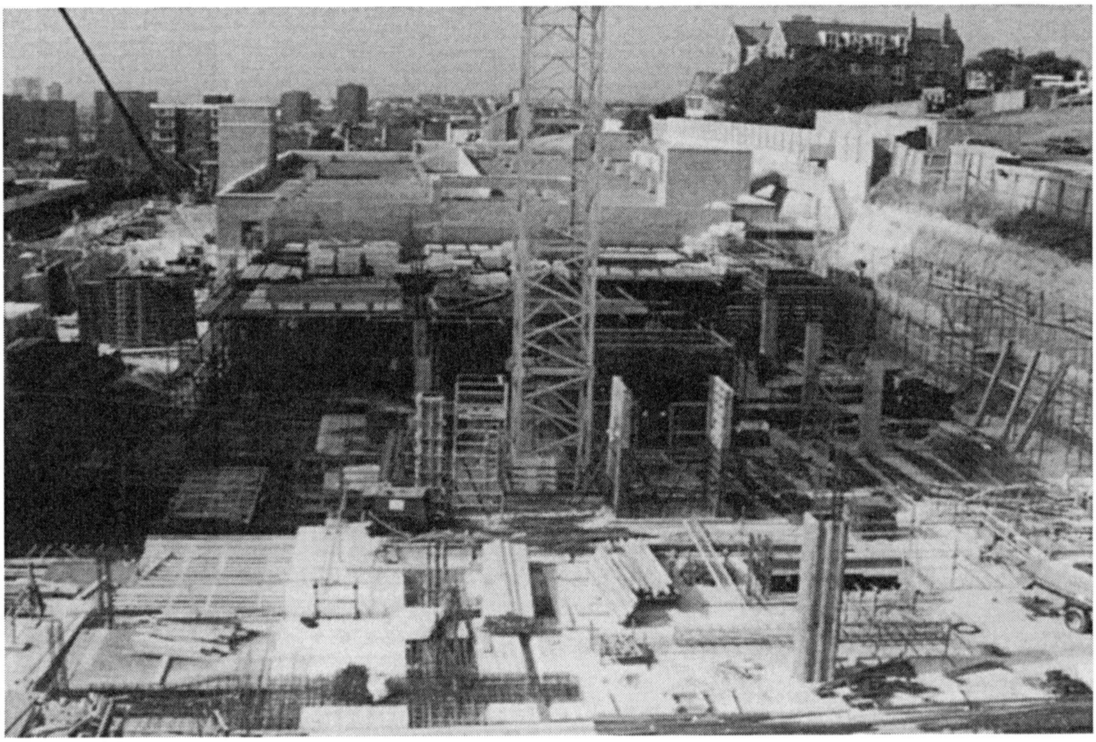

128. The new clinical block rises from the giant hole excavated in the chalk.

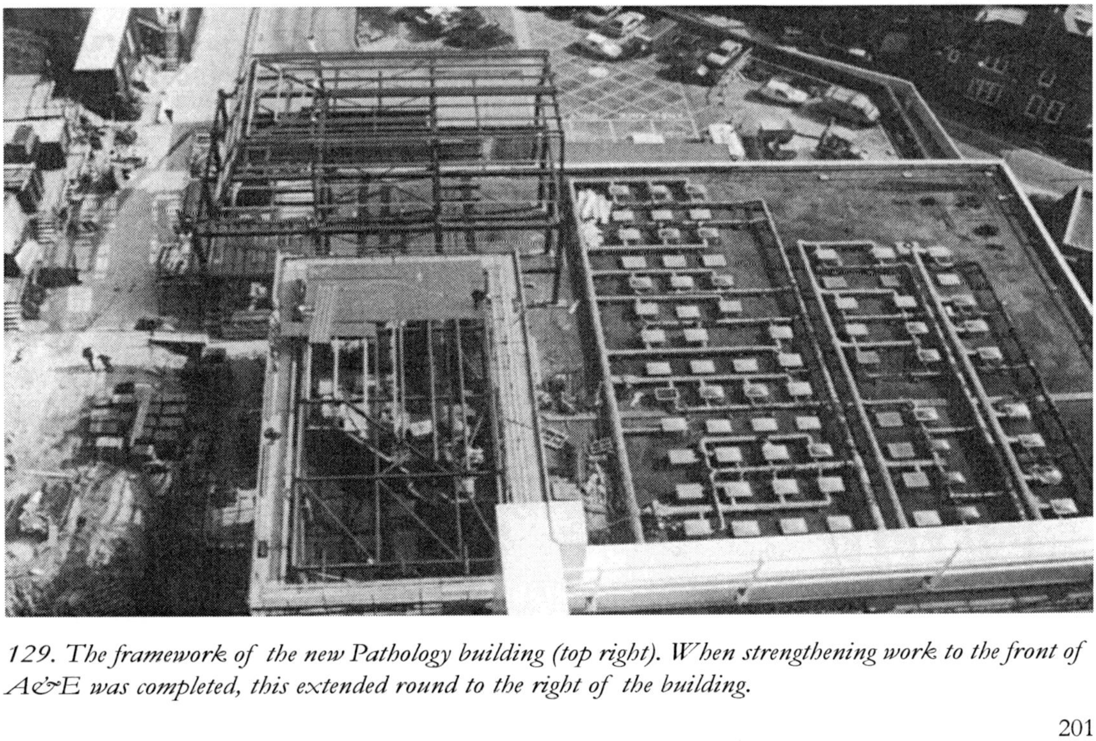

129. The framework of the new Pathology building (top right). When strengthening work to the front of A&E was completed, this extended round to the right of the building.

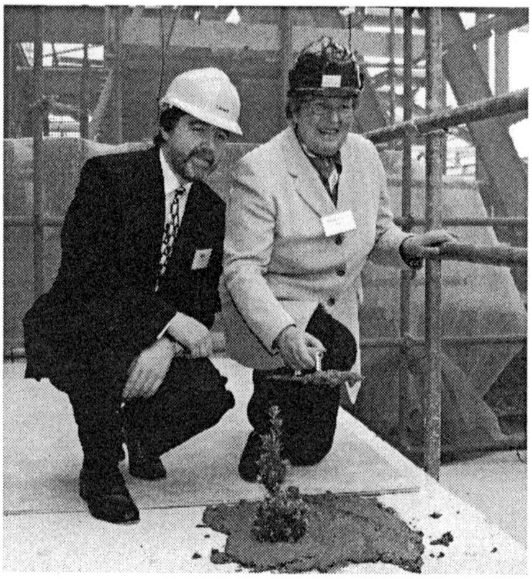

130. Baroness Emerton, watched by the managing director of the contractors, plants a yew tree in the final pour of concrete to mark the completion of structural work on the new clinical block.

were asked to refer patients to the hospital only where absolutely necessary.

The reduction in the A&E car parking space was more than compensated for a few months later when the new car park was opened by the chairman who was driven through a chequered banner across the entrance in an open top vintage Rolls Royce.

The 274 place car park built on the site of the old nurses' home was well lit and constantly monitored by CCTV cameras. It was hoped it would relieve some of the pressure on the site and the surrounding residential area. The only problem was that it was designed to accommodate 364 vehicles but at the time the local council had not given permission to use the 90 spaces on the top floor.

Meanwhile work had been progressing on the major hospital redevelopment. The observation ward, doctors' mess, resuscitation area and the endoscopy unit had been reduced to a pile of rubble from which the new clinical block building began to emerge.

The first major milestone was reached on the 4th December. Before an invited audience, which included representatives from every ward and department as well as former members of staff. Lord Egremont, a descendant of the hospital's founder, laid the foundation stone for the new clinical building in a ceremony described by the trust's chief executive, Stuart Welling, as marking the formal 'beginning of the work which will create a hospital for the 21st century.'

At the original stone laying ceremony in 1826, the site had been blessed by the vicar of St George's Church. On this occasion, in a significant sign of the changing times, there were inter-denominational prayers when the current vicar was joined by representatives of the Brighton Islamic Mission, the Brighton and Hove New Synagogue and the local Hindu community.

As well as these developments, there had been a great deal of other activity at the hospital throughout the year. In January, the chairman, Dame Audrey[1], officially opened the endoscopy unit in a vastly different environment following its move from Level 5 to Level 9 of the tower block. The development formed the first phase of the gastroenteroloy integrated patient care

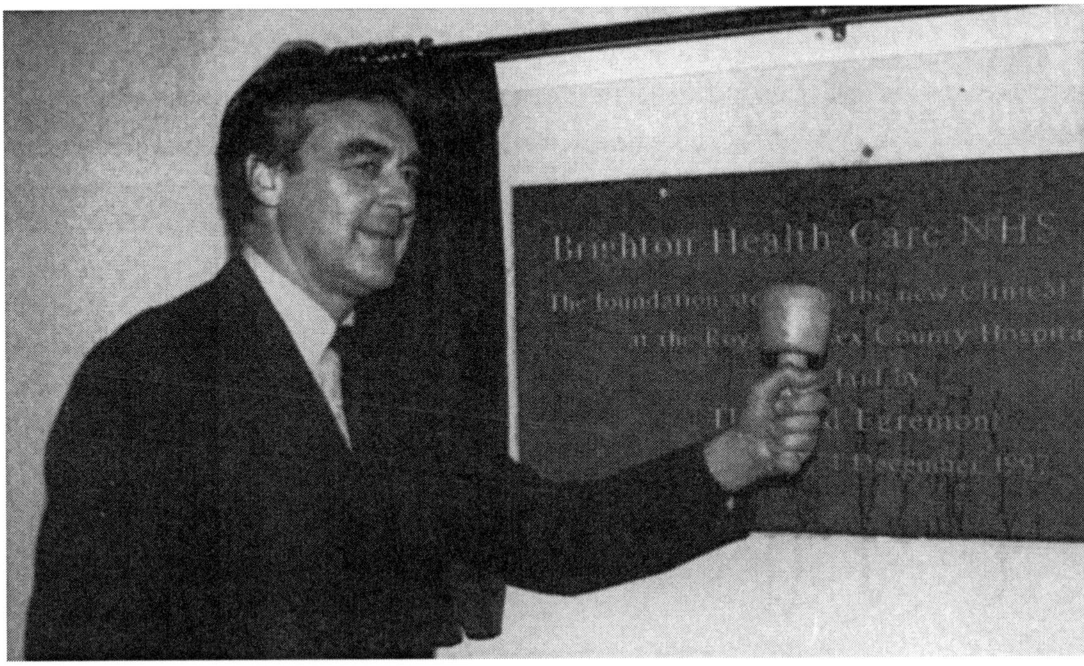

131. The Earl of Egremont with the stonemason's mallet that was presented to him as a memento after he laid the foundation stone for the new clinical building. He later cut a celebratory cake, a slice of which was sent was sent to every patient on Egremont ward.

project. The first area where all services were organised around the patient opened six months later in July, when former chairman Baroness Cumberlege returned to open the new centre for midwifery and neonatal care on Levels 11 to 14 of the tower block. These were transformed as the result of major upgrading work and refurbishment during the previous eighteen months. The centre contained six single rooms for post-natal women on Level 12 in place of the previous two. It also included the ante-natal clinic, which had been operating in a separate part of the hospital. The nursery for seriously ill babies on the Trevor Mann unit was doubled in size and an extra room was provided for parents who needed to stay in the unit with their baby.

The urology outpatient department moved to new accommodation on the lower ground floor of Sussex House. This enabled patients, who had previously needed to make two visits to the hospital, to have all necessary tests carried out there on the one day. The new department was officially opened by Australian Mark Little, the former Big Breakfast presenter and Neighbours star, who lived in Hove. He was presented with a replica penis used in the unit to help patients with erectile problems as a souvenir of his visit!

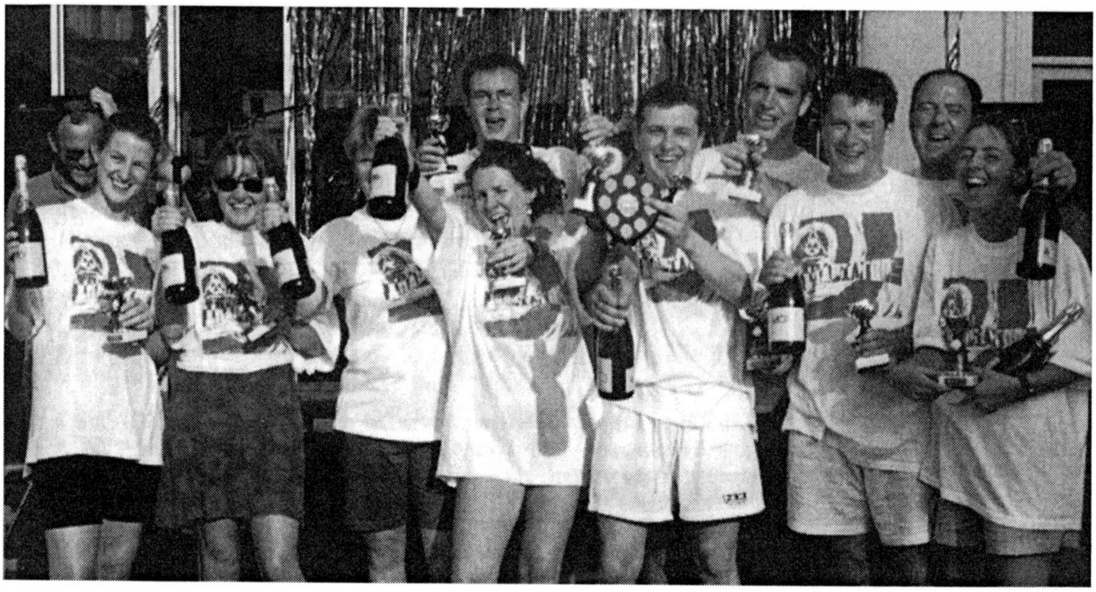

132. The County's X-Ray team won the trust's third annual Fun Day 'It's a Knockout' competition held in the grounds of Sussex House in 1997. The following year the event was linked with the revived Kemp Town Carnival and celebrated the 50th anniversary of the NHS.

Sussex House was also chosen as a new base for Coastway hospital radio. The charity had formerly operated from the Adur Civic Centre in Shoreham-by-Sea but had been forced to move because of ever increasing rent charges. The new studios, built with the aid of a £5,000 grant from the League of Hospital Friends, were launched with the aid of a host of celebrities from national, regional and local television and radio.

Sussex House also became the new venue for the trust staff and families third annual Fun Day. This featured an 'It's a Knockout' competition which had originated several years before as a County Hospital event held in the grounds of a cricket club in West Sussex. Another development for staff was a welcome improvement in catering facilities celebrated when the new food court was opened by celebrity cook Pru Leith in June.

There was good news and bad news for A&E the following year in 1998. The good news was that the extended and refurbished part of the department was due for completion at the end of March. All facilities were to be transferred there while the contractors worked in the remainder of the department. The bad news was that this would take nine months to complete and that the new area had only half the space of the already cramped conditions in which staff had been treating patients during the preceding twelve months Once again an appeal was made to the public to visit the department only for true accidents and emergencies.

Meanwhile, good progress had been made on the new clinical block. To mark the completion of structural work in March, a yew tree was planted in the final pour of concrete, an ancient ceremony originally meant to bring good luck and keep out evil spirits.

The topping out ceremony was followed by two official opening ceremonies for newly installed state-of-the-art equipment, which, like the new buildings, were moving the hospital towards the twenty-first century. A new CT scanner was opened on March 19th in a new department on Level 5 of the tower block. Costing £625,000, the new scanner combined even more advanced and sophisticated radiological and computer technology than its predecessor to provide high quality cross-sectional images of the body. It also made it possible to look inside blood vessels without invasive procedures.

In April two new gamma cameras were installed in the nuclear medicine department making it probably the most advanced in the country at the time. The department was the first in the south to be equipped with a gamma camera in 1970. This was replaced in 1972/3 and a second camera was installed in 1976. Both were replaced in the 1980s. The most important function of the larger of the two new cameras valued at over £300,000 was to support the planned new cardiac surgery centre.

One of the camera's benefits was that it enabled patients to be assessed for the risk of heart attack ahead of major surgery. The official opening was performed by Adam Faith who earlier in the week had presented two BBC television programmes on heart disease. The actor had previously visited the hospital in 1984 to launch the new trauma room in A&E and by coincidence a second £200,000 Traumex X-ray system for severely traumatised patients with multiple injuries was unveiled in June, one of only three such systems believed to be operating in the country.

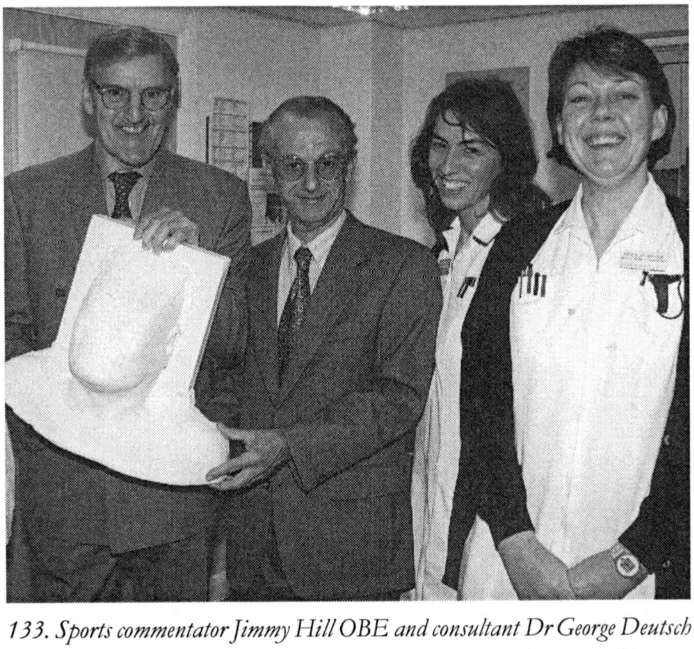

133. Sports commentator Jimmy Hill OBE and consultant Dr George Deutsch hold one of the Plaster of Paris moulds produced in the mould room and impression suite, a new addition to the Sussex Oncology Centre.

Not all the developments at the hospital during the year

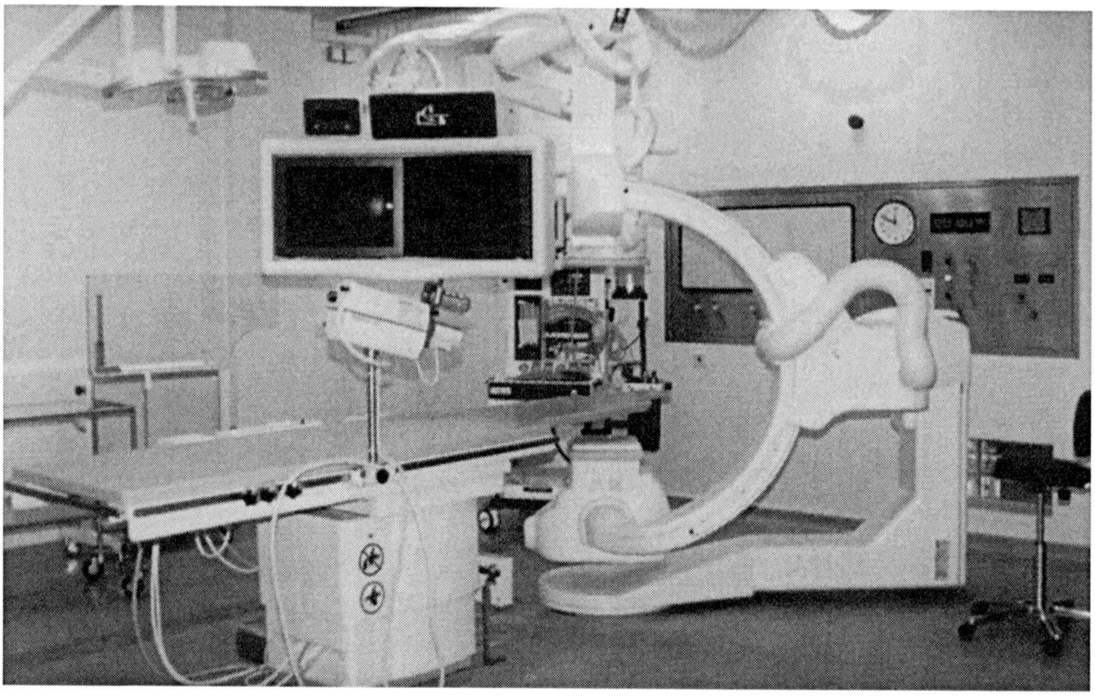

134. One of the hospital's new catheter labs that were also to be used by consultant interventional cardiologists from Worthing, Haywards Heath and Eastboune.

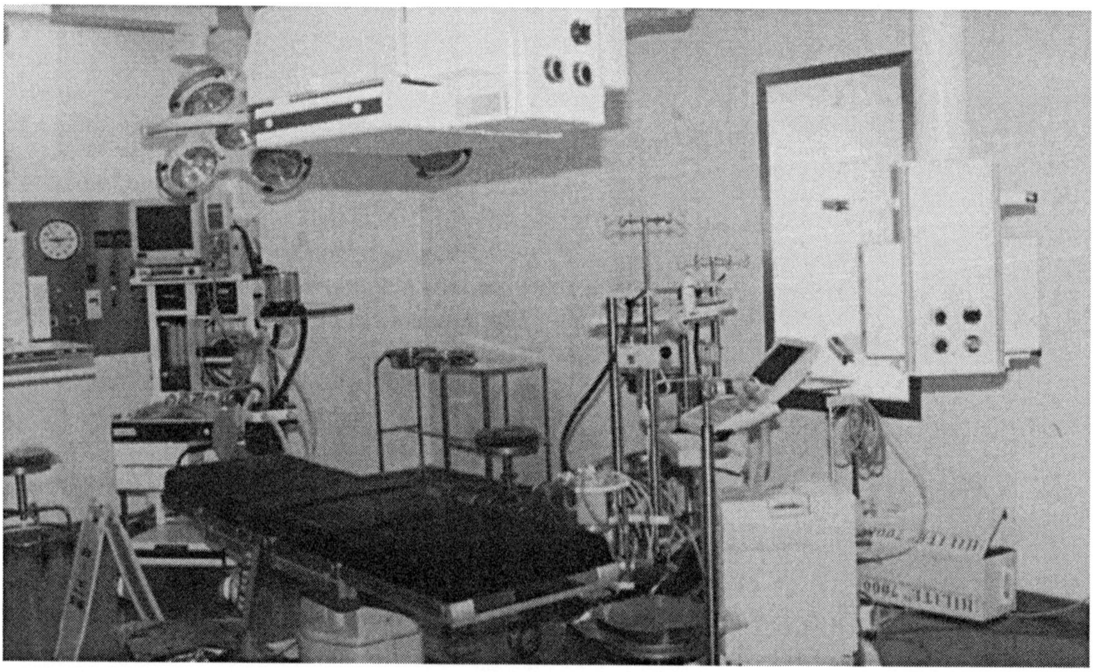

135. One of the two dedicated cardiac operating theatres in the new Sussex Cardiac Centre.

involved new technology. Egremont, the ear, nose and throat ward, for example, moved into a new era specialising in respiratory medicine and haematology.

Towards the end of the year a £120,000 new impression suite and mould room was opened in the Sussex Oncology Centre financed by the Sussex Cancer Fund. The technology remained the same but the new suite provided a welcoming and reassuring environment for cancer patients attending for the rather forbidding process of producing a plastic immobilisation mask that was essential for the precise positioning of radiation treatment to the head and neck.

In June 1998 the long-awaited cardiothoracic centre received its first patients. With two dedicated cardiac theatres, it was planned eventually to carry out six to seven hundred operations a year. At the same time, two new catheter laboratories became operational and for the first time Sussex patients were able to have their angioplasties performed by cardiologists in Brighton instead of travelling to London.

The Sussex Cardiac Centre was situated on Levels 6 and 7 of A Block (as the clinical block was known at the time). A few months later Levels 8 and 9 were opened. To avoid confusion with the tower block, these wards were known as 6A, 7A, 8A, and 9A. 9A was allocated to digestive diseases and marked another step forward in what had proved to be a somewhat complicated process of developing a pilot integrated patient care centre for gastroenterology. Originally it had been intended to develop the centre in its entirety in the main block but this had proved too difficult to achieve in the older building. The completion of Level 9A meant it was possible to provide all the 54 medical and surgical beds required there while Endoscopy was linked by means of a bridge between the two blocks.

Level 8A became the trauma and orthopaedic ward. Unlike digestive diseases, it had not proved possible to concentrate all the beds required in one place, or even on one site. As well as 56 beds in two wards in the new block, there were still 15 beds on Overton ward with a further 24 at Brighton General Hospital. However, the development did mean a further 10 beds became available to the speciality as well as new facilities that included physiotherapy and occupational therapy areas, cubicles for the isolation of patients, a large day room, a seminar room and an orthopaedic workshop.

Meanwhile the completion of the redevelopment in A&E allowed staff to move into the second part of the new department that had been nearly three years in the making. Among the benefits was the fact that there was no longer a disruptive major corridor going right through the centre of the department. Minor Injuries was situated adjacent to the waiting room, the major area was more central with a good control area and paediatrics had a dedicated area.

At the same time, significant changes had been taking place in intensive care. A new look ICU was linked by a bridge to the new cardiac centre in A Block. The area formerly occupied by coronary care and high dependency beds, now accommodated in A Block, was adapted and contained four single bedded intensive care bays and one two bedded bay. On the west side of the unit, five beds for cardiac patients and two post-surgical high dependency beds were planned.

There were other changes at the hospital during the year, the most notable being the realisation of a long-held dream of creating a diabetic care centre. In 1988 the diabetic department had moved from the crumbling York ward to Grant, a vast improvement, but still not ideal. A fund-raising effort with major contributions by the Lions and local branch of the British Diabetic Association raised £125,000, but just when it appeared possible to start work on a new centre in 1991 or 1992 the scheme was put on hold because of the trust's financial situation. In 1994, the chief executive offered consultant Dr Nick Vaughan the opportunity of a site at the rear of Main Outpatients and he immediately began setting out his vision for the new department. Fearing the original plan would resemble the Black Hole of Calcutta,[2] he finally persuaded the architects it should take the form of a light and airy central area doubling as a waiting room with consulting and treatment rooms with windows ranged round the outside. The dream eventually became a reality and the new centre opened in April 1999.

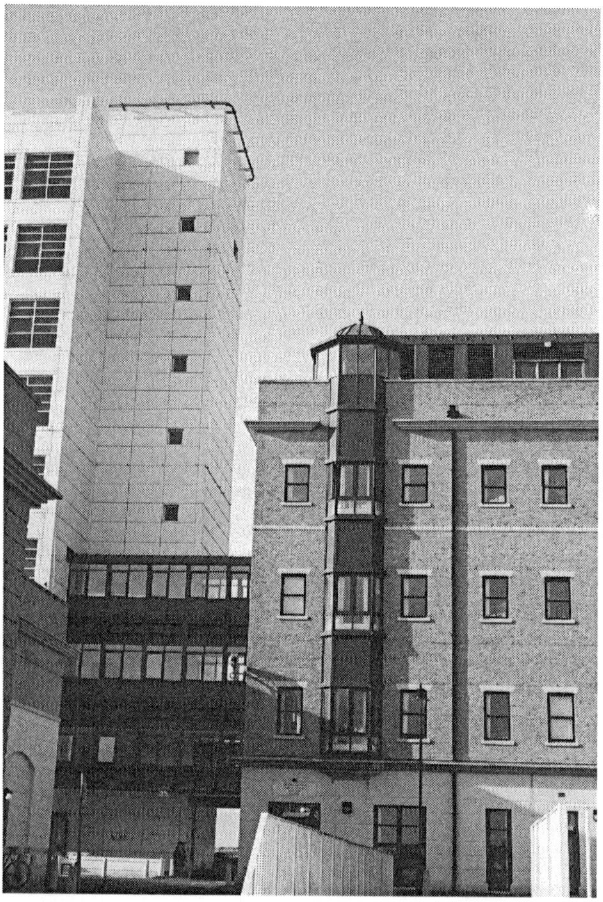

136. The new clinical block linked by bridges to the tower block's ICU and Endoscopy

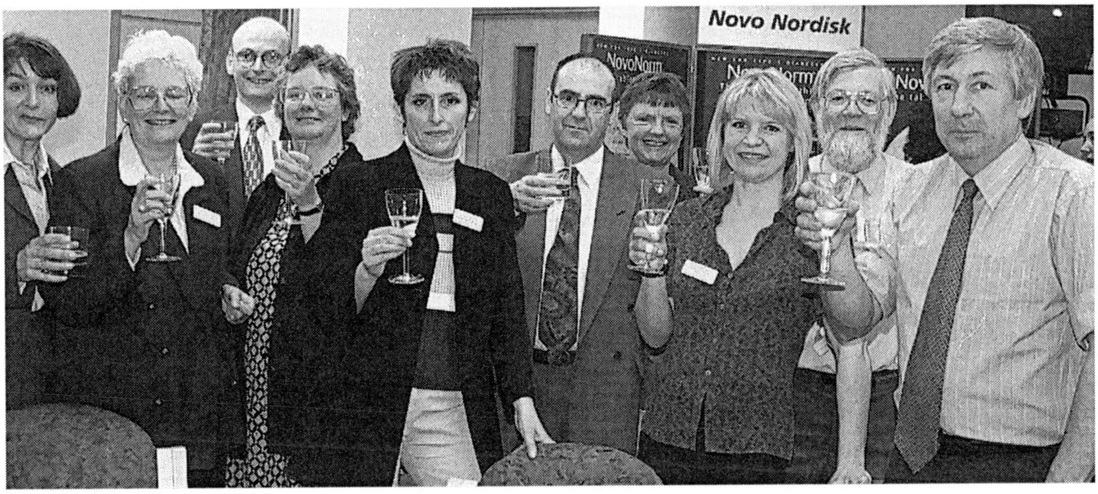

137. Consultant Dr Nick Vaughan (right) and staff and visitors toast the success of their long-awaited new diabetic care centre at an open day for interested local professionals in April 1999.

Grant ward was retained as an inpatient facility but the staff there rotated with those working in the new centre.

At its September meeting, the trust board approved proposals for naming new and existing buildings to make them more patient friendly. Level 6A in the new block became Roedean ward, Level 7A was named after consultant

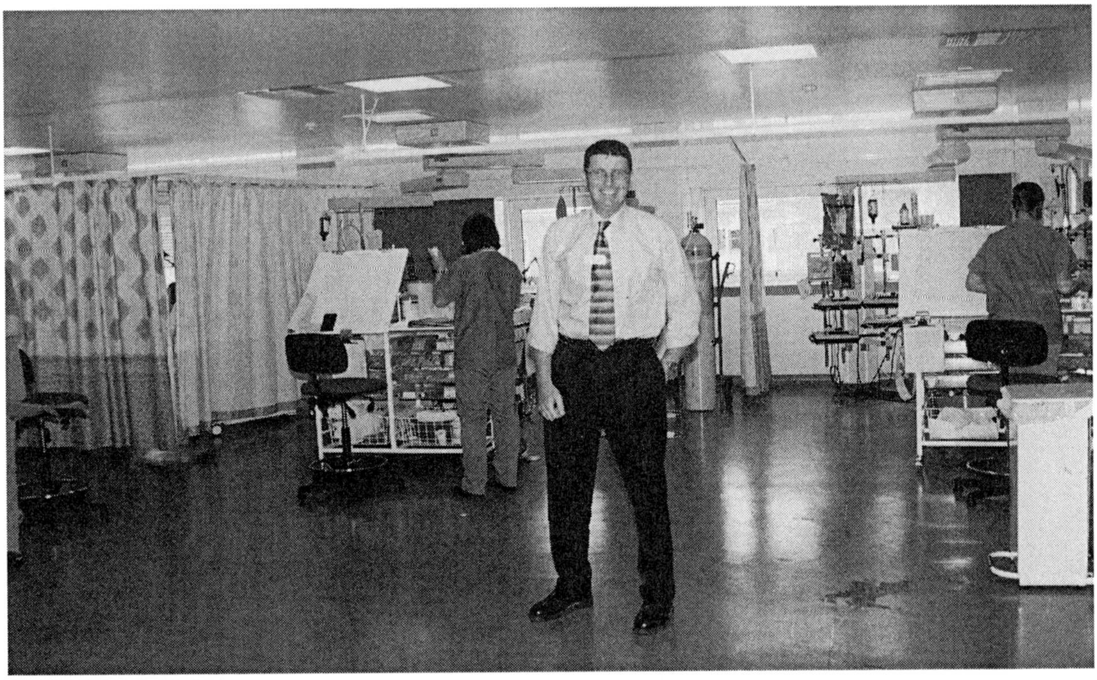

138. The Intensive Care Unit's head of nursing, Jim Valentine, in the new, uncluttered department.

cardiologist Professor Douglas Chamberlain[3], Level 9A became the Regency Digestive Diseases Centre, Level 9 in the tower block became Level 9 Regency OPD and Regency Endoscopy Unit, Level 10 in the tower became Level 10 Albion Ward (private patients) and Level 10 Lewes Ward (NHS cardiology), Level 11 was to be named after the first millennium baby. The new block was to be named later, possibly after the Royal personage opening it, the tower block became the Thomas Kemp Tower and the main building was named after its architect, the Charles Barry Building.

The year 2000 started fairly well with news that the council's planning committee had at last given approval to use the top deck of the new car park, although there were conditions attached to their decision. The protracted dispute regarding the top floor resulted from objections by residents whose homes overlooked the car park. At first the council suggested landscaping the area but this would have cost some £35,000, which the trust could not really afford, and also severely restricted the number of parking places. When it was discovered that the weight of the 31 planters suggested by the council was too great for the floor to bear, the number was cut to 13, which meant spaces would become available for 75 cars. However, other planning constraints restricted parking to between 8 am and 6pm and lighting was only permitted during these hours.

For pathology staff, January began even better. At last building work was complete and they were able to make the move to their purpose built new

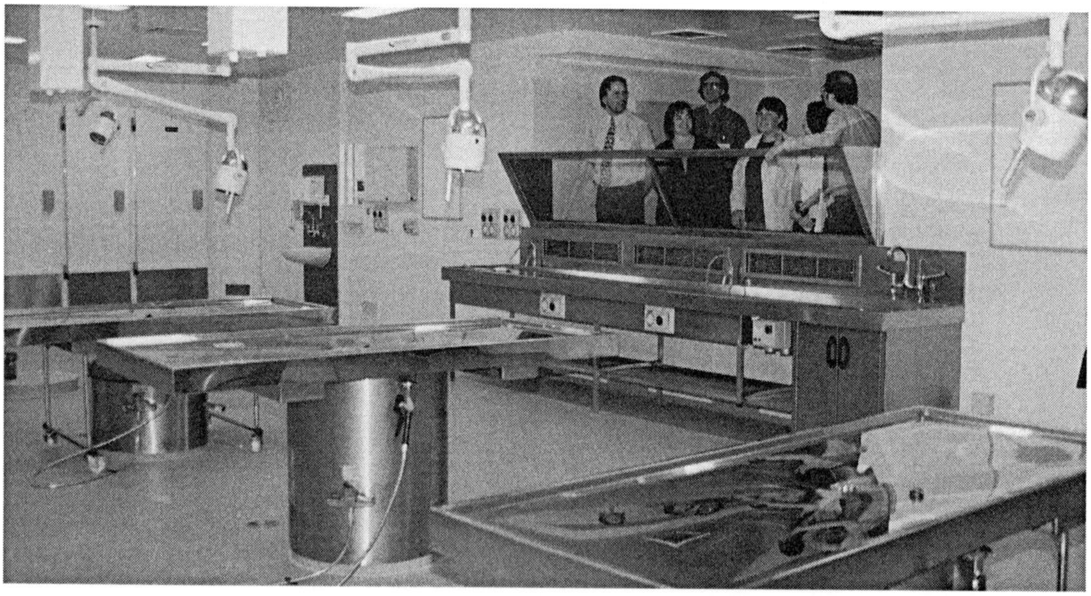

139. Visitors from the Pharmacy department view the new autopsy room and mortuary during an open day for staff.

department built over the orthopaedic department. Previously they had been scattered in different buildings on the County site – haematology staff just inside the entrance to the main building, pathology reception, phlebotomy and chemistry staff in the Stephen Ralli building. Histopathlogy, pathology stores and public health microbiology were in the Public Health Laboratory service building. Cytopatholgy was based up the hill at Brighton General. The new building would bring all these services under one roof. The only exception, the mortuary and autopsy room, was now located in new accommodation in A Block.

The business of moving into the new building, however, proved to be far from easy. Services had to be maintained whilst the change was taking place but there was a considerable amount of heavy equipment to be moved and there were no lifts in the old buildings. Sometimes procedures would be started in the new building then taken to the old one for completion. The way staff coped with this difficult situation was praised at the trust's board meeting that month.

In March staff and users celebrated the official opening of a new facility at the hospital, a branch library that had been established in Rosaz House[4]. As well as a collection of new books and all major medical journals, it contained computers and printers. Plans to establish a new education centre and library at the hospital had been under discussion for some time. The new facility was intended to go some way to providing a service with a professional librarian for hospital staff until the new centre became a reality.

Another library with a difference opened later in the year in the accommodation just inside the Barry Building vacated by Haematology. This was an equipment library containing a large collection of infusion devices. An audit had shown there were more than 450 devices including sixteen different types in use but there was no mechanism for tracking them, and no area accepted responsibility for their care and maintenance. No more than half were believed to be in use at any one time but

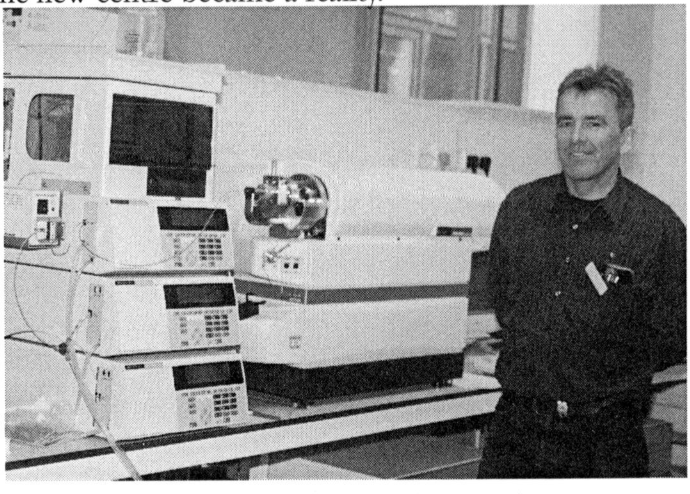

140. Dr Peter Sharp with a £200,000 Tandem Mass Spectrometer that replaced half a dozen machines in Chemistry used formerly for the analysis of drugs and metabolites. This was just one of a number of expensive new items of equipment provided in the new Brighton Pathology department.

until the new library was established there were often delays and difficulties locating equipment when it was needed, often at short notice.

Not all the developments during the year took place on site. The cardiac rehabilitation team, for example, normally provided a service in a large gym in the physiotherapy department in the Latilla building. The success of the Sussex Cardiac Centre had resulted, among other things, in a steady increase in demand for rehabilitation and the existing facilities were no longer able to cope with both surgical and medical patients. A solution to the problem was found outside the hospital. This new location for exercise sessions was at the David Lloyd Health and Fitness Club in the Brighton Marina complex – salubrious surroundings where patients had state-of-the art training facilities and were able to enjoy sea views while working out.

Nurses and nursing

The final years of the twentieth century also saw some significant developments in nursing. In 1997, nurse practitioners were introduced in the minor injuries area of A&E where long waiting times had been the norm. The decision to train staff as emergency nurse practitioners (ENPs) was an unqualified success. These specially trained nurses saw patients with a number of clearly defined injuries and complaints. They were able to examine them, diagnose, treat and discharge them without consulting a doctor, and also to prescribe a limited range of drugs. The result was that waiting times were reduced and waiting room aggression and the number of complaints in Minors dropped considerably. When details of the scheme were posted by a consultant on the Internet, it attracted considerable attention including enquiries from Iceland and Denmark. The Danes later sent a team to Brighton to meet the staff and learn more about the scheme and as a result two members of the A&E team visited Copenhagen to help set up an ENP training programme there.

The role of the nurse also changed in other departments. In 1998, Karen Booth, a nurse in the Trevor Mann Baby Unit, was appointed as the trust's first advanced neonatal nurse practitioner. This was believed to be the first appointment of its kind south of the Thames. In 1999, the intensive care unit appointed Denise Hinge as the trust's first nurse consultant whose first task was to set up an intensive care outreach team.

In 1997, the hospital appointed a Macmillan nurse in urology, believed to be only the second such appointment in the country, and another in palliative care. Brighton had led the way in the development of these specialist nurses. The trust had earlier appointed the country's first Macmillan breast

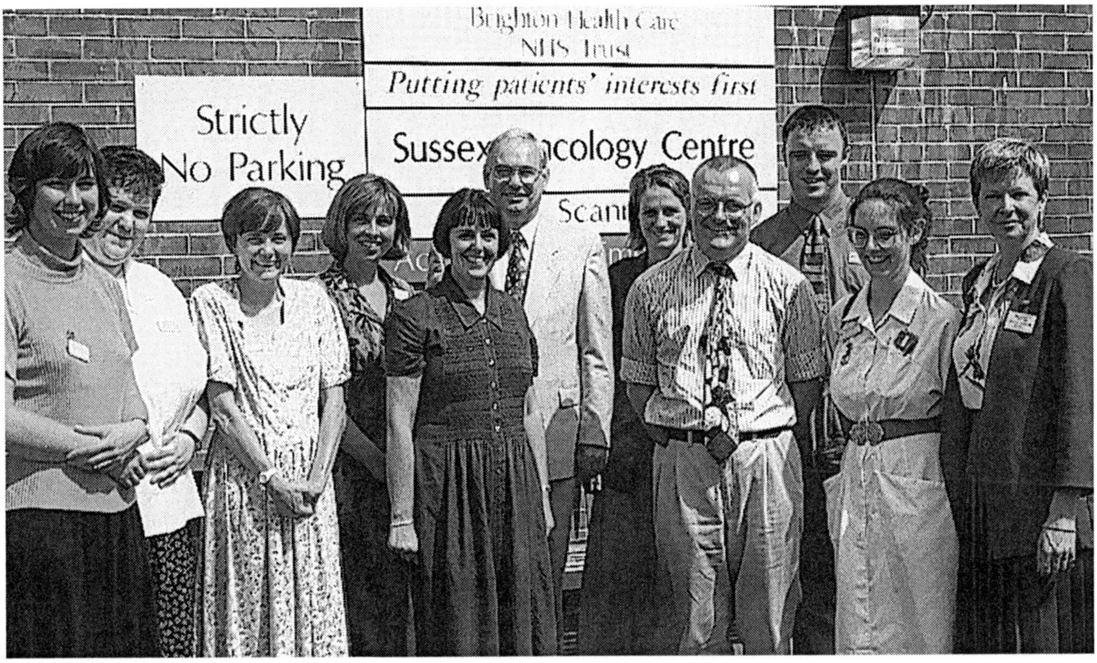

141. Kemp Town MP Dr Des Turner (centre) with seven of the hospital's eight Macmillan nurses and Macmillan director Loretta Tinkham (right). The Brighton MP was one of the first to respond when the Cancer Relief Fund invited all the 1997 intake of new Members of Parliament to meet Macmillan nurses in their constituencies and learn about their work.

care nurse followed later by several other ground breaking appointments. Funded initially for two or three years by Macmillan Cancer Relief, it was a condition that these nurses were eventually paid by the hospital. The two new appointments brought the total number in the hospital's Macmillan team up to eight which was believed to be probably the most comprehensive in the UK.

The latter part of the twentieth century witnessed continuing problems with a shortage of nurses nationally[5] and Brighton hospitals, including the County, were no exception. Nurses visited supermarkets (so-called Supermarket Sweeps) trying to encourage women to take up nursing or to return to nursing if their children were old enough; back to nursing courses were organised, nursing pools set up and schools visited. In 1998 well over 200 nurses left Brighton hospitals, many to follow careers outside nursing. In January 1999 there was some relief when the first nurses of the thirty who had been recruited in South Africa arrived. The majority of these worked at Brighton General but a small number, including two in renal and two in theatres, were employed at the County. Brighton General was probably the principal beneficiary of the 55 nurses recruited in the Philippines who arrived later in the year, but the County Hospital benefited too.[6]

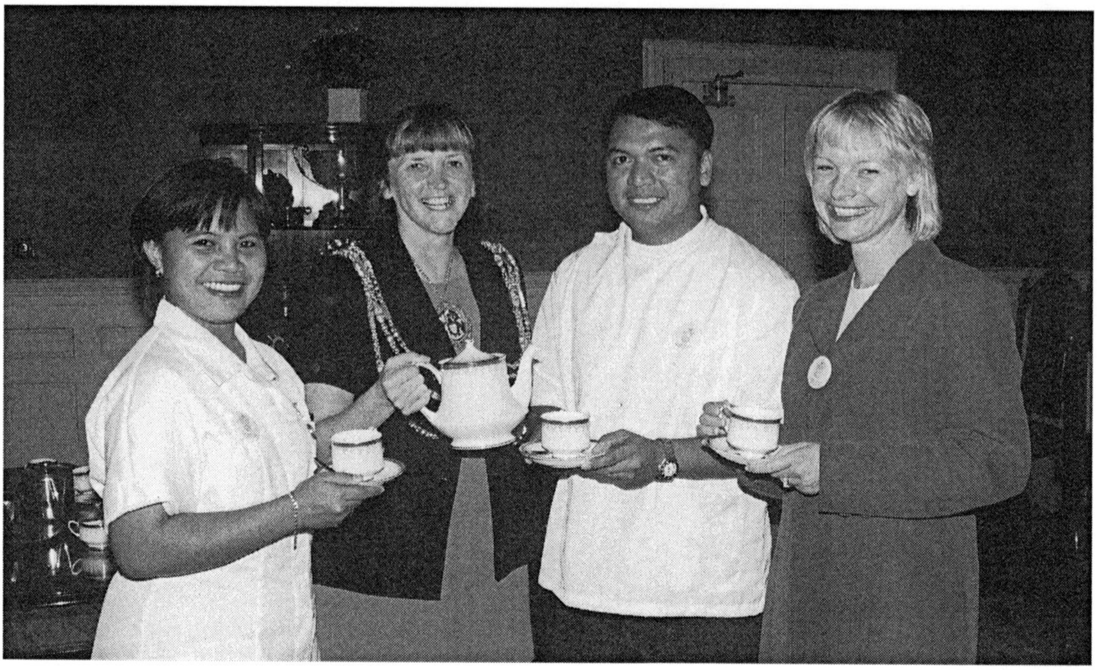

142. The first group of Filipino nurses to arrive in Brighton – including the group leaders Juliet P. Barcelo and Theodore Medran junior, who were accompanied by director of nursing Karen Parsley – were invited to tea by the mayor, Councillor Jenny Langston, in Brighton Town Hall.

In May 2000 a job fair at the Brighton Centre attracted more than 400 people. This was a new initiative to improve recruitment and cut the number of vacancies, not only on the wards but also in all hospital departments including imaging, pathology and physiotherapy. That month, too, advantage was taken of National Nurses Day to send teams of nurses into local primary schools prompted by research that showed that this was the age when ideas about future career choices are made.

The Millennium Bug

The months leading up to the end of the year were to some extent overshadowed by preparations for midnight on December 31st when the onset of the new millennium was expected to produce major problems with computers. Because some 85 per cent of computers allowed only two digits to indicate the year, they would be unable to differentiate between 1900 and 2000, the so-called Millennium Bug. As a result, on the stroke of midnight on the 31st December 1999 it was feared many computer systems would fail with disastrous effects on banks, air traffic control, telephone and power systems, prisons and, of course, hospitals. Contingency planning for the event began more than a year before but as the months passed a new possibility that particularly affected hospitals like the County emerged: major incidents arising from public order problems accompanying the millennium celebrations.[7]

To meet this possibility, access to the hospital was severely restricted. Only staff wearing identity badges bearing a photograph were allowed on site. A hospital control room was established and the bed bureau in the tower block manned from 10 pm for as long as necessary. This was the nerve centre for the night and was in radio communication with the police and with ambulance headquarters in Lewes. A full team was on hand to deal with any equipment breakdowns. All lifts were brought down to base level from about 11 pm on New Year's Eve to ensure nobody could be trapped in one. The only exception was a bed passenger lift manned by engineering staff that meant, for example, that a very ill patient could be moved to intensive care if necessary. Over 90 beds were emptied in case of a major incident.

Fortunately, the Millennium Bug didn't bite. Despite a heavier workload than usual, New Year's Eve passed relatively smoothly. There were foreseen delays transferring patients from A&E to the wards while the lifts were brought down to ground level and tested as a safety precaution. Although the department was busy, there were fortunately no major problems at the street party held in the Old Steine to be dealt with. Hospital admissions on New Year's Day were 40 per cent up on the previous year, but were predominantly for older people with respiratory problems such as asthma and chest infections. A&E attendances were up too, from 184 to 232. National forecasts of a flurry of millennium births were not borne out locally.

The first birth in the maternity unit did not take place until shortly before midday and a proposal to name the delivery ward after the first millennium baby seemed unlikely to go ahead because the parents were unwilling to go along with the suggestion.

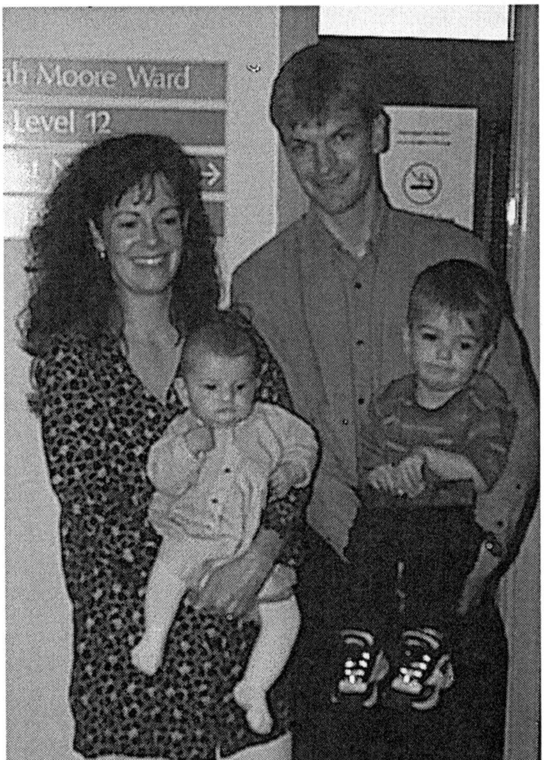

143. Brighton's first millennium baby Hannah Moore gave her name to Level 12. Held by her mother Sue she was joined at the naming ceremony by her GP father, Paul, and brother Luke.

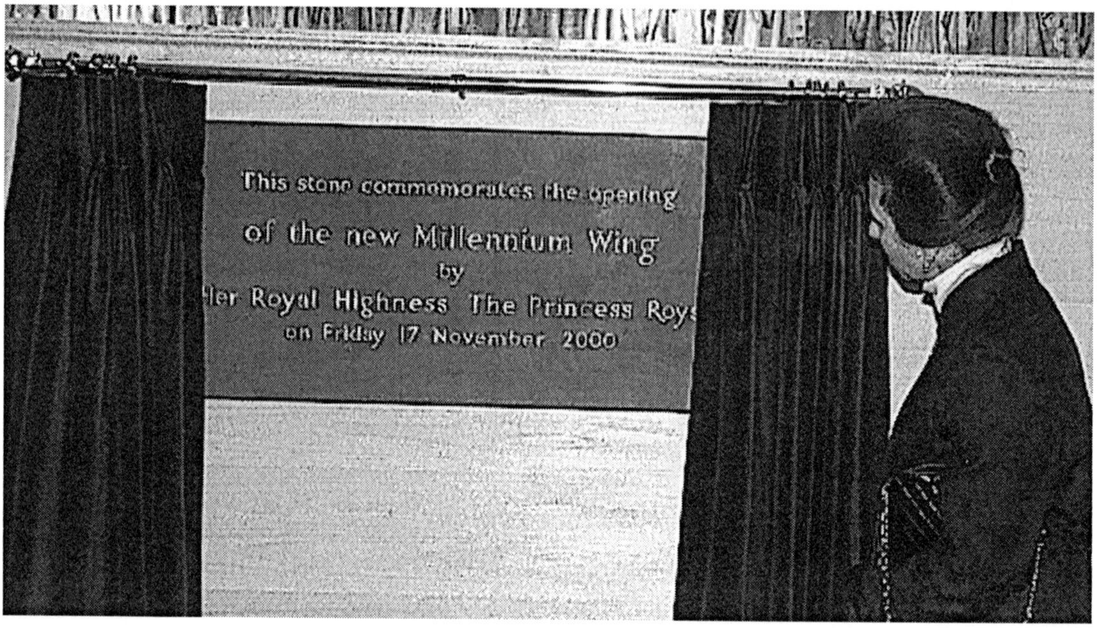
This stone commemorates the opening
of the new Millennium Wing
by
Her Royal Highness The Princess Roy
on Friday 17 November 2000

144. The Princess Royal admires the plaque, which she just unveiled. It was later placed on the wall outside the entrance to the new clinical building.

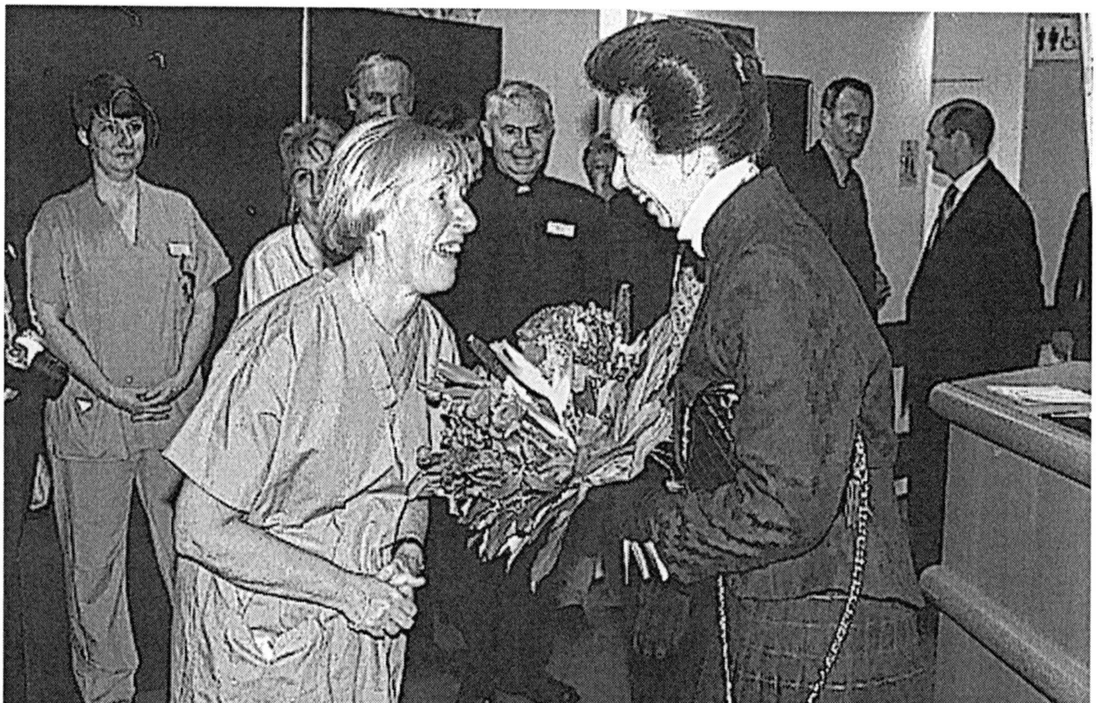

145. Ann Munro, the hospital's longest serving nurse, was chosen to present a bouquet to the Princess Royal at the official opening of the Millennium Wing.

There were four births on the day, including one at home. It was the latter birth that saved the day. This was in fact the first birth in the Brighton district at Ringmer, near Lewes. Baby Hannah Moore's father was a Newhaven GP, Paul Moore, who had once been a senior house officer at the hospital and worked on the ward that was to bear his daughter's name. His wife Sue had been trained as a nurse in Brighton. The ward was eventually named in May, the last official function undertaken by the retiring chairman, Baroness Emerton.

A Royal Occasion

The year 2000 brought must have been a welcome end to what many considered to be a decade of doubt and indecision. It was ten years since the consultants had invited the then health secretary to see for himself how Brighton hospitals were falling apart through lack of maintenance. Their campaign for a new hospital built on a greenfield site had not been successful. Even when approval for the redevelopment on the County site had been given in 1992, there remained what transpired to be the contentious issue of obtaining planning permission. It was not until 1997 that the new building was finally handed over by the contractors John Laing Construction Limited and this still had to be commissioned in stages. So it was not until Friday the 17th November that the new clinical block was officially opened by the Princess Royal and named the Millennium Wing.

Welcoming her, the new trust chairman Professor Michael Whiting said: 'Whilst there is much remaining to be done, this new development sets the standard for what is to come as the old and unsustainable is replaced by modern, efficient clinical space'.

What was still to come was a new renal unit to be built over the multi-storey car park, a new multi-disciplinary education centre, the complete refurbishment of the hospital's operating theatres and a new paediatric unit to replace the children's hospital in Dyke Road. Even then, the redevelopment would not be complete. At some time in the future, still to be determined, the original buildings in Eastern Road would have to be replaced.

18. A Teaching Hospital Once More, 2001 – 2003

During the next three years, 2001-2003, significant progress was made on the major redevelopment of the hospital. The new kidney unit and the work on the operating theatres were completed while work at last began on the long-awaited new education centre. More importantly, perhaps, the status of the hospital changed. After more than a century, it again became a teaching hospital, but this time as the major part of an undergraduate teaching hospital.

Two developments made this possible. One was the successful conclusion in 2001 of the long-running campaign for what was to become the Brighton and Sussex Medical School. Two years earlier prospects had looked bleak when Sussex University withdrew its support for the bid at the last moment. As recently as July 2000 there were tensions between the two universities involved, Brighton and Sussex. Then, according to Professor Richard Vincent, the mood changed. 'Since last October there has been remarkable energy and co-operation between the two universities,' he told a meeting of the Brighton Health Care board. 'Now we're fairly optimistic.'[1]

Three factors had prompted the change, he explained. The government's call for an extra 1,000 new undergraduate places, encouragement from the regional health authority and thirdly Southampton University who had been 'very enthusiastic to help develop the curriculum'. The medical school was to be formed in equal partnership between the two universities and NHS staff throughout the region. Students would be awarded a joint degree across both universities. The aim was for an annual intake of 128 students commencing in the autumn of 2003 who would have contact with patients during the first two years of the five year course through visits to hospitals and in the community. Much of the third year would be spent at the County and adjacent hospitals while the fifth would be 'a year of apprenticeship' with attachments in general and specialist hospitals and primary care sites throughout the region. A site for clinical teaching would be attached at the Royal Sussex County Hospital.

The following month it was learned that Brighton was one of the two successful bids to establish a new medical school.[2] Its importance to the County Hospital, which was to be the main teaching hospital, was underlined by the news that the £28.5 million venture would create around twenty new consultant appointments as well as twenty full-time teaching posts.

The second, closely linked, development was the announcement by health minister Hazel Blears in July that she had given approval for public consultation to take place on the Central Sussex Partnership proposals. For several months previously, there had been a great deal of discussion and debate about the best way to organise acute hospital services in Brighton and Hove, the Ouse Valley and Mid Sussex. The plan was establish 'one major university teaching trust, centred largely on the Royal Sussex County Hospital at Brighton and the Princess Royal Hospital at Haywards Heath, with all its clinical services co-ordinated under one management' [3]

As a result, the County would become the lead hospital in the new teaching hospital trust, but a number of changes between the way services were organised with its principal partner, the Princess Royal, were likely to have considerable repercussions on patients and staff. Proposals for reorganising A&E services published in a discussion document in 2001[4] had led to considerable debate, especially in Haywards Heath, but the greatest impact on the County was likely to result from a proposal to set up a single specialist service for breast care at Haywards Heath.

According to the discussion document, physical accommodation for breast care services in Brighton was unacceptable and access was poor. A *Sunday Times* survey made in the summer of 2000 had revealed that Brighton had the worst waiting times for breast treatment in the country. A more recent South East Breast Cancer Team report made following a quality assurance visit noted concerns about the waiting times for a first appointment and between diagnosis and treatment as well as the cramped conditions. The Nigel Porter Unit had been welcomed as a major improvement in Brighton's breast care service when it opened in 1993 but occupying less than 400 square metres it was considered, less than ten years later, to be too small.

In 2002 it was argued that the constraints on space there and in the adjacent Breast Assessment Unit impacted on their ability to meet current and future NHS targets. Against that, the report by the South East Breast Cancer Team had reported that despite its shortcomings Brighton offered excellent breast care services and that its clinical standards were among the best. So it was not surprising perhaps that the proposal to relocate to Haywards Heath met with vigorous opposition from women in the Brighton area, who would be the greatest number of users of the service. Women in the rural areas, on the other hand, were equally determined that the facilities should be provided at Haywards Heath. Both quoted the inconvenience of travelling fifteen miles or the inadequate parking facilities to support their arguments. It was also believed obtaining planning consent would present fewer problems in

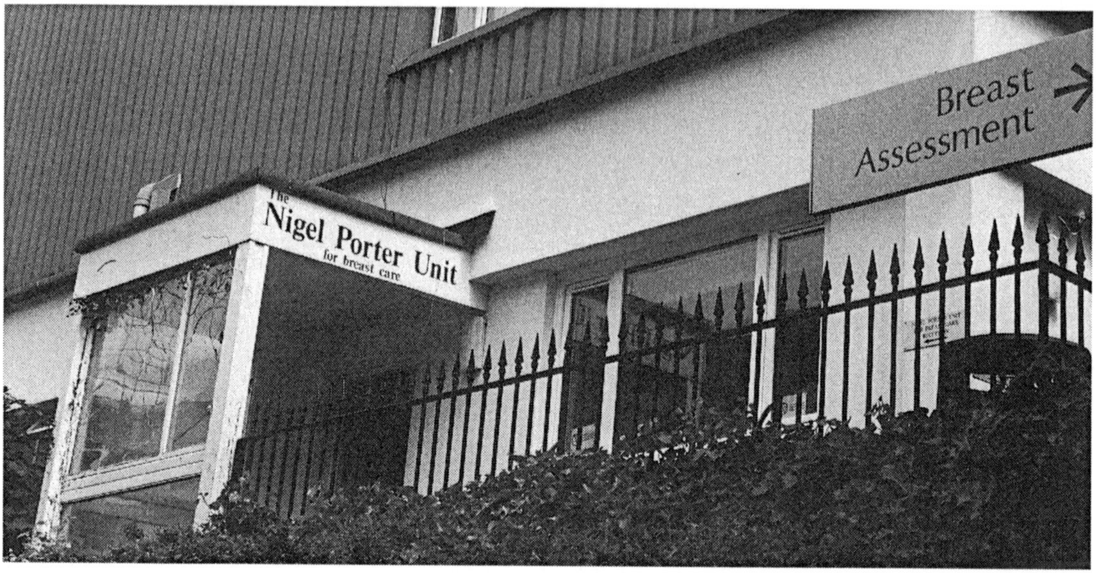

146. The breast care units based at the hospital: their long-term future was the subject of an emotional (unresolved) debate. Interim measures to improve the facilities were estimated to cost nearly £500,000.

Mid Sussex than in Brighton where there had been objections in the past to applications involving changes on the site.

To keep the service at the County, a new location would have to be found. Rosaz House was suggested but demolishing the property and constructing a new unit on the sloping site would be costly and take 24 months while the Princess Royal scheme would be cheaper and take only twenty months. Rising costs and increasing demands on government funding complicated the issue that, not surprisingly, proved difficult to resolve. Changes in the upper age limit for screening to seventy and on the number of X-rays from one per visit on each breast after the initial examination to two per breast also meant that steps had to be taken to meet the increased workload.

As an interim measure, it was decided to replace two temporary wooden buildings adjacent to the breast assessment centre. In December two large temporary buildings were dropped in position and a new processor installed which doubled the capacity for film viewing as well as making room for other facilities such as a filing room, toilets, showers, a staff room and an extension to the very small ultrasound room. Nevertheless, the £500,000 scheme did not solve all the problems. The small, cramped unit which had been the subject of a critical report by a Commission for Health Improvement team remained and the ideal solution that would allow the service to be retained at the County on the Rosaz House site still appeared to be some years off.

The beginning of the year saw a major shift in the way gynaecological services were organised in the trust with everything except day surgery moving to the County. Bristol Ward took over as the gynaecology ward and the colposcopy unit moved from Brighton General to the County's Main Outpatients building. In February it was learned that the Sussex House nursery would benefit from awards to twelve trusts that had been announced as a government package for improving childcare services. An allocation of £300,000 was made to extend the nursery raising the total number of places available to at least 55. A further £100,000 was awarded to meet the nursery's running costs.

Children benefited from another development that owed a great deal to the initiative of a team of staff from the children's hospital and the County. This concerned the hospital's magnetic imaging scanner introduced in 1994 and launched by the then health secretary, Virginia Bottomley. Beneficial although this was, it masked one major drawback. Space constraints meant that the new unit made no provision for scans to be carried out under general anaesthetic, an essential requirement for young children. As a result, there was a nine month waiting list for children and some still had to travel to London. To help mitigate this, children were brought from the Royal Alexandra Hospital by taxi to the County and returned following their scan by ambulance, a procedure that demonstrated that there were significant benefits to be obtained by providing paediatric services on the County site at some time in the future. In the meantime, thanks to a collaborative effort by the staff concerned at the two hospitals, a way was devised of simplifying the procedure by using the paediatric area of the A&E department for recovery although this still involved the transfer from the MRI unit on a specially equipped trolley carrying oxygen and a sucker accompanied by two porters, one of whom carried a telephone in case of an emergency. By means of this new procedure it proved possible to scan two children at each session instead of one as previously, the waiting list was reduced to four weeks and only one or two children a year, usually complicated cases, had to travel up to London.

This achievement was not the only one during the year that owed more to the efforts of staff rather than the expenditure of large sums of money. In September the maternity unit became one of only few large units nationally to achieve a UNICEF/World Health Organisation global 'baby friendly' award designed to promote and support breast feeding worldwide. The achievement owed everything to five years hard work by the maternity team during which Brighton's breast feeding rate increased from 56 per cent to 95 per cent consistently over two years.

The year 2001 also provided still more evidence of the way voluntary effort flourished and benefited the hospital. In March, patients and supporters of the vascular unit celebrated the opening of the Vascular Assessment Unit on Level 8 of the Thomas Kemp Tower. During the preceding twenty years the Sussex Stroke and Circulation Fund had purchased all the equipment in the unit. The charity had been set up in 1980 to fund research and provide equipment to help with the diagnosis and treatment of patients with vascular disease in Sussex. The new unit on Level 8 replaced the vascular laboratory set up by the fund in the Barry Building in 1992. Since then over £900,000 had been raised for vascular services at the hospital and the Princess Royal at Haywards Heath.

Another very supportive voluntary body was the Brighton Heart Support Trust. In the 20 years from 1987, more than £1.6 million was spent on new equipment, principally for the hospital's cardiac department. Much of this specialised equipment being computer based trequired upgrading or replacing on a regular basis.

By coincidence £900,000 was also the cost of the extended and modernised Sussex Oncology Centre, which was celebrated at an official opening in September by supporters of the Sussex Cancer Fund for Treatment and Research. Work on the north extension of the department started in the

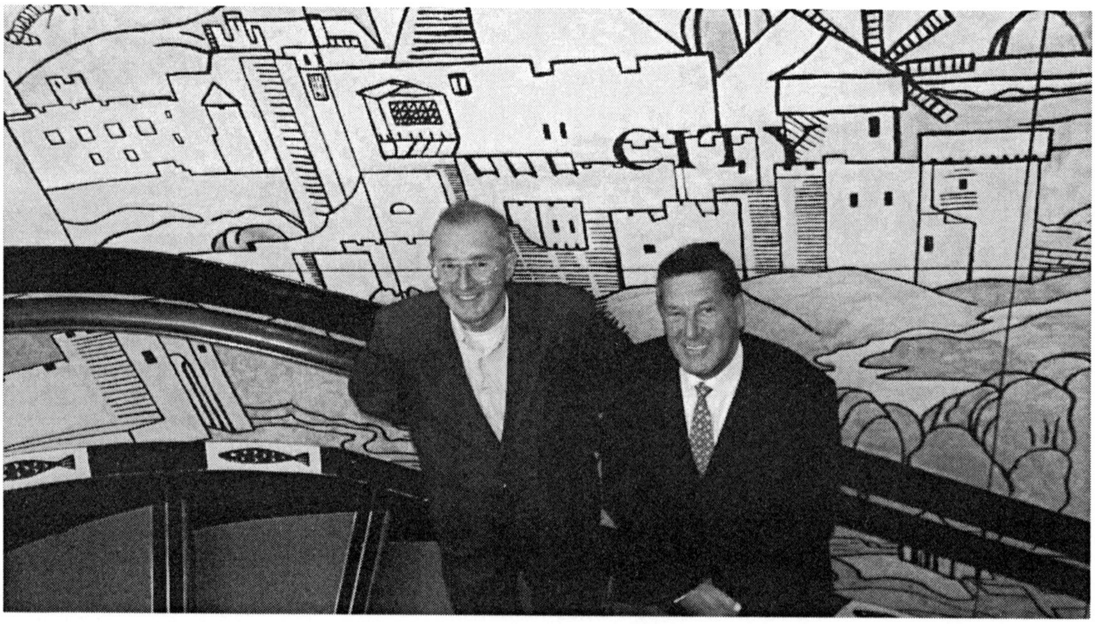

147. The impressive mural on the main staircase in the Barry Building was funded by the League of Hospital Friends, one of the many charitable bodies maintaining the tradition of voluntary support to the hospital. The artist, David Halliwell (left) is pictured with Friends' chairman, David Bowden.

previous year brought the total raised and spent by the fund since 1994 to well over £1 million including a dedicated new car park for cancer patients in Bristol Gate costing £170,000. The Friends of the Nigel Porter Unit gave £45,000 to meet half the cost of a new van for a mobile breast screening unit officially opened in June while the League of Friends provided £29,000 to pay for two vehicles to provide a transport service for patients and visitors between the main entrance, Oncology, A&E, the Millennium Wing and Sussex House.

Progress on major developments

The Brighton and Sussex University Hospitals NHS Trust became a legal entity in April 2002, and in same month there was what the chief executive described as 'a bit of a landmark', the first official opening ceremony to take place in the new trust. The ceremony marked the long awaited completion of the first phase of the redevelopment of the hospital, the Sterile Supplies Department (SSD) in the Millennium Wing.

Staff had expected to be working in their new building in September 1998 so that they would be able to cope with the demands of the new cardiac unit due to open the following summer. Instead they had to wait while the contractors finished their work. Then they had to wait while new contractors moved in to make a number of alterations due in no small part to new legislation that required higher standards that had outdated the original plans for the department which had been some six years in the making. The delays meant that staff had to continue to provide a service in poor environmental conditions with obsolete equipment that was always breaking down. Worst affected were those staff working at Brighton General in the original workhouse building built over 130 years before.

The opening of SSD was followed by events on the 24th April described by the chairman as marking 'a very special event in the history of the new trust'. In the morning the trust's board held its first meeting in the Sussex House boardroom. In the afternoon the directors and guests attended a commencement stone ceremony for its first new building and the beginning of the second phase of the hospital's development plan – the new Sussex Kidney Unit.

Consultant manager Dr Chris Kingswood told the guests how the renal unit had begun life in the 1960s when Lord Trafford saw a patient with renal failure. Although not a renal specialist, he hired a dialysis machine and treated the patient. News of the success of the treatment in Brighton spread, more and more people were referred and working together with Dr Paul

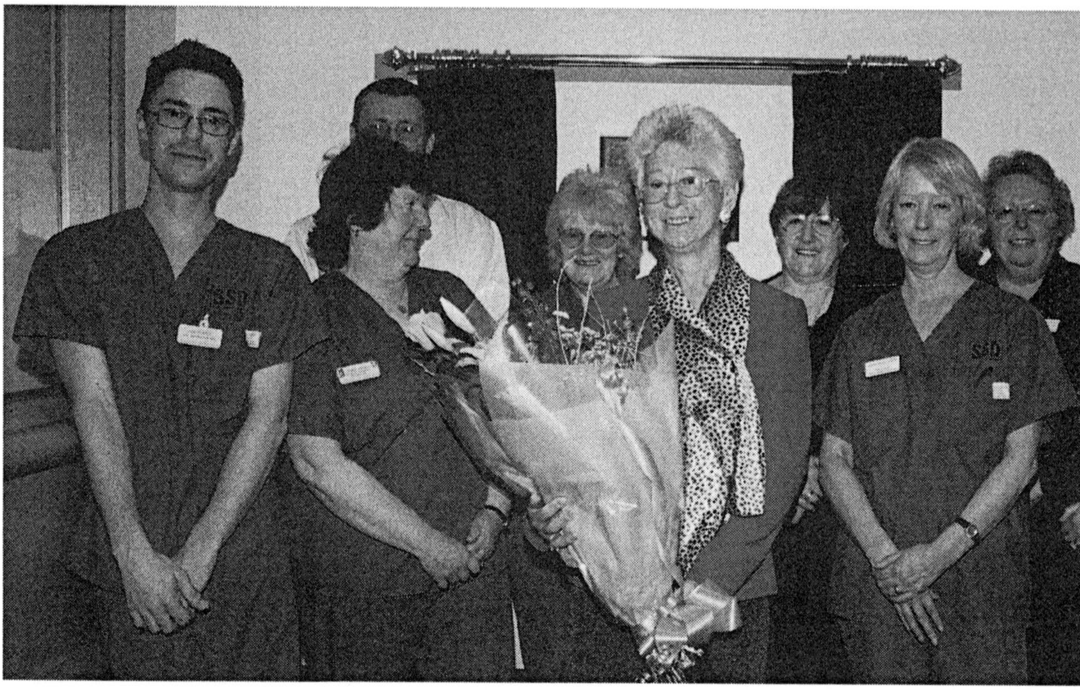

148. Former assistant manager June Williams, who had worked in the sterile supplies department at Brighton General Hospital, was chosen to open the new department at the County which she and her colleagues had helped to design.

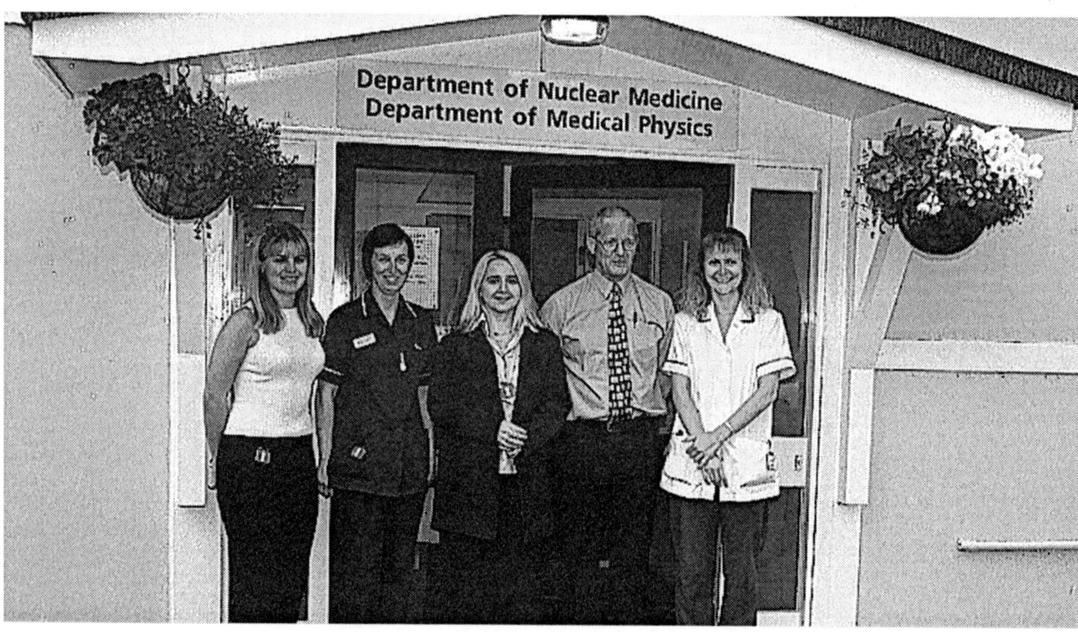

149. Lead consultant Dr Sabina Dizdaravic (centre) with some of the nuclear medicine team outside the welcoming entrance to their department, a more than 30 years old 'temporary' building in which £200,000 had been invested to help keep it going until its replacement in what appeared to be the far-off third phase of the hospital's redevelopment.

Sharpstone a new service was built up. Beginning life in the general medical wards, it opened in the first half of a 'temporary' prefabricated building in 1975. The new building was intended to replace that prefabricated building and free the space for the building of a new children's hospital on site.

Another department operating in a 30 year old prefabricated building was not so fortunate as renal. By 2003 it had become cramped and dingy; in wet weather rain came in through the windows of the nuclear medicine department and up through the floor. However, like most of the buildings facing Eastern Road, it was unlikely to be replaced until the third phase of the redevelopment which was several years off and a way had to be found of keeping the old building going in the meantime. This was achieved thanks to an investment of £200,000, which was spent on a complete external repair. The building was reroofed and all external timber, windows and fascia panels were replaced. As well as new flooring and redecoration, new seating was provided and a new fire alarm system installed.

The first stage of the redevelopment of the hospital's operating theatres was completed during 2002. Theatres 1 and 2 were refurbished to provide laminar clean air ventilation for orthopaedic joint replacement and Theatre 6 was refurbished for general surgery emergency work and gynaecology. Work on Phase 2, an £11.8 million scheme, began in September 2003. The theatres in the Thomas Kemp Tower had been opened over thirty years before as part of the original uncompleted development of the hospital. Some of the equipment was still in use in 2003. As part of the project, it was intended to replace all the equipment in the department to bring it up to current standards. The cost was approximately £1.5 million for the equipment and a further £1 million for new instruments.

Theatres were not the only part of the tower block to be upgraded during the year. Thanks to a successful bid for £850,000 for modernisation money available nationally, the maternity department was redecorated and provided with new facilities. These included a breastfeeding room on Level 12, new en-suite shower rooms on Levels 11 and 12 and extra toilet and shower facilities. Additional equipment provided included an increased width operating table, ultrasound scanning and diathermy equipment and eight electric birthing beds, seven neonatal resuscitation cots and anaesthetic monitors and a replacement deluxe birthing pool. A new £113,000 CCTV security system was the single most expensive item provided in the scheme.

There was yet another historic day for the hospital on the 29th May with the groundbreaking ceremony for the new education centre carried out by Professor Jon Cohen, dean of the Brighton and Sussex Medical School

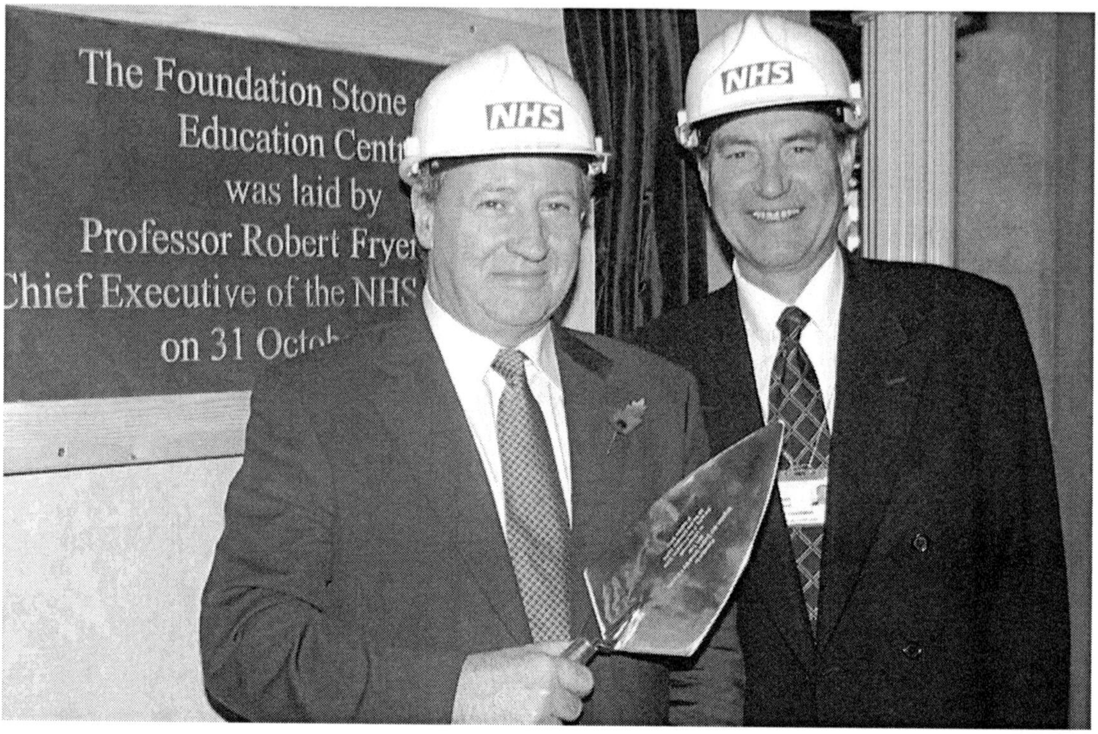
The Foundation Stone
Education Cent
was laid by
Professor Robert Frye
Chief Executive of the NHS
on 31 Oct
NHS
NHS

150. Professor Bob Fryer, chief executive of the NHS University, who unveiled the foundation stone at the long-awaited new education centre with trust chairman Professor Michael Whiting.

which had received its first 136 undergraduate students at the end of September. The new £10.2 million centre, he said, would be the clinical heart of the medical school.

The former chairman of Brighton Health Care, Baroness Emerton, was one of the guests at the stonelaying ceremony on the 31st October. The new building, chief executive Stuart Welling told the guests, would be named the Audrey Emerton Building in recognition of what he described as 'her extensive contribution to education nationally and the development of local healthcare.'[5] The former director of medical education, consultant Dr John Hartley, recalled that at one stage during the ten year process of planning the building, it had been a choice between building the centre or a new cardiac centre. The development of the medical school provided the final boost for the project, which would provide the training base for the new students. When completed it would also provide educational and training facilities for all trust and local health economy staff in a five storey building that would include a 190 seat lecture theatre, an 80 seat lecture hall, a clinical skills training room, six seminar rooms, 12 training rooms, a multi-disciplinary library and a 170 cover restaurant.

The major developments at the hospital came at a time when unfavourable media attention on the NHS generally – and the County Hospital was no exception – seemed to be the order of the day. Brighton Health Care had fared badly when the NHS performance ratings published in the summer of 2001, for example, revealed that waiting times for an outpatient appointment and appointments to see a breast surgeon failed to meet national targets and that some A&E patients were enduring trolley waits of more than twelve hours. Staff, in particular, welcomed the publication of good news to balance the negative press publicity and reports on new developments of major schemes were of some help. Figures published in *The Times* in November provided a welcome boost when they showed that the hospital was among the best in the country for cardiac bypass surgery and for the treatment of fractured femurs and stroke patients. During the same month, the trust's patient advocate, Penny Dunman, was presented with a national award by health minister John Hutton for 'setting the gold standard in patient centred services', which she hoped 'would be a turning point for Brighton'.[6]

However, good news reports like these, were almost as nothing compared with the one that filled many pages in the press and was featured on national television in January 2002. It not only made the front page of one of the tabloids, but also earned the comment in the *Sun* newspaer 'Isn't it wonderful to read an NHS success story?'

The story concerned a patient, 39 year old Carina Marong from Hangleton. She was so grateful for the care she received she returned to the hospital together with her husband, father and baby to hold a press conference, where they faced a battery of TV and press cameras to recount their story.

Carina was 37 weeks pregnant in August 2001 when she was admitted to the County and diagnosed with TB meningitis, a rare condition which, consultant neurologist Dr Angus Nisbet said, the hospital might expect to see only once in every four or five years and was universally fatal if not treated promptly. She gave birth to her second daughter, Sophia, on the 25th August and was also diagnosed with Hodgkin's lymphoma, but was too ill to start anti-cancer treatment.

In mid-September she slipped into a coma. According to consultant oncologist Dr David Bloomfield, her meningitis had robbed her of all meaningful movement. 'The only control she had was with her eyes. Although we were hopeful for the best, her chances of major recovery seemed slight'.[7] However, Carina did slowly improve. She awoke from her coma in October – a very emotional moment for the staff on Solomon ward, according to

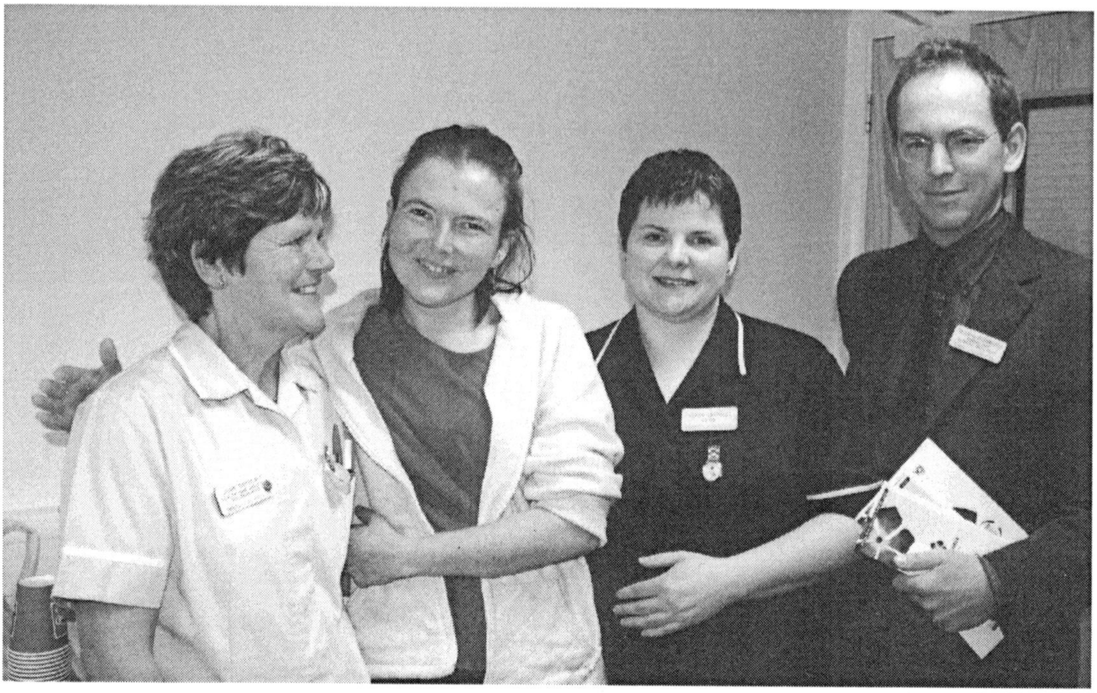

151. Carina Marong, whose NHS good news story was featured in national newspapers and on TV, with Solomon ward staff and consultant oncologist Dr David Bloomfield when she returned to the hospital to thank them for saving her life.

the ward sister. But she awoke with no recollection of the previous twelve months and was amazed to find herself the mother of a baby daughter she knew nothing about. She told the press conference:

> I missed the first six weeks of my baby's life but I could have lost so much more. The staff in the hospitals could not have been more gentle, caring and tolerant. They were utterly professional, yet totally human, and without them I could not have coped with this experience.[8]

Her father added: 'Carina was lucky to be in the right hospital with the necessary expertise at the right time.'

Progress report on major developments

Whilst much of the attention during 2001-2003 was focused on the major developments and stories like that of Carina Marong made the national headlines, a considerable number of lesser, but nevertheless important, developments were taking place. Traditionally, reliance had been placed on the London teaching hospitals for specialised surgery and procedures for patients from Sussex, but steady progress was being made in making the County more self sufficient. The development of cardiac surgery and the changes in the MRI unit are two examples of how this was being achieved. There was less publicity, however, for another important development in local haematology services.

Early in 2002, the trust appointed its first haematology nurse specialist, a ward sister on the haematology and bone marrow transplant unit at St George's Hospital in Tooting. Her appointment opened the way to develop haematology services in Brighton where local patients had to travel to London for treatment, sometimes twice a week. By July she had trained another nurse and opened a small four-bedded unit off Egremont Ward where they were able to treat day cases. In less that six months they successfully dealt with 200 patient episodes, including more than 80 blood transfusions.

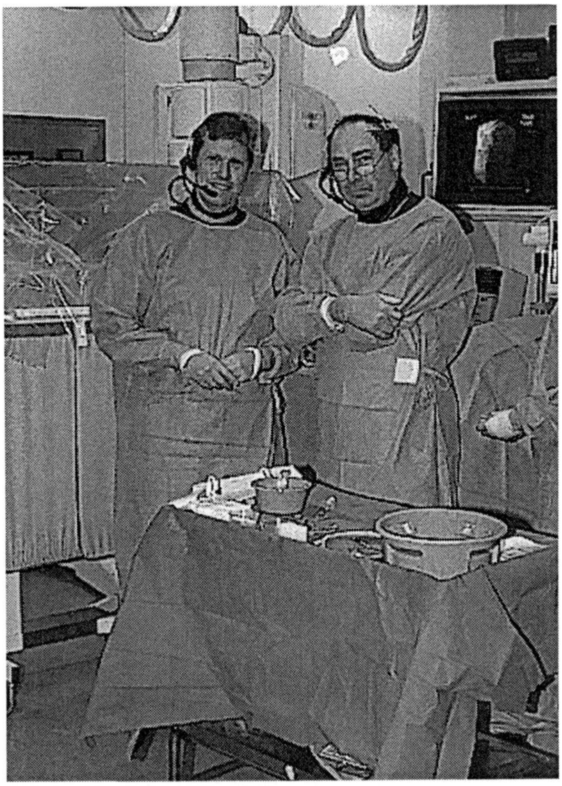

152. Consultant cardiologists Dr Steve Holmberg and Dr Mark Signy wearing microphones as they are about to 'go live' and perform a complicated angioplasty, which was broadcast from the hospital to an audience of consultants and specialist registrars in London.

In June 2003, cardiologists won high praise when they demonstrated their angioplasty skills to a London audience. A morning session in the Brighton catheter laboratories by four consultant cardiologists was beamed live to the Hilton Park Lane hotel to an audience of consultant colleagues and senior registrars at the London Intervention 2003 meeting. At the same time as performing some difficult procedures, the cardiologists also had to respond to questions from their London audience. When the Sussex Cardiac Centre opened, 50 interventions a month were planned and 87 were actually carried out. In the month before the live demonstration, 392 cases were dealt with.

In August, the Sussex Cancer Centre (formerly known as the Sussex Oncology Centre) unveiled its state of the art £1 million linear accelerators that had been installed during the three years since receiving a £7 million award for refurbishing the department. In order to maintain the service without interruption, the existing machines that were nearing the end of their useful life had been kept running while a new department was being built. This involved moving many tons of chalk from the hillside to accommodate new lead and concrete bunkers specially designed so that no radiation could escape.

At the unveiling, lead consultant Dr Geoff Newman told his audience that a major benefit of the new more powerful linear accelerators was that they were able to deliver radiation 'to treat a banana'[9] explaining that formerly the accelerators only showed rectangular shapes which did not conform to the shape of the tumour. To overcome this, radiographers had to alter the shape by inserting heavy lumps of lead. This was no longer necessary because the new machines produced a beam matching the size and shape of the patient's tumour.

Nursing and nurses

Nursing vacancies in the trust hit a three year high in March 2002 and the County suffered in common with the other trust hospitals. Staff shortages at the time affected a wide range of staff, including radiographers and physiotherapists. The chief executive told the board there were four main reasons for the situation: the cost of living locally, expensive housing, career development and working conditions. Nurses at the County in particular suffered from an upsurge in emergency work: on some wards bed occupancy exceeded one hundred per cent! In the circumstances, it was hardly surprising sickness levels were up and turnover was increasing. The situation would have been even worse but for the successful recruitment of nurses from South Africa and the Philippines.

A number of new measures were taken in an attempt to deal with the situation and at least one taken earlier bore fruit. This was a scheme to second health care assistants (HCAs) who possessed few or no formal qualifications to Brighton University. Perhaps at first this contributed to the shortages at the hospital but in the longer term it guaranteed an increasing supply of qualified nurses, the first of whom began work in October. By then, despite having nearly 280 nursing vacancies in the trust, forty health care assistants had been funded to train at the university, with a total of 25 in the current academic year.

In September, after an absence of several years, cadets returned locally to mark the start of a new scheme organised in collaboration with the Brighton, Hove and Sussex Sixth Form College (BHASVIC) and South Downs Health trust. While not simply nursing cadet as in earlier years, the new scheme was for health care cadets. Their placements would include areas such as Pathology and X-ray as well as working on the wards although it seemed likely nursing would probably be the main beneficiary. When the

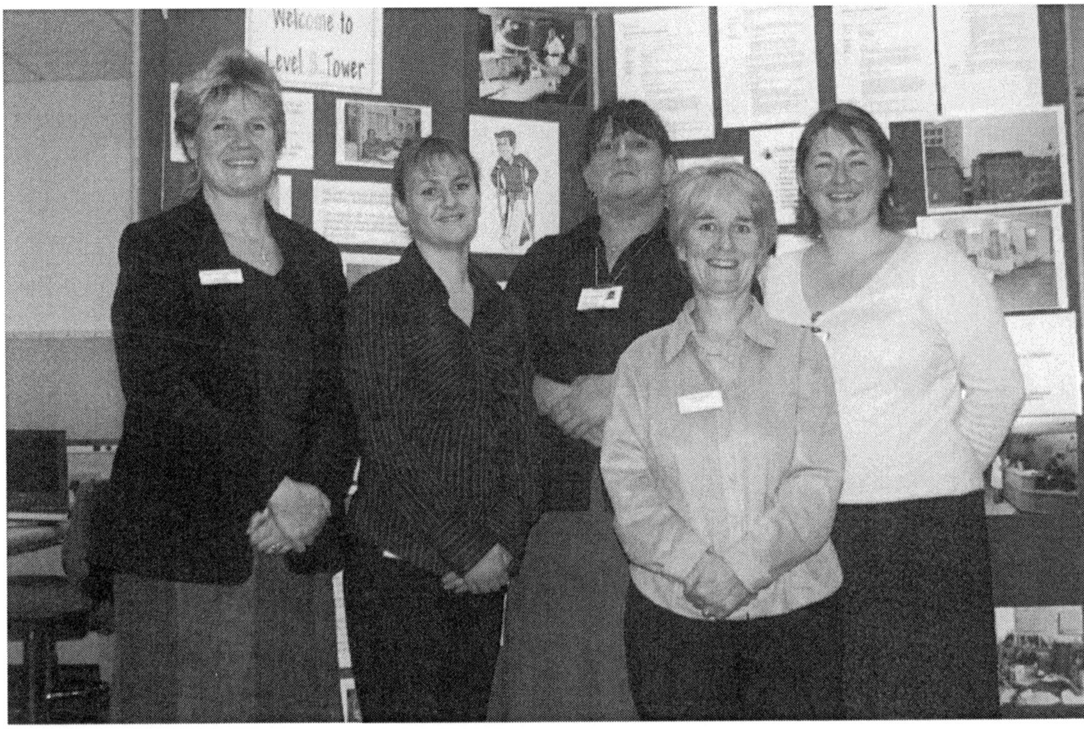

153. Ward managers and senior nursing staff who met applicants at a successful open day they organised in an effort to recruit more staff.

first group of nine 16 to 18 year olds graduated the following July, one had already begun her nursing diploma course at Brighton University. Two had taken up HCA posts on Vallance Ward and one in the fracture clinic. Others were waiting for the results of interviews. South Downs Health had also employed one cadet as a nursing assistant and the Princess Royal had appointed another as a porter in X-ray. To mark the success of the scheme, 30 cadets were enrolled for 2003/4 in two groups of 15, which included an advanced group with sufficient GCEs to undertake A Level or university courses.

In October 2003, four new overseas nurses were working on the wards at the Sussex County. They were part of a group of eleven who had been recruited to do three to six months supervised work in trust hospitals by a County Hospital sister, Liz Johnson, who had undertaken the role of adaptation nurse co-ordinator. Earlier, in September, ward managers on two areas of the hospital – orthopaedics and cardiac – organised an event to boost recruitment to Level 8A East and West, Overton Ward and the cardiac department. Fifteen interested people visited the hospital and two more telephoned. Six posts were offered following interviews to some of those attending on the day and six others were offered interviews to be held later.

Two notable nursing developments occurred during the latter part of the year. Following a year's work, two former County nurses who had been appointed to a job-share post in the Claude Nicol Centre established a ground-breaking new sexual health clinic for young people living in the area.

Meanwhile two sisters in the renal unit completed a course at Brighton University enabling them to prescribe a list of medications and became the trust's first nurse prescribers.

19. *More Developments, More to Come, 2004 – 2007*

The three years from 2004 to 2006 saw the completion of several major developments beginning with the Sussex Kidney Centre. In February 2004 staff and patients moved into the new £12 million unit which contained a 36 bedded inpatient ward, twelve more than in the old unit, and six high dependency beds. The ward was named after Lord Trafford. Built on two floors over the North car park, the new renal unit also contained 41 dialysis stations, compared with 21 in the old building, a home dialysis centre, a peritoneal dialysis department, a large outpatient department and several other attractive facilities.

The standard and finish of the new unit so impressed a visiting team from NHS Estates that its members requested copies of the design drawings which they planned to use as a template for future renal developments in the NHS.

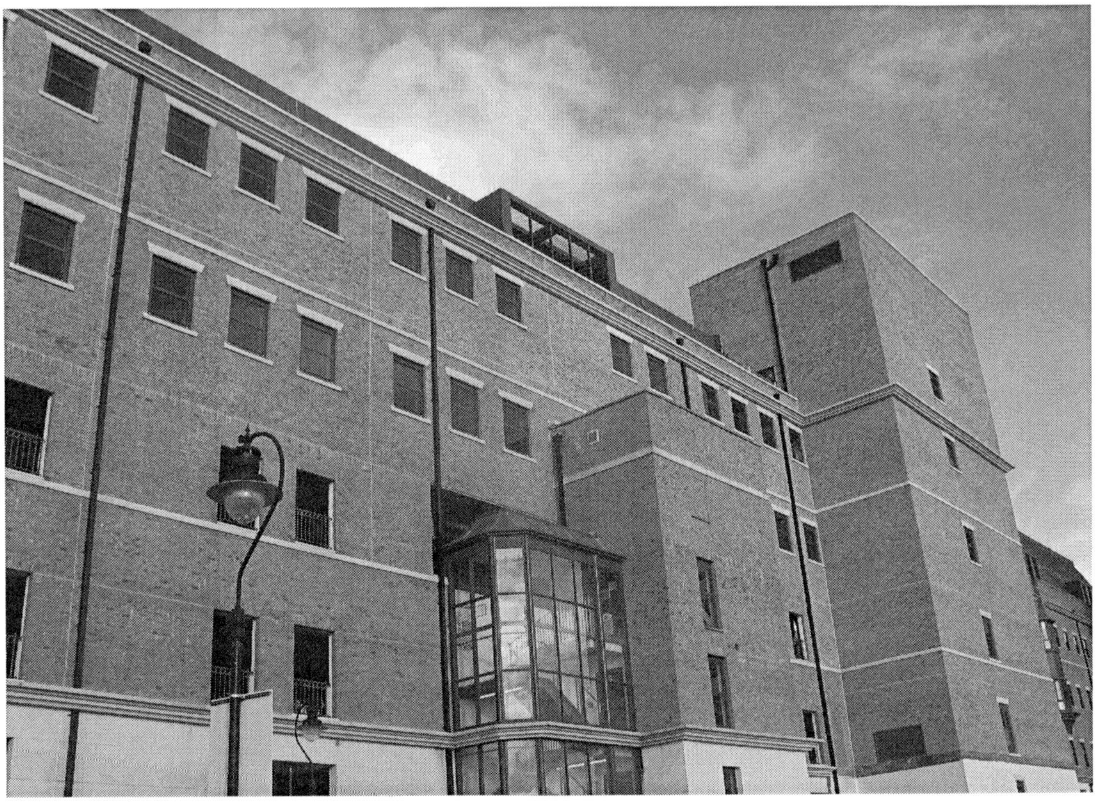

154. The Sussex Kidney Centre built above the North Car Park.

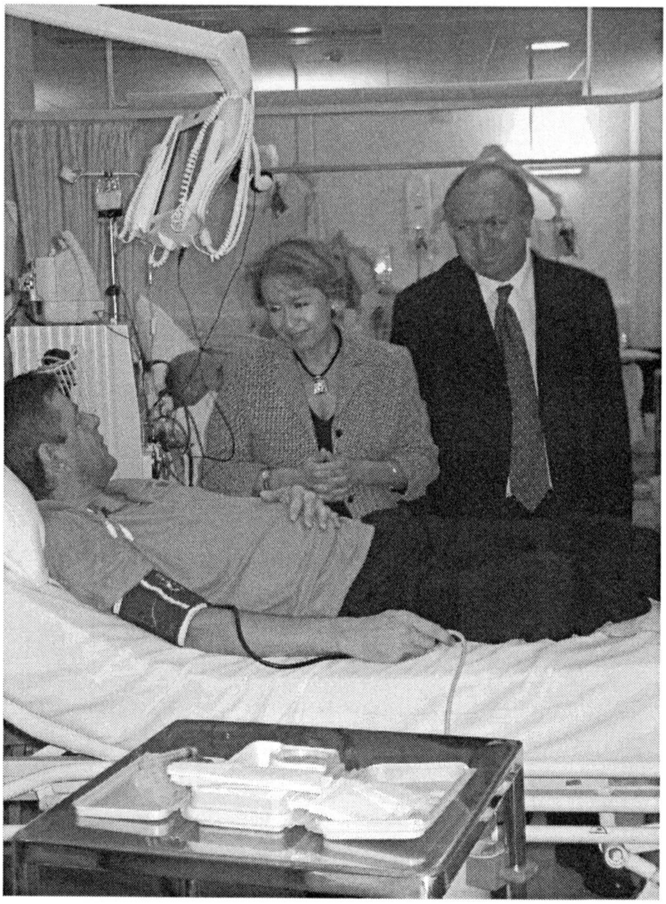

155. Health minister Rosie Winterton chats to a patient on the new kidney unit during a visit with local MP David Lepper.

Much of the equipment for the unit was bought by charitable donations. These included £250,000 from the Sussex Kidney Development Fund, £16,000 of which was donated by *The Argus* Appeal. £73,000 was donated by the Sussex Kidney Trust, £50,000 by the Trafford Trust and £25,000 by the South East Kidney Patients' Association. The Friends of Brighton and Hove Hospitals donated twenty electrically operated therapy chairs costing £38,000.

A media launch on the 5th March was filmed and featured in regional news programmes by the BBC and Meridian Television. There was further media coverage for the official opening at which, disappointingly, last minute changes had to be made. Health minister Rosie Winterton, who was to have performed the opening ceremony, was prevented from attending by pressing parliamentary business. Former chief executive, Stuart Welling, who had retired the previous week, stepped into the breach and unveiled a plaque with the aid of seven-year-old Tom Anson, the son of Rachel Anson, a sister in the unit's outpatient department. Later in the year, however, the minister made amends and toured the unit meeting patients and staff and commenting, at the end of her visit: 'The £12 million investment that's gone into making this wonderful unit has provided an excellent service for patients and a pleasant atmosphere for staff and patients.'[1]

During the year, work was completed on two schemes that increased the number of scanners in operation at the hospital. Following the conversion of an observation ward in A&E, a second CT scanner was installed on Level 5 of the tower block at a cost of £1.19 million. Later, in September, work was completed as planned, despite encountering major difficulties, on a £3.36 million MRI scanner scheme. This was intended to replace a 1994 scanner by one that was more technologically advanced and also to install an additional scanner provided through Cancer Network Improvement Funds.

This was a complex scheme which required significant redevelopment of the imaging department that included providing a proper facility for administering general anaesthetics, a new reception and waiting area and offices. In addition, two walls had to be demolished in order to install the new electro-magnets, each weighing between one and two tonnes.

An unexpected problem arose when water, that was believed to have been trapped above the ceiling following an earlier repair to the leaking roof, escaped and damaged the copper-lined Faraday cage which was intended to keep out radio frequency signals that would interfere with images produced by the scanner. As a result, the cage had to be returned to the factory for repair, which delayed the installation of one of the scanners.

Despite this, and the major chaos and disruption experienced during the build, the service to patients was maintained throughout, the scheme was completed on schedule, and the chief executive of the NHS, Sir Nigel Crisp, officially opened the refurbished department during a visit to the hospital on September 24th.

A fifth major development completed during 2004 created a new home for medical records and active X-rays from the hospital and others managed by the trust. A rundown warehouse, conveniently situated close to the hospital on the Freshfield Industrial Estate, that needed a new roof, cladding and windows was given a new lease of life at a cost of £750,000, almost a third of which was spent on a two tier racking system.

Although the completion of the new education centre had been programmed for November, it was not actually ready for use until the summer of 2005, fortunately in time for the arrival of the first 136 medical students for their attachments to the hospital's clinical firms. As well as the education and training facilities, the new building also contained a spacious new library that replaced previous facilities based inconveniently at Brighton General Hospital and in Rosaz House on the County site. The old health authority library at Lewes and the city health promotion library were also transferred to the new accommodation.

Work on the new-look Barry Building was also completed in 2005. The £2 million scheme was not, despite appearances, simply cosmetic. First, extensive work was carried out renewing the roof of the building and making

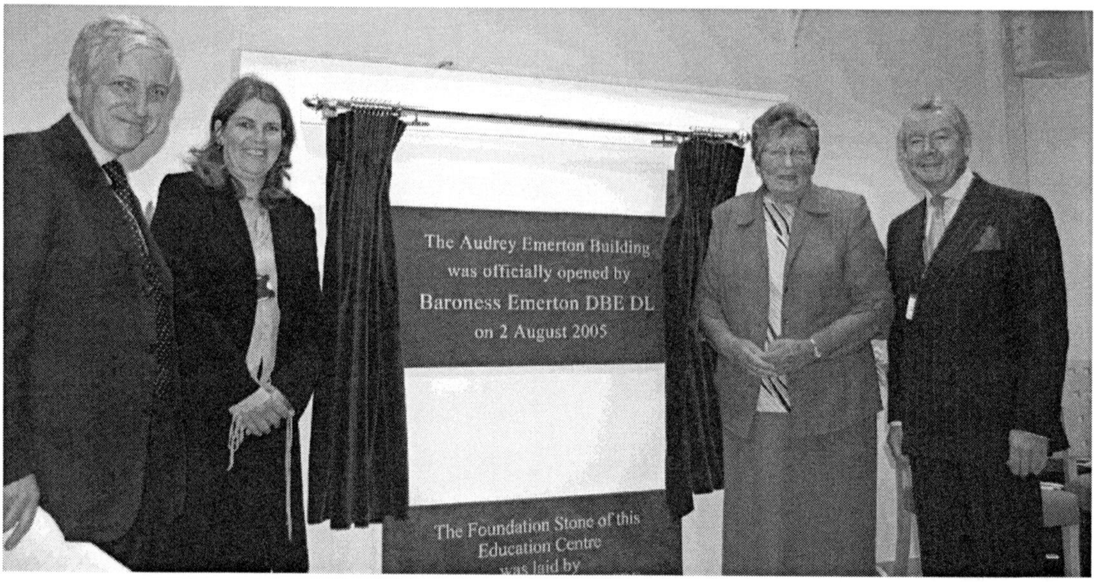
The Audrey Emerton Building
was officially opened by
Baroness Emerton DBE DL
on 2 August 2005
The Foundation Stone of this
Education Centre

156. Baroness Emerton and Trust chair Glynn Jones (right) at the unveiling of a commemorative plaque at the official opening of the new education centre together with Professor Jon Cohen, Dean of the Medical School and medical education director, Julia Montgomery.

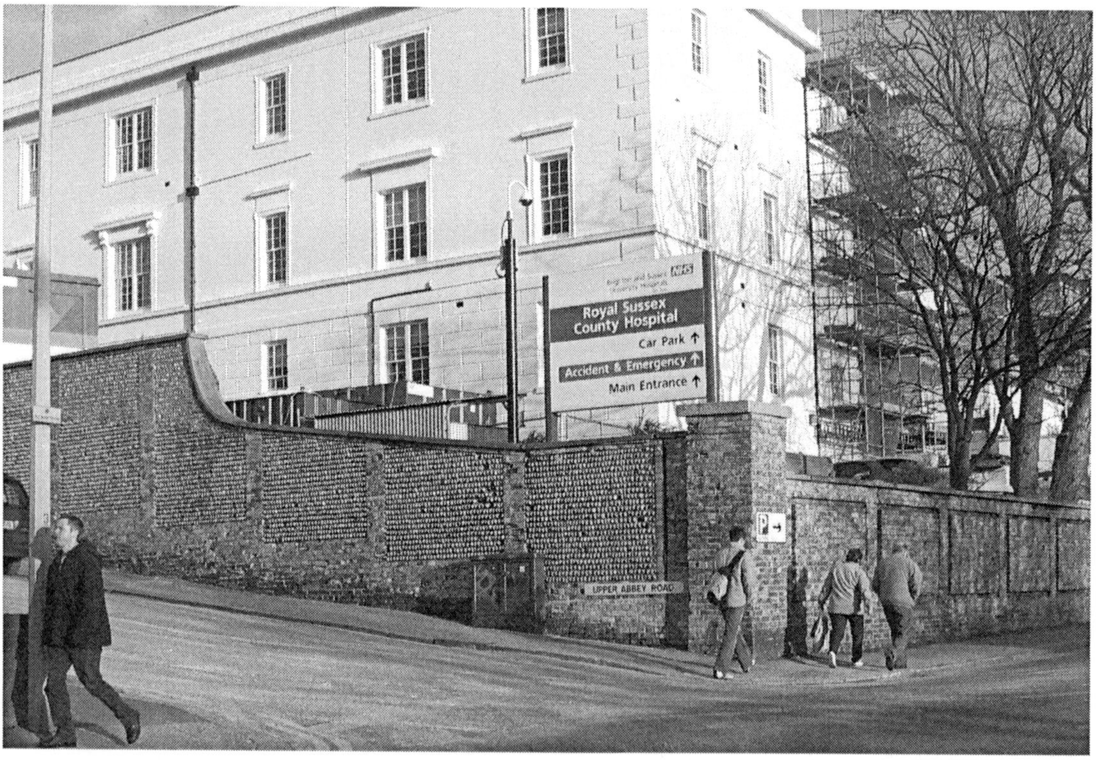
NHS
Royal Sussex
County Hospital
Car Park
Accident & Emergency
Main Entrance
UPPER ABBEY ROAD

157. A new coat of paint protected the fabric of the Barry Building.

it watertight. This was followed by the installation of new windows and repairs to gutters and pipework. Finally, the perished exterior rendering was painted to provide a plastic coating, which also helped to make the old building waterproof. The scheme was followed by similar work on the adjoining Jubilee Building, which was completed by the end of the year.

The main theatres redevelopment scheme entered its final phases in the spring of 2005. The refurbishment of theatre 3 was completed, so too was the construction of the new theatre 7, which left only theatres 4 and 5 remaining to be upgraded. Before this work began, however, work got underway on Level 4 to provide a new patient reception area, new entrance lobby, porters' lodge, offices, teaching, training and on-call rooms.

The completion of the final major development during this three year period led to the opening on the 21st September 2006 of the £4 million state of the art purpose built clinical research and investigation unit which had been built on the roof of the linear accelerator building. A joint project with the Brighton and Sussex Medical School, the new unit contained a 40-seat lecture theatre, a 9-bed trolley bay, laboratories and interview and clinical rooms providing a dedicated facility for research into conditions such as cancer, diabetes and heart disease.

The unit occupied the upper two floors of the new building and the medical school was also associated with a development on the lowest floor for which the Sussex Cancer Fund had provided £450,000. The new spacious facility for the Sussex Cancer Centre expected to open in the spring of 2007 provided increased facilities for chemotherapy patients necessary because of the demand for treatments was expected to increase at an annual rate of some sixteen per cent. Moreover, the shifting focus towards outpatient treatment, which could require some patients to be in the unit for several hours, necessitated the provision of additional facilities such as toilets and a kitchenette.

Other developments

A number of other schemes, not strictly part of the capital development programme, were completed between 2004 and 2006. Pride of place went to the £1 million new interventional radiology suite opened in September 2006. The centrepiece was a new machine capable of taking a 3D rotational angiogram of a patient's blood vessels – one of only three of these pieces of high tech equipment in the country. Producing clearer and more accurate images than earlier machines, its principal uses included detecting and treating narrowing of the arteries in the legs or kidneys caused by vascular

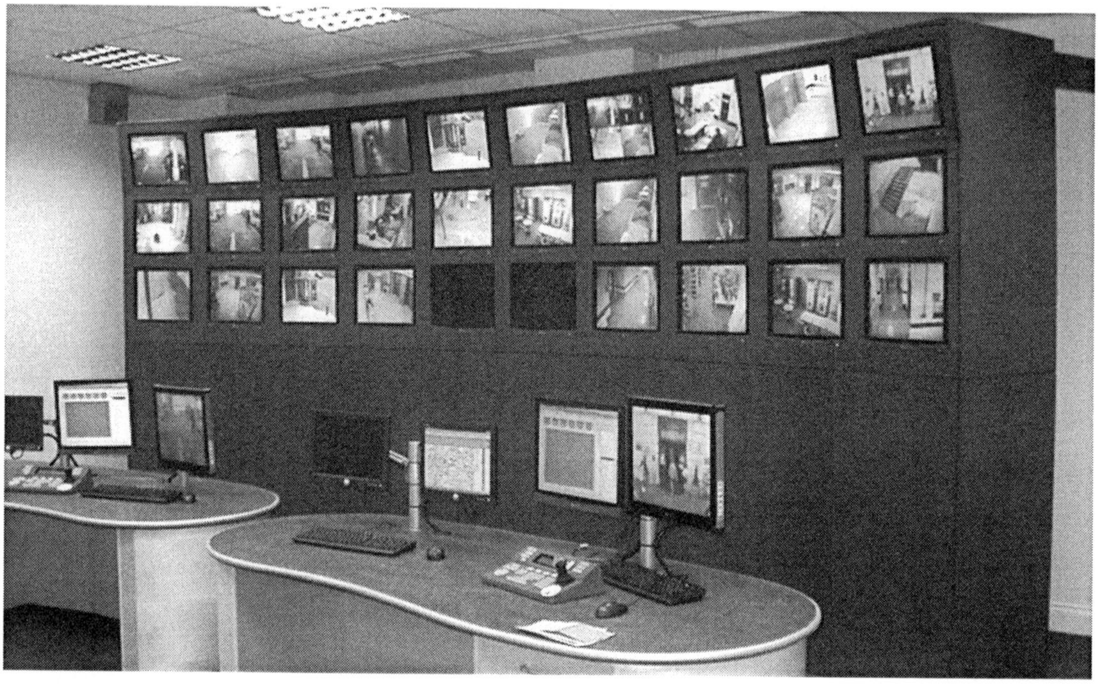

158. The huge panel of screens in the new security control room.

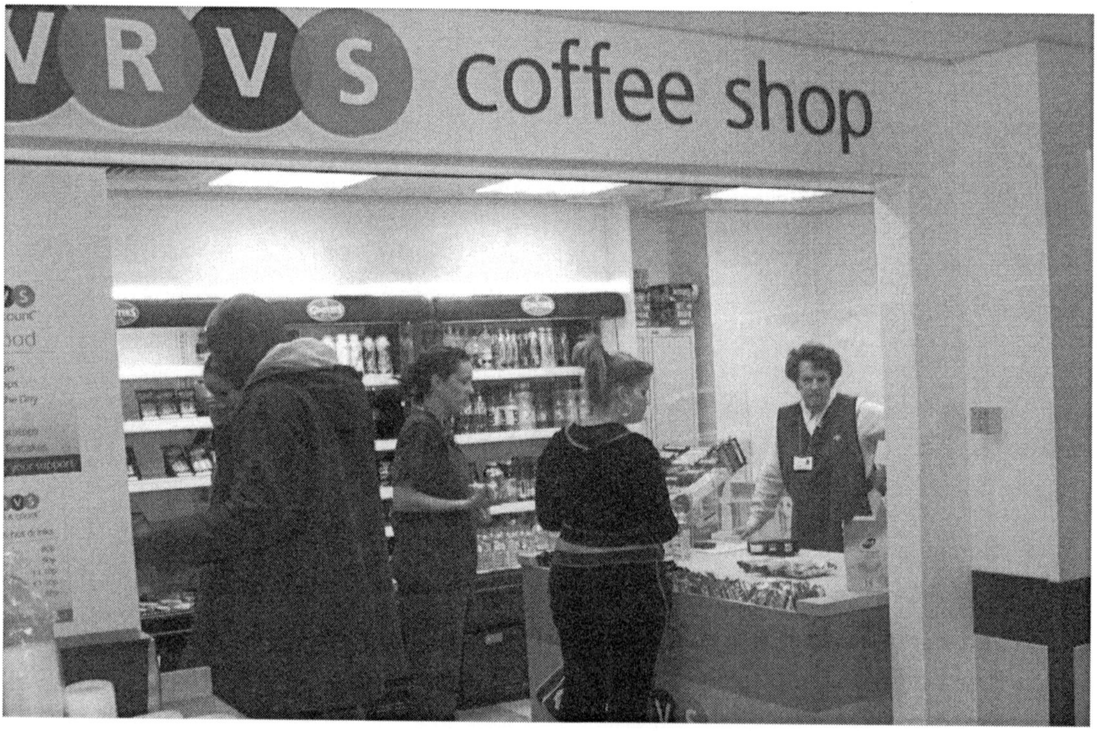

159.The new WRVS coffee shop in the A&E department.

diseases and guiding the placement of stents to relieve the symptoms of patients with cancer of the oesophagus, bile duct or bowel. As part of the development of the old angiography suite, a three bedded bay was created for patients before and after the procedure.

Earlier in the year, the hospital unveiled its new security control room situated on Level 4 of the tower block underneath A&E. The original purpose-built security control room was built in A&E in 1994 when it was realised there was a need for a full-time security presence at the hospital, and especially in A&E. There were twelve cameras in this original CCTV system recording on VHS tapes that had to be changed every twelve hours. A new control room was provided in the Phase I development in 1999 where security staff monitored 64 cameras and numerous personal attack alarms and the following year digital recorders were installed to replace the tape recording system.

By 2005, the CCTV system had grown to 175 cameras but there was no more space for further developments, principally the need for 32 additional cameras to monitor the proposed new children's hospital. The space occupied by the control room was also needed to permit the construction of a new urgent care centre at the front of A&E. The new department boasted 200 cameras compared with 12 in the original 1994 control room and included a brand new state of the art recording and picture management system designed to protect staff, patients and visitors by deterring and detecting crime and anti-social behaviour, a growing problem locally and nationally.

Thanks to the continuing financial support of the WRVS a £40,000 upgrading of two of their coffee shops was completed in 2005, first in A&E then the Level 8 food court in the Millennium Wing, which was opened in June. The following year the WRVS provided a further £35,000 to meet the cost of a makeover to their coffee shop in Main Outpatients. At the same time, the trust funded the establishment of a new coffee shop just inside the entrance to the Barry Building using space created by moving the volunteers' office and the discharge lounge.

Noteworthy developments during these three years that owed much to staff and did not require new buildings included the introduction in February 2006 of a new dedicated ambulance for the Brighton Baby Emergency Service Transfer Team.

Led by the hospital's lead neo-natal consultant, Dr Cassie Lamb, the team had set up a pilot scheme two years earlier using emergency ambulances to move infants requiring neonatal care that could not be provided in the hospitals where they were born. Their declared aim at the time, however, was for an adapted ambulance specially equipped for emergency neonatal care. On February 27th, their dream became a reality and their new ambulance, which would allow the team to carry out difficult treatment during transit, made its first journey from the Sussex County to the Princess Royal Hospital at Haywards Heath crewed by one of the six specially trained ambulance personnel in neonatal care.

Meanwhile, staff in the Sussex Cardiac Centre were continuing their pioneering work in the catheter laboratories. In June 2005 the hospital hosted the 3rd Left Main Stem Intervention meeting. Five invited experts from around the UK and Europe helped by the local interventional cardiology team performed a procedure using less invasive techniques on five patients with narrowed arteries. These would usually have been dealt with by coronary artery bypass surgery.

Most of the UK's leading exponents of interventional cardiology had gathered for the day to hear a variety of lectures on the progress of the new technology at the conference centre on the seafront. While they were there, they were able to witness a live transmission of the procedures being carried out at the hospital.

In November 2006, the centre hosted a workshop for consultants and senior registrars who visited Brighton to hear lectures and see live demonstrations, this time of another new technique being pioneered by a number of institutions in the country, including the Sussex County.

In 2006, the nuclear medicine department learned that it was one of the two runners up for the prestigious Ammy Award for the nuclear medicine department of the year. The award by GE Healthcare acknowledged that over the previous two years the department had undergone a metamorphosis becoming a fully fledged university department offering advanced diagnostic and therapeutic services, teaching and research.

The Sussex Cancer Centre was also named as an award winner during the year, this time an exceptional care award from the Cancer Network Patients' Forum. It was given to acknowledge the efforts of staff who gave up their free time to organise a series of welcome evenings for new cancer patients. These were designed to show them the department and its equipment and answer their questions. In this way they hoped to overcome the apprehension of many newly diagnosed patients faced with the prospect of undergoing radiotherapy. Typical of the responses from those attending was one from a patient who said: 'I'm not looking forward to the treatment, but now I can cope.'[2]

Trials and tribulations

It is perhaps in the nature of things that negative publicity often tends to overshadow many of the achievements of hospitals, and the County was no exception during this period.

In September 2001, the government published the first performance ratings for NHS trusts providing acute hospital services. In spite of achieving six of the nine key targets set out in the NHS Plan, Brighton Health Care was given three months to achieve improvements in the other three areas. Failure it was told, could lead to the replacement of the trust's chairman and chief executive, a situation which earned it the label of 'a failing trust' in the local media.

Thus began a period extending over several years when the trust was criticised for failing to reach the highest standards in the government-set targets. Despite earning two out of a possible three stars the following year (the only trust in Sussex to achieve this) and being listed as one of the country's top forty performing teaching and major district hospital trusts for the third year running in 2003, the ratings continued to give rise to concerns in a number of areas.

Although the ratings covered the whole trust, there was one area that always gave rise to concern, the County Hospital's A&E department. One of the original three areas in which the trust 'significantly underachieved' was trolley waits of over 12 hours. Subsequently there were failings to see, treat or discharge patients within four hours of arrival. Although reorganisation within the department was to bring some notable improvements, the underlying problem was not of its own making.

Throughout (and even in 2007) the hospital suffered from the problem of what was perhaps euphemistically called considerable numbers of 'delayed discharges', patients ready to leave hospital for whom no alternative accommodation such as a nursing or rest home place was readily available[3]; indeed this is a problem existing in the health service since its earliest days when the situation was called, perhaps more realistically, 'bed blocking'.[4] The lack of available beds elsewhere in the hospital to which patients could be transferred from A&E was perhaps the principal reason for its failure to meet the national targets.

Another reason was that Brighton's A&E always suffered from the arrival of unduly large numbers of patients who could well have been dealt with in their GP surgeries, by visiting a pharmacist or by ringing NHS Direct.[5] The situation was complicated, too, because it had to be seen against a background of rising attendances, a national phenomenon, and which, in 2004 in Brighton, was at the rate of 7 per cent per year.[6]

Despite all these difficulties, staff in the department made radical changes in 2004 that brought about remarkable improvements in performance. By means of a Meet and Treat system, nurses were able to deal with the majority of patients with minor injuries and illnesses without recourse to other professionals; also a clinical decision unit (CDU) led by a senior nurse was established to track all patients requiring longer periods of care or investigation ensuring they were taken into a more appropriate environment.

The success of the trust's A&E departments was judged to be 'the most improved in the UK' and earned a special reference in Professor Sir George Alberti's report presented to the prime minister and to the secretary of state for health in October 2004. The following month health minister Rosie Winterton visited the Brighton department and added her congratulations to the staff there.

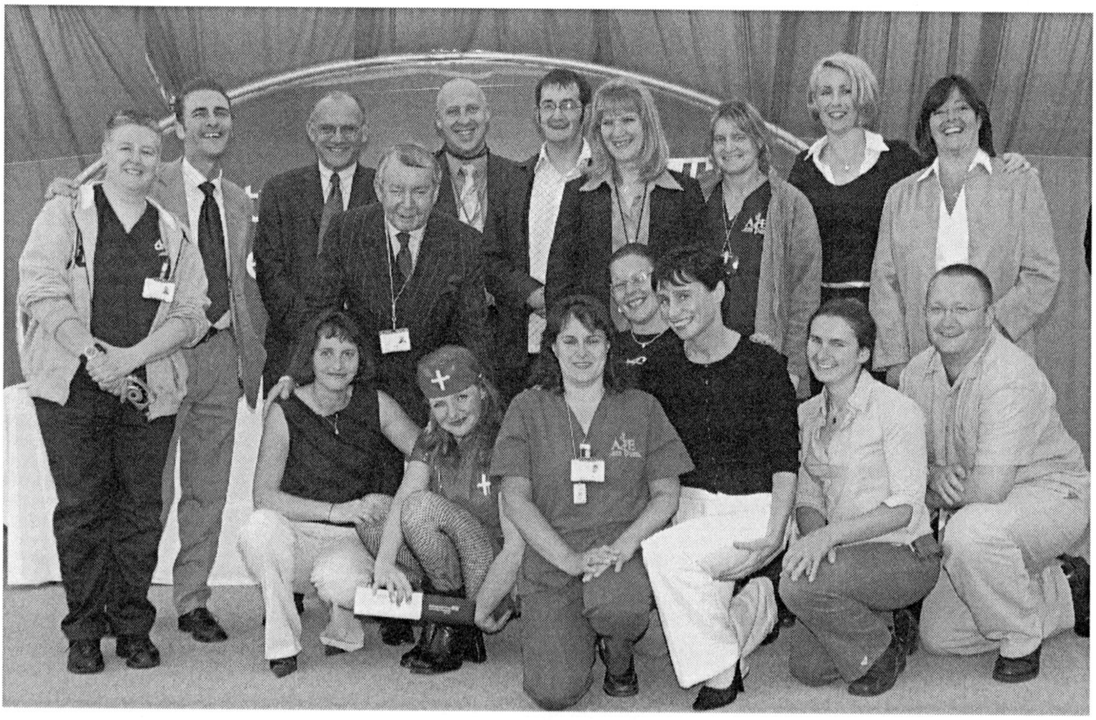

160. The hospital's award-winning A&E team joined by colleagues from the Princess Royal Hospital celebrate their success with chief executive Stuart Welling and chairman Glynn Jones (3rd and 4th from left).

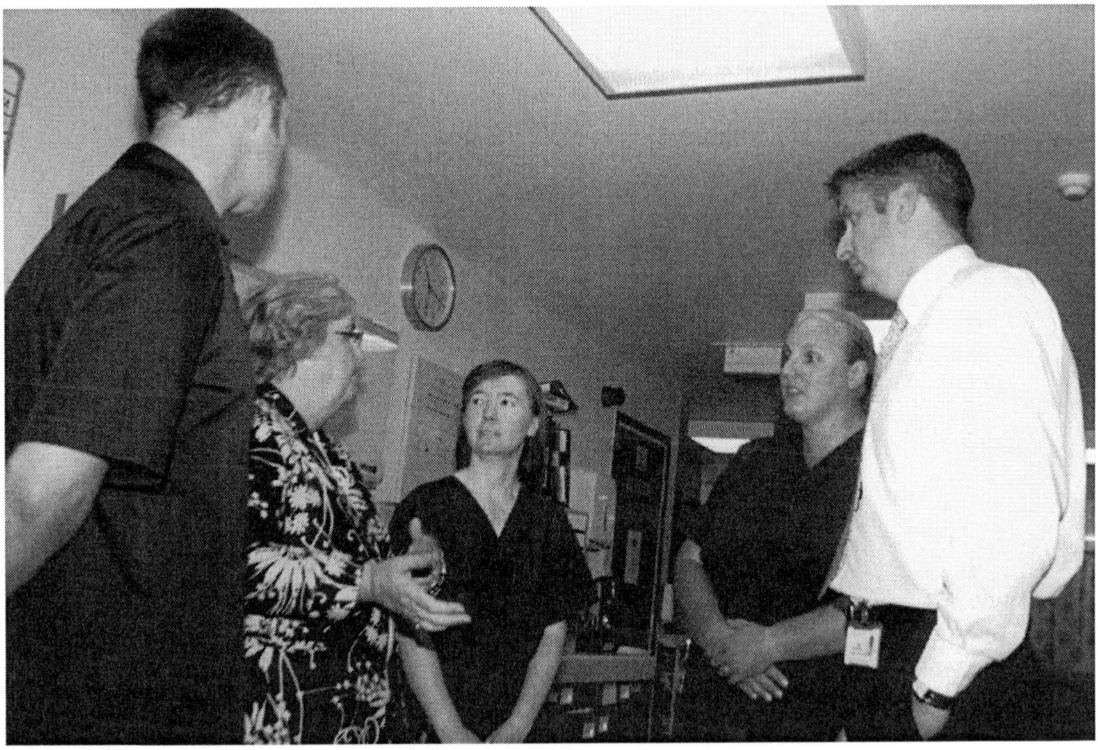

161. Chief nursing officer Professor Christine Beasley discusses the infection control plan with matron Jim Valentine (right) and three members of his ICU nursing team.

The national and local media also gave a great deal of coverage to a national problem from which the Sussex County was not exempt: the rising number of hospital acquired Infections (HAIs). Specialist hospitals like the County were especially vulnerable in this respect suffering from numbers of very sick patients with intravenous lines, for example in intensive care and the kidney unit. But here, too, staff responded to the situation and earned praise from the Department of Health's chief nursing officer, Professor Christine Beasley, who visited the hospital in September 2006

In July 2005 the BBC screened a Panorama programme called *Undercover Nurse* filmed at the hospital, which came as a shock to staff and public alike. The scenes shot secretly over a period of three months of elderly patients on Peel and Stewart Ward made for uncomfortable viewing for everyone concerned – patients' relatives and staff – and led to widespread criticism of the hospital in the media.[7]

In fact the trust was already aware, through complaints received the previous autumn from relatives and patients, that there were problems on the ward. An internal investigation led to a number of changes, culminating

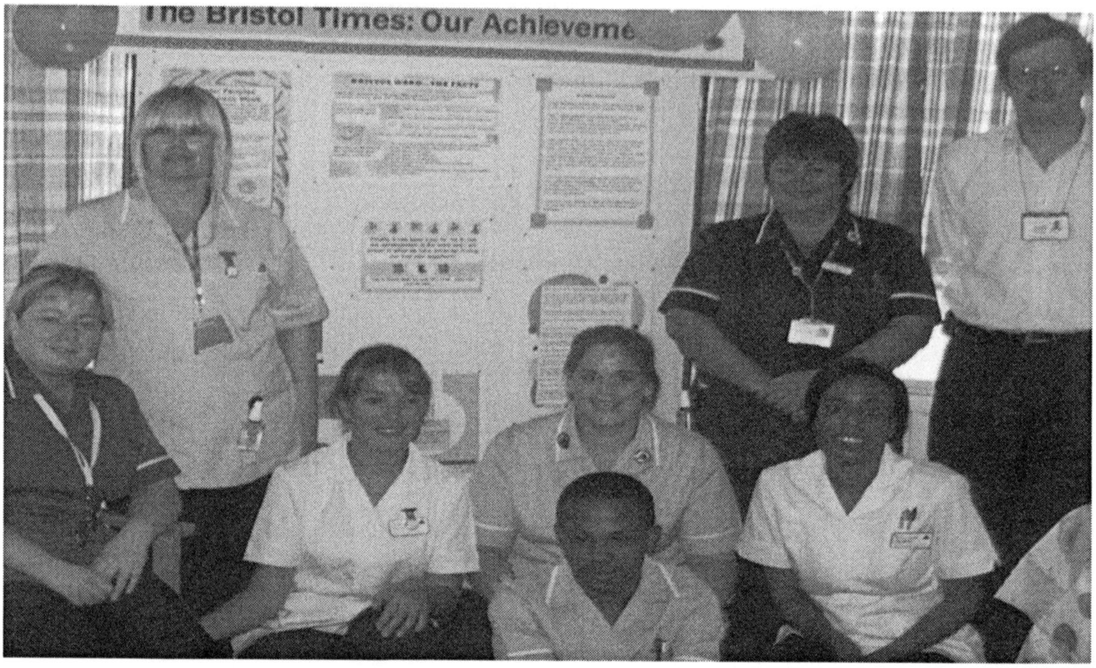

162. Bristol Ward celebrated its successful first year as an elderly care ward in 2006.

in the appointment of a new ward manager and, as a result, things had improved considerably by the time the programme was screened.[8] Led by the new ward manager, the improvements continued and the following year the nursing team's efforts were recognised in the annual staff achievement awards where they took first place in the category nominated by staff and patients.

Evidence that improvements had indeed taken place – and an indication that the problems had been confined to one ward – came less than a year later in the results of a survey into hospital care for the over-50s carried out by Dr Foster, an independent authority on healthcare in the UK, compiled for Saga Health Care. This study looked at 223 hospitals in England, 25 in Scotland and 17 in Wales. The Royal Sussex County was judged the second best hospital in the South East and nationally was placed 26th out of the 265 hospitals surveyed.

Possibly a contributory factor was the success of staff on Bristol Ward. They began a new role as a short stay elderly care ward in July 2005, receiving patients from A&E, the medical assessment unit (MASU) and outlying wards at the hospital. More than 600 patients passed through the ward in the first year, earning so many plaudits from them that the team were able to celebrate their success with an anniversary tea party in 2006.

Nurses and nursing

Even before the Panorama broadcast, all wards in the trust except paediatrics and maternity had been asked to identify two older people's champions, a trained nurse and a health care assistant. The plan was that they were to have special training into the care needs of older people before returning to their wards with a view to challenging practice, a proposal first put forward in the National Service Framework for Older People, published in 2001.

The scheme was launched at Sussex House in November, and the following year each ward and department displayed photographs of the volunteer nurses who had undertaken the responsibility of helping to improve care where necessary, acting as advocates for their older patients and highlighting gaps in services.

However, the biggest change in nursing at the hospital took place in June 2004 when, after a gap of thirty years, in response to a national initiative, matrons returned to the wards.

Unlike their predecessors at the hospital, these modern matrons were appointed to various departments and specialities, such as Imaging, Renal, Medicine and Surgery. To ensure they were highly visible, it was decided they should wear distinctive purple uniforms. Their role was to drive up standards of patient care, ensure the cleanliness of the ward and the quality of nutrition for patients, and also provide leadership for the nursing staff.

Their position within the organisation was described in a paper setting out a proposed new management structure for the trust in November 2005: 'ward managers will report to modern matrons who will in turn report to the divisional senior nurse'. When the new structure came into being in 2006, three divisions were set up named Elective Services, Emergency Services, and Specialist Services. The senior nurse in each division took the title of associate director nursing services and formed part of a management team together with a general manager and a consultant, the clinical director.

No doubt the retired nurses attending the 60th anniversary meeting of the Nurses League in October 2006 would have found it hard to reconcile these changes with their experiences working at the hospital, perhaps with a matron and hospital secretary in charge, or when they trained in the hospital's own training school.

Ward transfers and closures

In 2004, a scheme known as Streamlining Beds that planned to make major changes in bed use was launched. The changes were intended to make

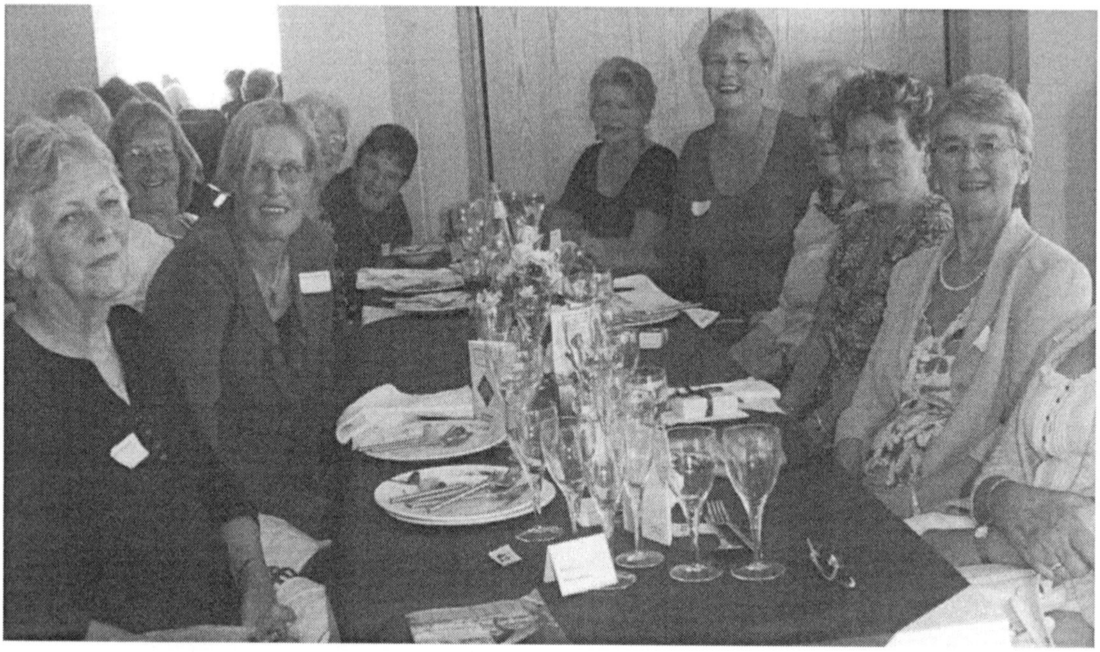

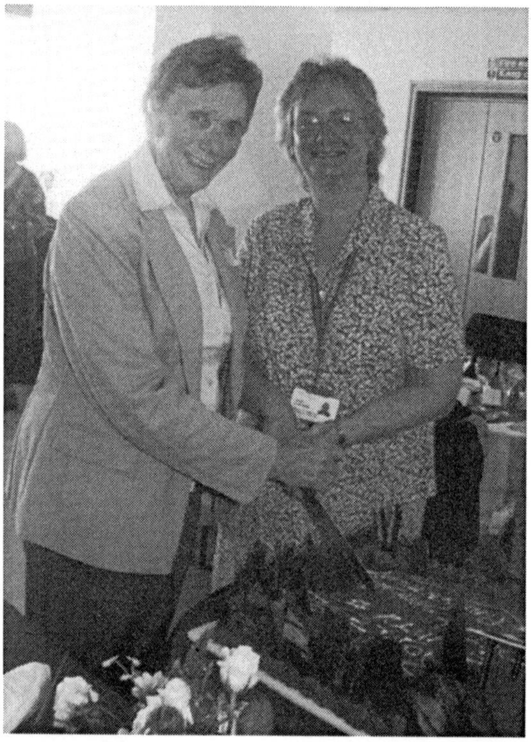

163. Celebrating the Diamond Anniversary of the hospital's Nurses' League at which treasurer Lilian Emberley and secretary Janet Cheesman cut the decorated cake.

more efficient use of beds, improve patient care, overcome the problem of delayed discharges and help to meet performance targets. The first step involved closing beds in Ward E2 at Brighton General Hospital and placing the patients in community settings while wards E3 and E3A were transferred to the Sussex County. During August, urology in Peel and Stewart was relocated to Level 8 in the Thomas Kemp Tower.

Then, in October, a consultation document was published called *Best Care, Best Place*. Among the proposals in this document were that A&E services should continue to be provided at the Princess Royal in Haywards Heath and at Brighton, but that the Sussex County would deal with all those patients requiring major abdominal surgery and that those suffering from major trauma would also be referred to Brighton. The Princess Royal Hospital, on the other hand, would undertake all routine orthopaedic work.

A purpose designed neurology and neurosurgery department with extra intensive care beds was also proposed for the Sussex County.

The practical effects of *Best Care, Best Place* were soon seen after consultation ended in February 2005, July being set as a target date for the changes in orthopaedics. Elective work on Level 8A East in the tower was moved to the Princess Royal for the acute phase of treatment; Level 8A East was to receive trauma activity from Haywards Heath and also from Overton Ward at the County. Overton Ward and Bristol Ward were scheduled to receive acute elderly care patients from Brighton General.

It was planned to transfer acute HIV and AIDS beds to Howard 2 Ward from the Elton John Centre at Brighton General: day care and research were to be transferred to the Patients' Hotel in Sussex House which in turn would move to the Elton John Centre (although, in the event, the Patients' Hotel was closed after the HIV/AIDS move took place).

A calendar presented to the trust board in May included details of other changes affecting the County. Jowers Ward electives were to move to Haywards Heath and majors to Level 8 in the Millennium Wing. Jowers was to receive gynae from Bristol Ward whose breast inpatients were to move to Haywards Heath. July 18th was set as the provisional date for these moves, subject to a sufficient reduction in beds occupied by delayed transfers of care.

More changes followed in 2006 as a result of a situation that bore uncanny echoes to 1922: once again finance was the problem, and bed closures were seen as the solution. On this occasion, however, the closures were permanent.

Although financial problems had continued to plague the various managements of Brighton hospitals from the outset of the NHS, in the last year of its existence Brighton Health Care earned its award of two stars in the annual performance ratings because of its success in achieving seven of the nine key targets, including financial management. Mid Sussex Hospitals, on the other hand, achieved six of the targets and only one star, the important difference from the Brighton result was that it 'significantly underachieved' in financial management. In the following year, 2002, the two trusts in effect became the new Brighton and Sussex University Hospitals Trust and the prospect of financial difficulties reared its head: in a message to staff in July the chief executive, Stuart Welling, said: 'Our new trust faces many challenges, not least the inherited financial deficit from the old Mid Sussex Trust.'[9] At the September meeting of the trust board the finance director forecast an overspend of over £5 million at the end of the financial year, half of which he attributed to spiralling charges for agency nurses. As if this was not bad enough, adding the £4.1 million overspend by Mid Sussex, he said, meant an extra £9 million was needed if the trust was to break even.

So began a steadily worsening financial situation. Added to the inherited problem from Haywards Heath were the heavy additional heavy costs of sending some patients to private hospitals and of employing expensive agency nurses in order to meet government performance targets. By 2005 the situation had deteriorated to the extent that, faced with a projected £13.6 million deficit, a 'Turnaround Project' was launched with funding from the Department of Health. Thus the stage was set for solutions that included staff reductions and ward closures.[10]

In March 2006, a programme to shed around 325 posts across the trust was announced, although it was hoped to achieve this without involving 'wholesale redundancies'. In September staff consultation on the proposed closure of 109 beds was completed and a staff briefing gave details of how the hospitals would be affected. According to this, many of the wards closing at the County were 'among the oldest in the trust with cramped and inadequate facilities', first Stewart and Peel wards, then beds on Grant Ward by the 3rd November and 16 cardiology beds on Baily Ward by 27th December, the patients moving to 'better facilities in the Millennium Wing'.[11]

The new children's hospital

When the Sussex Maternity and Sussex Throat and Ear hospitals were closed and their services transferred, they were fully integrated and became part of the County Hospital. However, although it was being built in the centre of the County Hospital site, it was agreed that the Royal Alexandra Hospital for Sick Children should nevertheless retain its own separate identity. For this reason, a detailed account of the development would appear to be more appropriate to a possible forthcoming history of the children's hospital. Nevertheless, it was inevitable that from the outset, by reason of its physical presence alone, building the new children's hospital would impact on everyday life at the County.

Although highly regarded and much loved locally, the children's hospital in Dyke Road built in 1881 was acknowledged to be no longer suitable for the provision of modern paediatric medicine: its fabric was in poor condition and there were sound clinical reasons for providing all its services on the admittedly cramped County site. The opportunity to achieve this was provided by the decision to build the Sussex Kidney Centre over the North car park. Accordingly, in 2002, Brighton and Hove's city planners agreed that following the completion of the kidney unit a new children's hospital could be built on the site previously occupied by the renal department.

The first indication of how the County Hospital would be affected when work began in May 2004 was given in the trust's publication *Watch This Space!* published in March. Firstly, the Level 4 corridor from the Barry Building to the Thomas Kemp Tower had to be demolished to make way for the new Alex. To replace this, while building work was going on, a new high level link bridge was to be built with its entrance adjacent to the Sussex Ear, Nose and Throat department terminating at Level 5 of the tower. To make way for a site construction building for the contractors, it was planned to demolish the engineer's house then being used by junior doctors. The junior doctors would be housed in a new building behind the Jubilee Block, which would also accommodate the Estates and Facilities departments and provide a new post room.

2007 and beyond

The new children's hospital duly opened in 2007 and Glen Court was converted to provide accommodation for the parents of children being treated as in-patients and also for parents of babies receiving treatment

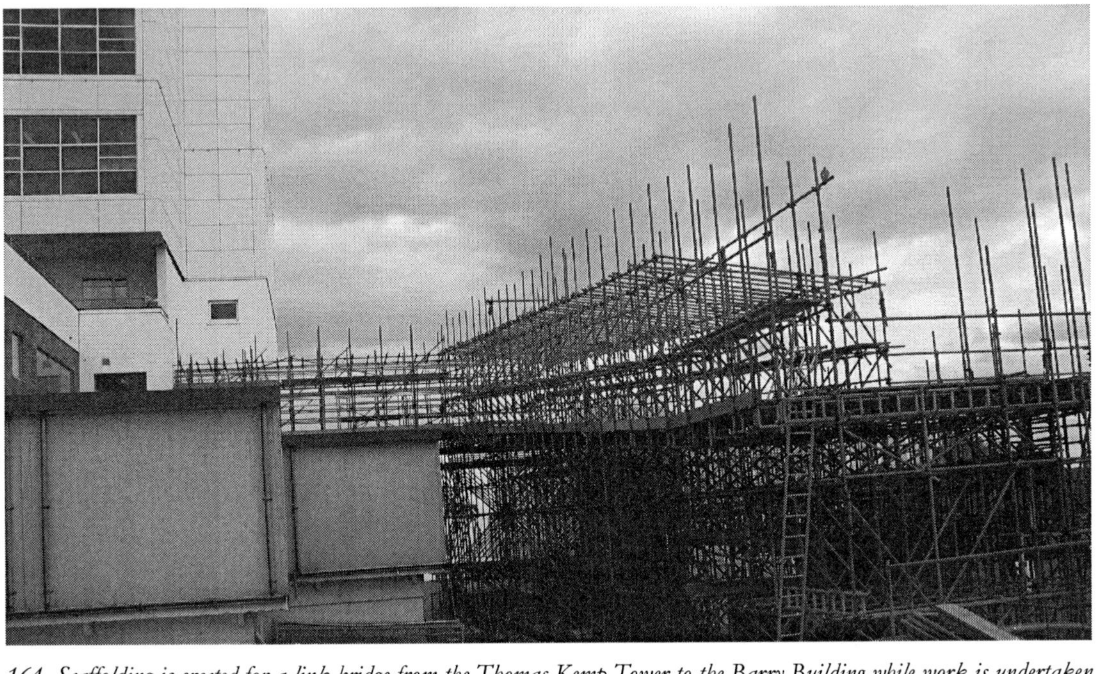

164. Scaffolding is erected for a link bridge from the Thomas Kemp Tower to the Barry Building while work is undertaken to build the new children's hospital.

on the Trevor Mann Baby Unit. Other projects for the year included the completion of the £1.2 million Urgent Care Centre, a £750,000 scheme to install a new switchboard and the upgrading of sanitary facilities on the remaining wards on the Barry Building.

Between 2008 and 2011 it was planned to continue the upgrading of the Barry Building wards and to extend the Trevor Mann Baby Unit by an extra 20 cots in order to allow more Sussex parents to have their babies treated in the unit. The reconfiguration of Level 5 to allow greater flexibility for the use of Accident and Emergency and the Medical and Surgical Assessment Unit was also under consideration.

The earlier suggestion to demolish Rosaz House and provide new facilities for breast care services on the site no longer featured in the Estates Strategy for 2008 to 2011. Instead there were plans to develop Rosaz as a Macmillan Resource Centre for patients and to provide an off-site provision for breast care services at Preston Park.

Long term plans for Phase 3 of the hospital's redevelopment included a £45 million scheme to transfer neurosciences and neurosurgery from Haywards Heath and a £30 million scheme to extend the Sussex Cancer

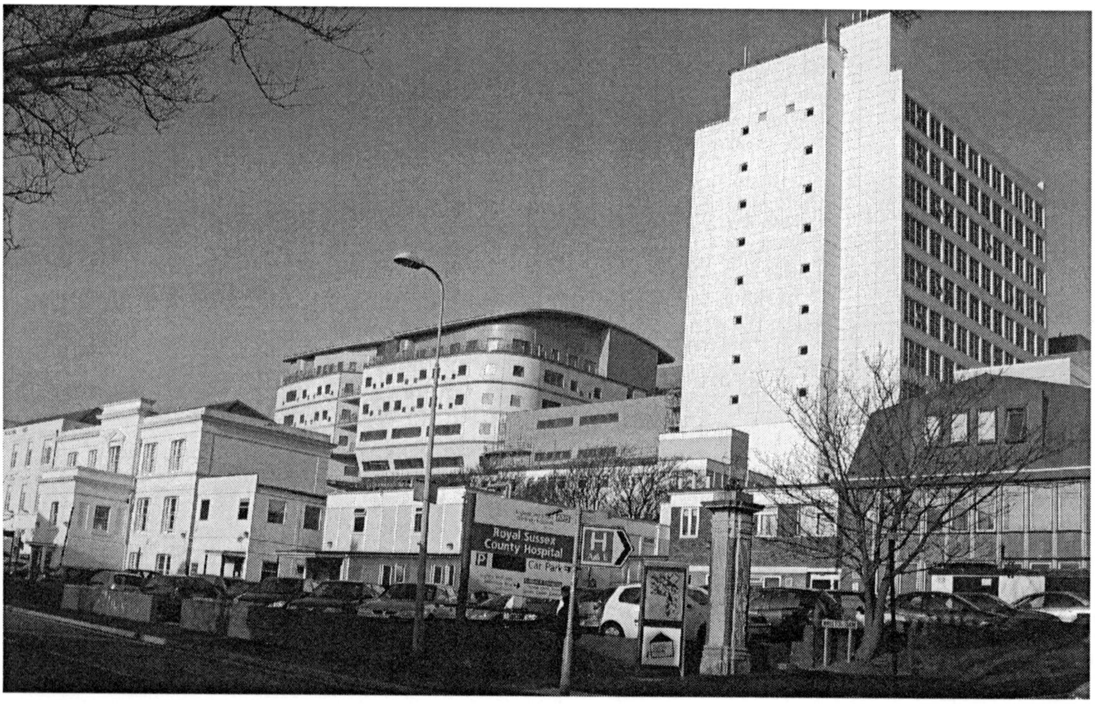

165. The changing skyline of the Royal Sussex County at the beginning of 2007with the new children's hospital in the centre of the site adjacent to the tower block.

Centre. Redeveloping the south side of the hospital campus was expected to cost £150 million.

According to a briefing on the Estates Strategy issued in 2004, the proposal, following discussions with the city council, was for a building consisting of five floors rising from the Eastern Road level to Level 10 of the tower block. This would be the same height as the new children's hospital and one floor lower than the Millennium Wing. The outline planning application included a new front entrance to the hospital and low level parking in an underground car park.

The history of the hospital shows only too clearly how plans for the development of the Royal Sussex County Hospital have frequently altered over the passage of time. And only time will tell how the face of the hospital along Eastern Road will finally appear in 2012 – 184 years after the opening of the original Barry Building.

NOTES

All unattributed quotations are taken from the official hospital records such as minutes and annual and other reports.

Chapter 1. Introduction

1. Relhan, A. *A Short History of Brighton, with Remarks on is Air and an Analysis of its Waters*, 1761. Interestingly, another edition was published in 1829, the year after the Sussex County Hospital opened.
2. Holmes, E. *Seaward Sussex: The South Downs from End to End*, 1920.
3. Musgrave, C. *Life in Brighton*, Faber and Faber, 1970, pp. 56-8.
4. Awsiter, J. *Thoughts on Brighthelston Concerning Sea-Bathing and Drinking Sea-Water with some Directions for their Use*, 1768.

Chapter 2. From Dispensary to Hospital

1. There are many different spellings of Brighthelmston.
2. Musgrave, C. p. 247.

Chapter 3. The Early Years

1. Risley, M. *The House of Healing*, London, 1961, p. 134-5.
2. Woodward, J. *To Do the Sick No Harm*, London, 1974.
3. Abel-Smith. B. *The History of the Nursing Profession*, London, 1960., p. 5
4. Porter, R. *Disease, Medicine and Society in England*, 1550-1860, CUP, 2nd ed., 1993. p. 33
5. Cartright, F.F. *A Social History of Medicine*, Longman, 1977, p. 50-2
6. Cameron, H.C. *Mr Guy's Hospital, 1726-1948, Longmans Green, 1954.*
7. Birch, C.A. *The Medical History of Hastings*, 1980.
8. Durr, A. *Co-operation in Early Nineteenth Century Brighton*, Brighton Polytechnic History Workshop, August 1982.
9. Blaker, N.P. *Reminiscences*, 1906.

Chapter 4. Growth and Development, 1830 – 1856

1. Woodward, J. *To Do the Sick No Harm*, London, 1974.
2. Woodward, J. *op cit.*
3. Berry, Sue. *Urban Development, 1750-1914 in An Historical Atlas of Sussex* (eds. Leslie, K. and Short, B.), 1999.
4. Short, B. *Population Change, 1801-1851. An Historical Atlas op cit.*
5. Musgrave, C. p. 262
6. Ellis, C. Hamilton, The *London, Brighton and South Coast Railway*, 1960.
7. Ellis, C.Hamilton. *op. cit.*

Chapter 5. The Jubilee Years

1. Possibly this was a reaction to allegations of abuse nationally. In 1894, thirty letters on outpatient abuse were published in the *British Medical Journal* in a period of six months. See Abel-Smith's *The Hospitals in England and Wales, 1800-1948,* p.176.
2. Quoted a magazine dated March 1896. (See note 4, chapter 6.)
3. *Brighton Gazette*, 2 September 1897.

Chapter 6. Staff and Patients, 1830 – 1900

1. *An Illustrated Handbook on Brighton and its Environs*, published in 1850, quoted in *Brighton Health Bulletin,* January 1983.
2. Woodham-Smith, C. *Florence Nightingale*, 1820-1910. London, 1950, pp. 57-8.
3. Quoted by Brighton surgeon H.J. McCurrich in his presidential address at the opening of the centenary session of the Brighton and Sussex Medico-Chirurgical Society in October 1946, who added 'The stench of gangrene and putrefaction in the surgical wards must have been overpowering.'
4. According to Mr Crawford, the resident house physician, the problem was not the fireworks but one of the metal mortars used to discharge the rockets, which burst among the spectators. This would account for the fact that the injuries dealt with at the hospital included seventeen compound fractures and many severe contusions. Mr Crawford also referred to 'the Rottingdean omnibus accident' when 20 injured were attended by the resident medical staff. (Quoted in a magazine article describing a visit to the hospital, March 1896. The archived copy of the article does not give the name of the magazine).
5. Hovell, B.C. *The Hull Royal Infirmary, 1782-1982,* 1982, pp. 23-5; Railton, M. and Barr, M. *The Royal Berkshire Hospital, 1839-1989.* 1989, p. 103
6. Hone, J. *The Life of Henry Tonks*, London, 1939.
7. Hone, quoting from Tonks' biography, *Wander Years.*
8. In an interview with a reporter from the *Sussex Daily News* published in March, 1934.
9. Morton, H. *How to Become a Nurse: and How to Succeed*, London, 3rd edition, 1895.

Chapter 7. Urgently in Need of Money, 1900 – 1914

1. In the article in an unidentified magazine published in March 1896, the writer also described how an eighteen month old child, 'the victim of a very sad accident' was being nursed by a sister adding: 'one for whom, but for this Hospital, the necessary efforts for its recovery would have been impossible.'

Chapter 8. Called to the Colours: The First World War, 1914 – 1918

1. Clifford Musgrave in *Life in Brighton*, quotes extensively from the *Brighton Gazette* to present a picture of life in the town during the Great War.
2. *Sussex Daily News*, 11 September 1916.
3. Musgrave, p.374.
4. Musgrave, p.375.

5. Abel-Smith, *The Hospitals*, p.252.
6. See, for example, Joyce Collins, *Dr Brighton's Indian Patients*, published by Brighton Books Publishing, No.2 n.d..
7. Musgrave, p.370.
8. *Sussex Daily News,* 13 December 1917.
9. 1 March 1918.
10. *Sussex Daily News,* 19 March 1915.
11. *Sussex Daily News,* 25 April 1918.

Chapter 9. An Uneasy Peace, 1919 – 1929

1. 11 October 1919.
2. 12 August 1922.
3. *Sussex Daily News*, 8 September 1922.
4. *Brighton Herald*, 7 October 1922.
5. *Sussex Daily News*, 12 September 1922.
6. *Sussex Daily News*, 15 September 1922.
7. Abel-Smith, *The Hospitals*, p.284.
8. Abel-Smith, pp 287-288.
9. Abel-Smith, pp 289 and 303.
10. *Sussex Daily News* 12 September 1922 but not the only occasion on which this was alleged.
11. *Brighton Herald*, 23 September 1922.
12. *Brighton Herald*, 14 October 1922.
13. *Brighton Herald*, 21 October 1922.
14. *Brighton & Hove Her*ald, 25 November 1922.
15. *The Hospital*, 22 January 1921.
16. *Sussex Daily News*, 26 and 27 November 1920.
17. *Evening Standard*, 1 June 1922.
18. *The Star*, 1 June 1922.
19. *Daily News*, 2 June 1922.
20. *The Daily Telegraph*, 2 June 1922.
21. *Sussex Daily News*, 13 June 1922.
22. *Brighton Hospitals Bulletin*, May and September, 1971
23. *The Nursing Mirror and Midwives Journal.* 10 April 1920.
24. For the background to the complex situation and debate regarding registration and national nursing shortages see Abel-Smith, *A History of the Nursing Profession.*
25. *Sussex Daily News*, 12 January 1922.
26. *Sussex Daily News*, 7 October 1922

Chapter 10. The Thirties

1. Bernhard Baron, was born in Russia of humble parentage. He was taken to Russia by his father while a small boy where he obtained work in a tobacco factory and unable to afford lodgings, slept in one of the tobacco sheds. Coming to Britain, he bought Carreras, a small tobacco business, where he eventually made his fortune. His early struggle led him to become a great supporter of the poor and an enthusiastic supporter of the Labour Party, making considerable contributions to its election funds in 1924 and 1929. His gifts to charity amounted to about £2 million, including well over £740,000 to hospitals. Before his death he set aside over £750,000 creating a trust for the benefit of hospitals and for homes of orphaned and crippled children.
2. *The Nursing Times and Midwives' Journal*, 25 April 1931
3. Dr R.W. Windle, The Latilla Story, *Brighton Hospitals Bulletin*, February 1968.
4. *The Nursing Times*, 14 January 1939.
5. Val Brown, *Women's Hospitals in Brighton and Hove,* The Hastings Press, 2006, p. 155.
6. *Brighton Hospitals Bulletin*, February 1968.
7. Abel-Smith, *A History of the Nursing Profession, p. 150.*
8. M.I. Sankey: *Thank You, Miss Hunter, 2001*, p. 11.
9. 14 January 1939.
10. M.I. Sankey, p. 14.
11. *The Nursing Times*, 19 January 1939.

Chapter 11. The Second World War

1. *Sussex Daily News*, 6 September 1939.
2. *Sussex Daily News*, 9 September 1939.
3. *Brighton Hospitals Bulletin*, February 1968.
4. *Sussex Daily News*, 19 February 1941.
5. The War in East Sussex, *Sussex Express and County Herald*, August 1945.
6. David Rowland, *War in the City*, Vol. 1, Finsbury Publishing, 2005, p.61.
7. Rowland gives the number of dead as eight children and six adults; he says official records do not clearly state the details, but many suffered appalling injuries. Timothy Carder in *The Encyclopaedia of Brighton* says four children and two adults died and twenty others were injured.
8. M.I. Sankey, *p. 39.*
9. *Sussex Daily News*, 17 September 1940.
10. *Brighton Herald*, 19 October 1942.
11. *Australian Woman's Weekly*, 28 November 1942. The article told of two such operations, the second carried out by McKenzie, a New Zealand surgeon in a field ambulance in Egypt and concluded: 'Beresford's action was the first time a live shell had thus been removed and McKenzie's speedy work on a similar extraction adds a new chapter to surgery.'
12. *Brighton Herald*, 1 June 1949.

13. *M.I.Sankey, p. 37.*
14. *The Hospital*, July 1944.
15. *Sussex Daily News*, 26 January 1945.
16. *Brighton Herald*, 23 March 1940.

Chapter 12. An End to Uncertainty, 1946 – 1947

1. Yeo, G. *Nursing at Barts*, Alan Sutton Publishing, 1996, p. 83.
2. *Nursing Times*, 3 April 1948.
3. *Brighton and Hove Herald*, 15 December 1947,
4. The Open University, *Caring for Health: History and Diversity*, 1985, pp. 72-3.
5. *Sussex Daily News*, 20 October 1947.
6. *Sussex Daily News*, 5 July 1948.
7. *The Hospital*, October 1932.
8. Dr S.J.Firth, *Report on Co-Ordination of Local Hospitals as a Single District Hospital*, 17 February 1947.

Chapter 13. An N.H.S. Hospital: The Early Years

1. Carder, T. *The Encyclopaedia of Brighton*, 1990, 58 (a)
2. Dale, A. *The History and Architecture of Brighton.*
3. *Brighton Hospitals Bulletin*, May 1967.
4. According to theatre superintendent Sylvia Stenning writing in *Brighton Hospitals Bulletin*, June 1967.
5. Kenneth Ross, who was a young volunteer on Vallance Ward at the hospital in the early 1950s, in an email to the author, February 2007. Mr Ross, who eventually enjoyed a long nursing career at Brighton General and other local hospitals, said that at the time the County would not accept males for training.

Chapter 14. A New County Hospital – Or a New Site?

1. *Brighton Hospitals Bulletin*, August 1971.
2. Progressive patient care was one of a number of new ideas being trialled at the time and involved moving a patient during recovery from high intensity nursing and observation into a quieter environment, ideally including dayrooms, to which a patient could go as they recovered. The system was ideally suited to the new racetrack wards but it was not always successful, even in these.
3. *Brighton Hospitals Bulletin*, November 1966 and January 1967.
4. *Brighton Hospitals Bulletin*, April 1969.

Chapter 15. The Debate Ends and a Decision is Made

1. Thatcher, M. *The Downing Street Years*, Harper Collins, 1993.

2. The options were scored for quality of care (including benefits of linking specialties on one site, accessibility), design (engineering, building and environmental factors) and building and running costs. Option 1 contained two additional variations using a Department of Health 'off the shelf' design, cost being a major factor. Option 2 also had a variation using the 'off the shelf' design.

Chapter 16. First Steps Towards a New County, 1992 – 1996

1. Kate Goddard, who was appointed outpatient sister in 1992, in a communication with the author, 16 December 2003, following her retirement as outpatients and medical records manager.
2. *Brighton Health Care Bulletin*, August 1994.
3. The Wilde Clinic, offering free, confidential advice for gay and bisexual men, was opened in the Lawson Unit by broadcaster Simon Fanshawe in November 1998.

Chapter 17. Towards the New Millennuim, 1997 – 2000

1. Dame Audrey Emerton, a professional nurse and former regional nursing officer who had been made a DBE in 1989, was awarded a life peerage in the New Year's honours list for her 43 years' service to the NHS and the St John Ambulance.
2. Dr Vaughan interviewed for *Brighton Health Care Bulletin*, May 1999.
3. Other consultants recognised in this way since the introduction of the NHS were surgeon Nigel Porter (The Nigel Porter Unit), physician Lord Trafford (The Trafford Department of Renal Medicine) and paediatrician Dr Trevor Mann (Level 14 Trevor Mann Baby Unit).
4. Library facilities were previously available at the Sussex Postgraduate Medical Centre situated at Brighton General Hospital. A new multi-disciplinary educational centre to replace it at the County Hospital was considered essential to secure ongoing approval for junior doctor training and also for the training and development of staff generally.
5. It was not only the UK that was experiencing problems with the shortage of nurses. When a team from Brighton visited South Africa to recruit nurses they found themselves competing not only with five other NHS trusts but with the United States as well. (*Brighton Health Care Bulletin*, February 1999).
6. When wards at the General were later transferred to the County, the Filipino nurses accompanied them.

5\. As part of Brighton's celebrations, the Steine was closed for a big street party, virtually cutting the town in two.

Chapter 18. A Teaching Hospital Once More, 2002 – 2007

1. *Brighton Health Care Bulletin*, March 2001.
2. The other successful bid involved collaboration between the universities of Hull and York.
3. *New Trust News, a Central Sussex Hospitals Consultation Update,* July 2001.
4. *Strengthening Hospital Services Across the NHS in Central Sussex.*

5. *BSUH Bulletin*, November 2003.
6. *Brighton Health Care Bulletin*, December 2001.
7. All quotations from *Brighton Health Care Bulletin*, February 2002.
8. She was later treated at Hurstwood Park and Southlands Hospital.
9. *BSUH Bulletin*, September 2003.

Chapter 19. More Developments, More to Come, 2004 – 2007

1. *BSUH Bulletin*, December 2004.
2. *BSUH Bulletin*, February 2006.
3. For example, there were 108 patients ready for discharge blocking beds in the trust in September 2002, including 20 in E2 Ward at Brighton General Hospital. In February 2007, despite continual efforts to eradicate the problem, 65 patients were blocking beds in the trust (*The Argus*, 6 February 2007.)
4. In 1951, for example, Brighton hospitals suffered from the problem of having acute beds blocked by chronic sick patients.
5. About 30 per cent of patients who could have been dealt with in this way and need not have attended A&E, according to associate director Janet Cheesman. (*BSUH Bulletin*, June 2006)
6. Figure given by general manager Gill Dewey to the trust board (*BSUH Bulletin* January 2005).
7. Regrettably, shortcomings in the care of elderly patients in hospitals appears to have been an ongoing problem. See for example, Barbara Robb, *Sans Everything, A Case to Answer* (1967); Martin, J.P., *Hospitals in Trouble* (1984); even in 2007, the Healthcare Commission, as a result of its investigations of conditions in 23 hospitals, reported in its report, *Caring for Dignity*, that eight hospitals including Barts and the West London Trust were issued with formal warnings for failing to treat older patients with dignity. This was followed by the scandal of Maidstone and Tunbrige Wells hospitals where 90 elderly patients died following *C.difficile* infection and 'staff at every level allowed patients to lie in squalor'. (Quoted in *The Observer*, 14 October 2007).
8. Chief executive Peter Coles in an interview with the BBC after watching footage of the film prior to its screening.
9. *BSUH Bulletin*, September 2002.
10. The trust was not alone in experiencing financial difficulties. A survey published by the *Health Service Journal* revealed that almost half of English acute trusts were not confident about meeting their year-end financial targets, with London and the South East trusts the most pessimistic. (Quoted in the *BSUH Bulletin*, March 2004.)
11. Although the move did offer the prospect of better conditions for the patients, it should be said Baily had been upgraded and although it was a mixed ward, it was not really cramped like most of the others such as Peel and Stewart.

INDEX

Bold figures refer to illustrations; titles of published works and newspapers are in italics.